Infection Prevention and Control
in Healthcare Settings

Infection Prevention and Control in Healthcare Settings

Edward Purssell
Anglia Ruskin University
Essex, UK

Dinah Gould
Independent Consultant
London, UK

WILEY Blackwell

This edition first published 2023
© 2023 John Wiley & Sons Ltd

The right of Edward Purssell and Dinah Gould to be identified as the authors of this work has been asserted in accordance with law.

Registered Offices
John Wiley & Sons, Inc., 111 River Street, Hoboken, NJ 07030, USA
John Wiley & Sons Ltd, The Atrium, Southern Gate, Chichester, West Sussex, PO19 8SQ, UK

For details of our global editorial offices, customer services, and more information about Wiley products visit us at www.wiley.com.

Wiley also publishes its books in a variety of electronic formats and by print-on-demand. Some content that appears in standard print versions of this book may not be available in other formats.

Library of Congress Cataloging-in-Publication Data
Names: Purssell, Edward, author. | Gould, Dinah, author.
Title: Infection prevention and control in healthcare settings / Edward
    Purssell, Dinah Gould.
Description: Hoboken, NJ : Wiley-Blackwell, 2023. | Includes
    bibliographical references and index.
Identifiers: LCCN 2022040057 (print) | LCCN 2022040058 (ebook) | ISBN
    9781119842590 (paperback) | ISBN 9781119842576 (Adobe PDF) | ISBN
    9781119842613 (epub)
Subjects: MESH: Cross Infection–prevention & control | Infection
    Control–methods | Disease Transmission, Infectious | Microbiological
    Phenomena | Health Facilities
Classification: LCC RA643 (print) | LCC RA643 (ebook) | NLM WC 195 | DDC
    362.1969–dc23/eng/20221027
LC record available at https://lccn.loc.gov/2022040057
LC ebook record available at https://lccn.loc.gov/2022040058

Cover Design: Wiley
Cover Image: © Fotomay/Shutterstock

Set in 9.5/12.5pt STIXTwoText by Straive, Pondicherry, India
Printed and bound by CPI Group (UK) Ltd, Croydon, CR0 4YY

C9781119842590_161222

Contents

Foreword

The events of recent years have shown the ever-present danger of infection, and the need to act decisively to counter the threat posed by dangerous micro-organisms. This includes new or emergent organisms, those which have remained ever-present, and existing organisms that are evolving alongside ourselves to be more pathogenic or resistant to antimicrobials. At the same time, healthcare is changing, with more invasive and immunosuppressive treatments, and a population with more older people and those living with chronic illnesses or conditions. It is also important to understand the relationship between the environment and disease, for example the effects of climate change and deforestation on the patterns of infections in different areas.

However, the often cited need to 'follow the science' is complicated by the inconvenient fact that much about infection control remains unknown or untested. Furthermore, it is wrong to treat all micro-organisms equally, with most being harmless to humans, and only a small number having the ability to cause disease. Healthcare is also delivered in a variety of different settings and contexts, and infection control solutions that are suitable for hospitals are often not helpful in community or home settings.

This book aims to bridge the gap between complex infection control manuals and simpler books which take a mechanistic approach by explaining the practice and rationale behind infection control practice. We draw extensively on original material and seminal works, applying the principles to practical examples. This is important because while many of the details differ according to organism and setting, and change over time, most of the underlying principles do not. Microbiology and infection control are dynamic subjects because of the constant evolution of micro-organisms and changes in people and the environment in which we live. This presents both challenges and opportunities, which this book discusses throughout.

The authors of this book are highly experienced academics and clinicians, who are grounded in the everyday work of clinical practice as well as research and academia. This means that they understand both the science and the complexity of actually delivering healthcare in a variety of different settings. They have worked in general adult areas, gynaecology, paediatrics and hospice care. By explaining the principles behind practice recommendations, they hope to empower healthcare professionals and those in their care to safely adapt these principles to meet the needs of individual patients.

Rose Gallagher MBE
Professional Lead Infection Prevention and
Control/AMR and Nursing Sustainability Lead

Preface

The impetus to write this book arose through the experience of teaching infection prevention and control. Discussions with students, educationalists and newly qualified practitioners suggested the need for a new book that would prepare nurses and other practitioners to work in a range of different clinical settings and contexts, applying principles to practice. Today more than ever, practitioners need to develop the skills of critical appraisal. Recommendations for infection prevention may have to be adjusted according to the specific organism, patient group or clinical setting but the underpinning principles remain the same.

Practitioners need to consider key questions when they apply evidence-based guidelines to practice. What are the recommendations? Are they sensible? Can they be applied in a specific clinical setting? What adaptation, if any, is indicated? Updating is a further consideration. Healthcare is constantly changing: faster patient throughput, increased use of venues outside hospital for patients requiring acute care, new treatments and a population that is becoming older with concomitant increase in the number of people living with chronic conditions and increased exposure to invasive procedures.

The complex interplay between environment, micro-organisms and populations has implications for patterns of infection: climate change, deforestation and the emergence of 'new' infections such as HIV and SARS-CoV-2 can have profound effects on human health. SARS-CoV-2 has brought home the ever-present danger of infection and the need to act swiftly and decisively to counter the threats posed not just by existing infectious agents but also by emergent and re-emergent organisms alongside the global threat of antimicrobial resistance.

Against this backdrop, education to promote safe practice will never be complete: continual review and updating must be ongoing. We saw the need for a fresh approach to infection prevention designed to foster critical thinking and an appreciation of evidence-based practice to enable practitioners to take an informed approach to 'evidence' related to infection prevention and its applicability to their specific client groups and clinical settings.

The authors are experienced academics and clinicians grounded in the everyday work of clinical practice as well as research and academia. They understand the science and complexity of delivering healthcare in a variety of different settings, with clinical experience in general adult areas, sexual health, paediatrics and continuing care. By explaining the principles underpinning recommendations for practice, they hope to empower healthcare professionals to safely adapt these principles to meet the needs of individual patients.

1

The Chain of Infection and Main Groups of Micro-organisms Causing Infection

The Scope of Microbiology

Microbiology is the scientific study of organisms too small to be seen with the naked eye. They are ubiquitous and many perform essential ecological functions, for example breaking down the molecules of dead animals and plants which then re-enter the ecosystem. Some micro-organisms tolerate extreme conditions where other organisms would not survive (e.g. high temperatures) while others cause disease and are medically important.

Chain of Infection

The Chain of Infection is an epidemiological model applicable to all *pathogens* (micro-organisms able to cause disease). It comprises a series of events that must occur before pathogenic micro-organisms can spread and describes interactions between the pathogen, its host and the environment. Links in the chain are shown in Figure 1.1. Breaking a link in the chain can prevent infection.

Reservoir

The reservoir is where the pathogen lives and multiplies. Possible reservoirs include people (e.g. patients, nursing home residents, health workers and those visiting healthcare premises). They may show signs and symptoms of infection or be asymptomatic because they are mildly infected, incubating the infection or recovering from it. Two people affected by the same organism may present differently and many organisms are carried asymptomatically. For the classic

Infection Prevention and Control in Healthcare Settings,
First Edition. Edward Purssell and Dinah Gould.
© 2023 John Wiley & Sons Ltd. Published 2023 by John Wiley & Sons Ltd.

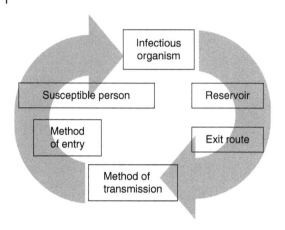

Figure 1.1 The chain of infection.

communicable diseases of childhood (e.g. measles, mumps, rubella) and influenza, other people are the reservoir. Inanimate surfaces and objects (e.g. clinical equipment, clothing) can operate as reservoirs and are sometimes described as *fomites* (Box 1.1).

The environment operates as a reservoir for infections in premises where healthcare is delivered (Box 1.2). It is also the source of infections acquired in the community (e.g. tetanus, legionnaire's disease). Animals are reservoirs for a number of infections including rabies, Ebola disease, Lyme disease and exotic emerging infections such as monkeypox (MPX virus) and zika virus.

Box 1.1 Fomites

Fomites are defined as inanimate objects that can operate as vehicles for the transmission of an infectious agent. In healthcare settings, they include patient care items (e.g. bedclothes, bedpans, urinals) and environmental surfaces. They often give rise to outbreaks of infection because disinfection has not been undertaken or undertaken poorly.

Source: Adapted from Kanamori et al. (2017).

Box 1.2 Environmental Reservoirs for Healthcare-Associated Infection

In premises where healthcare is delivered, drains and sinks can become heavily contaminated with micro-organisms and have been identified as reservoirs when outbreaks occur. Problems are compounded when sinks in clinical areas are used for non-clinical purposes (e.g. to empty washbowls). Innovations to reduce risks include sinks which self-disinfect with chemicals or heat and 'waterless wards' where conventional sinks and plumbing are removed from patient care areas.

Portal of Exit

The portal of exit is the path taken by pathogens to escape from the reservoir. Respiratory pathogens (e.g. colds, influenza) are released in coughs, sneezes and spluttered speech. Enteric pathogens causing food-poisoning escape in vomit and faeces. Skin scales and dust can provide a portal of exit for some bacteria, including those frequently causing healthcare-associated infection (e.g. *Staphylococcus aureus*).

Mode of Transmission

The mode of transmission describes how the pathogen spreads (Table 1.1).

Transmission can occur by direct contact between surfaces such as hands and fomites and via contaminated food and water (e.g. cholera, typhoid). Houseflies (*Musca domestica*) breed in faecal material. Their feet become contaminated with micro-organisms which can be transferred to open wounds. This type of zoonosis is called *mechanical transmission*. It has been documented as a means of spread for *Clostridioides difficile*, methicillin-resistant *S. aureus* (MRSA), *Escherichia coli* and *Salmonella* spp. (Davies et al. 2016). Biological zoonotic transmission occurs when the pathogen lives and multiplies inside a vector. The infectious agent causing malaria (*Plasmodium* spp.) lives inside female mosquitoes (*Anopheles* spp.). Infection is transmitted when the mosquito bites a human host.

The air-borne route is an important mode of transmission for respiratory pathogens and the classic communicable diseases. The 2020 COVID-19 pandemic stimulated renewed interest in air-borne transmission. Conventionally, it was thought to occur via two distinct routes: droplet and air-borne transmission (Table 1.2).

Droplet transmission was proposed according to the findings of research dating from the 1930s that described the theoretical behaviour of particles according to their size (Wells 1934). From this work it was concluded that respiratory secretions are spread in two distinct ways according to their dimensions. According to this school of thought, droplets are thought unlikely to remain air-borne for long

Table 1.1 Modes of microbial transmission.

Direct contact
Indirect spread via fomites
Air-borne spread
Contaminated food and water
Inoculation via skin or mucous membranes
Vertical transmission from mother to foetus
Zoonotic spread from animals

Table 1.2 Respiratory transmission.

Term	Definition	Implications for practice
Droplet	Transmission by large droplets, diameter >5 μm transported via turbulent air flow generated by violent expiratory events (e.g. coughing or sneezing)	Most likely at close range with pathogens deposited on the conjunctivae or mucous membranes of new hosts
Air-borne/ aerosol/droplet nuclei	Transmission via inhalation of small respiratory droplets, typically <5 μm	Remain air-borne long enough to transmit the pathogen over distance and does not depend on face-to-face transmission. Pathogens are deposited deep in the respiratory tract as far as the alveoli

periods. Instead, they fall through gravity because of their relatively large size and their period of infectivity is correspondingly brief.

Aerosols were thought to remain suspended for much longer because of their minute size, depending on environmental conditions (e.g. humidity, turbulence, ventilation) (Tang et al. 2021). It has now been suggested that the distinction between air-borne, aerosol/droplet nuclei and large droplet transmission should be replaced by a unique non-contact air-borne transmission mode (Drossinos et al. 2021).

For many pathogens, there is more than one mode of transmission. Norovirus is spread by droplets released when vomiting occurs, by direct and indirect contact and by eating contaminated shellfish (Hassard et al. 2017). Many viruses responsible for respiratory and gastrointestinal infections can probably also be spread by fomites contaminated with body fluids (Boone and Gerba 2007).

Portal of Entry

The portal of entry is the route taken by pathogens to gain access to the tissues of the new host. The micro-organisms responsible for influenza and the classic communicable diseases are inhaled. Enteric pathogens gain access by ingestion. The urogenital tract is the portal of entry for urinary and sexually transmitted pathogens. Inoculation via skin and mucous membranes is the mode of entry for pathogens causing surgical site infection. Needlestick injury allows access for pathogens causing blood-borne infection: the viruses responsible for human immunodeficiency disease (HIV) and hepatitis B and C. Vertical transmission from mother to foetus occurs by two possible mechanisms: from the maternal to foetal circulation via the placenta (e.g. congenital syphilis) and via the contaminated birth canal (e.g. congenital gonorrhoea). Some pathogens are transmitted vertically via both routes (Box 1.3).

Box 1.3   Vertical Transmission: Group B Streptococcal Infections in Neonates

One in four women carry Group B *Streptococcus* vaginally without symptoms. It can infect the amniotic fluid before delivery or be acquired during passage down the birth canal, causing neonatal meningitis, pneumonia and septicaemia. Very low-weight babies are at greatest risk of developing severe infection and mortality can be as high as 30%. Infection is either early onset (during the first week of life) or late onset occurring when the infant is between a week and six months old (Heath and Jardine 2014).

Women who are carriers can be identified by screening. Vaginal or rectal swabs are taken at 35–37 weeks gestation. Women who test positive should receive antibiotics during labour or earlier if the membranes rupture before labour commences to avoid the risk of neonatal infection.

Intact skin and mucous membranes are usually good barriers against many potential pathogens but are overcome by the invasive procedures commonly undertaken during healthcare (Stamm 1978).

Interaction Between Host and Pathogen

The immune status of the host, size of the infective dose and virulence of the pathogen are key determinants of infection. This is a complex area currently receiving scientific scrutiny. A key question is why when two people are exposed to the same pathogen, one succumbs but often the other does not.

Some individuals are more susceptible than others. Genetic variation can play an important part. People with sickle cell disease and thalassaemia have inherited innate immunity to malaria. Susceptibility to the same pathogen can also vary between individuals. The likelihood of contracting tuberculosis and HIV appears to be influenced by genetic factors. Immunity can be acquired throughout the lifespan through exposure to infection or vaccination. Some infections are species specific. Few domestic animals are susceptible to viruses able to cause the common cold, for example. Norovirus is a human pathogen but humans are not susceptible to the related feline calicivirus.

Infectious Dose

The infectious dose is the number of organisms required for infection to occur. It varies widely and is much lower for some pathogens than for others (Schmid-Hempel and Frank 2007). It has been estimated that in the case of SARS-Cov-2, the infectious dose could be as few as 100 virus particles (Karimzadeh et al. 2021). In general, the larger the infective dose, the more likely it is that the pathogen will be able to overwhelm the host immune system. Exposure to a patient with tuberculosis who is exhibiting a productive cough generating prodigious amounts of sputum is much more likely to result in infection than exposure to an asymptomatic patient. The frequency of exposure is also important. People who have multiple sexual partners are more likely to develop sexually transmitted infection and their risk of contracting more than one type of sexually transmitted disease is greater.

Some individuals and situations operate as super-spreaders (Box 1.4). Risky behaviours very likely to result in the transmission of respiratory infection between members of the public have also been reported, particularly in relation to COVID-19; risk is likely to be heightened through exposure to people who are inebriated or emotional.

Super-spreading occurs when a single individual infects a disproportionately large number of contacts (Wong et al. 2015). The outbreaks of Ebola disease 2014–2015 in Guinea and Sierra Leone, the outbreak of Middle Eastern respiratory syndrome (MERS) in 2015, severe acute respiratory syndrome (SARS) in 2003 and more recently the 2020–2021 COVID-19 pandemic have increased interest in super-spreading.

Virulence

Virulence is the ability of a pathogen to cause disease. Severity of the resulting infection is greater if the pathogen is highly virulent and the potential host is exposed to a large number of organisms (infective dose). Virulence factors are the properties of a pathogen that increase its ability to invade potential hosts, colonise them and evade the host defences. Morphology influences virulence.

Pili are minute hair-like processes that enable bacteria to attach to the surface of the host cell. Piliated strains of *Neisseria gonorrhoeae* enable the bacteria to attach to the cervical epithelium. Non-piliated strains are less likely to cause infection.

Box 1.4   Factors Likely to Contribute to Super-Spreading

- Individual behaviour, e.g. particular tendency to generate spluttered speech
- Number of susceptible victims present
- Air flow (respiratory infections)
- High population density (opportunity for spread by direct and indirect contact is increased)
- Specific environmental conditions – the outbreak of Ebola disease in 2014–2015 was associated with traditional burial customs that placed family members of the deceased at risk through contact with body fluids
- Examples of situations likely to promote super-spreading are:
  - hospitals
  - prolonged contact with members of the same household
  - mass travel (aeroplane)

A mucus capsule surrounding the bacterial cell wall helps prevent desiccation for some bacterial strains. Some of the earliest epidemiological investigations exploring the spread of healthcare-associated infection established that strains of *Klebsiella* with mucus capsules were more likely to cause outbreaks than non-encapsulated strains because they could survive desiccation, remained viable for longer on hands and fomites and were more easily transmitted (Casewell and Phillips 1978).

Some bacteria release enzymes that increase their *pathogenicity* (ability to cause disease). Haemolysins are enzymes that destroy red blood cells. *S. aureus*, streptococci and enterococci release haemolysins. Cytotoxins released by *Salmonella* kill cells by destroying proteins. *S. aureus* releases collagenases. These enzymes destroy the protein collagen present in connective tissue. The damaged collagen forms a protective wall around the bacteria, resulting in the formation of an *abscess*. Abscesses contain dead *neutrophils* (pus), cellular debris and live bacteria protected from *phagocytosis* by neutrophils in the tissue fluid of the host.

The structure of bacterial cells can also increase virulence. For example, *Mycobacterium tuberculosis* has a tough, waxy coat that protects it against host defences, including phagocytosis. Many bacteria have numerous virulence factors. Group B *Streptococcus*, which can cause serious infection in pregnant women, neonates and older people, is protected from phagocytosis by its outer polysaccharide coat, pili which enable it to attach itself to host cells and ability to release an enzyme (C5a-ase) that allows it to evade the host immune defences by preventing the migration of neutrophils to the infected site.

Main Groups of Micro-organisms

The main groups of micro-organisms are shown in Table 1.3.

Table 1.3 Main groups of micro-organisms able to cause disease.

Bacteria
Viruses
Fungi
Protozoa
Mycoplasmas
Rickettsiae
Chlamydiae
(Parasitic worms – infestations)

Bacteria

Bacteria are the oldest known group of cellular micro-organisms, thought to have appeared four billion years ago. They are found everywhere but most are *saprophytes*. They live on dead organic matter and play a vital role in degrading complex organic molecules and recycling them into simpler ones used by other organisms to support metabolism. Many species of bacteria are commercially important, for example making wine. The characteristics of bacteria are the same as those of all living organisms (Table 1.4).

Approximately 50 species of bacteria cause disease in animals, plants and humans but virulence is highly variable. For example, *Yersinia pestis*, the pathogen responsible for plague, always causes very serious infection. In contrast, some bacteria called *opportunists* do not attack healthy tissues and are likely to cause serious infection only in people who are already sick and whose immune systems are compromised. Bacteria responsible for many healthcare-associated infections (e.g. *Klebsiella* spp., *Escherichia coli*, *Pseudomonas* spp.) are opportunistic.

The normal *commensal flora* is made up of bacteria and other micro-organisms living harmlessly in or on the body, for example on the skin or in the gastrointestinal tract. They receive nourishment and shelter from the host and in return protect the host from other invading pathogens in a reciprocal arrangement. Commensal micro-organisms can cause infection if they are transferred to a different anatomical location (Table 1.5).

Endogenous (self) infection results in the transfer of micro-organisms from one anatomical site to another on the same person. Transfer of *E. coli* from the perineum to the urinary tract of the same individual is an example. *Exogenous (cross) infection* occurs when micro-organisms are transferred between different people, for example on the hands of health workers or via fomites. Infection prevention and control strategies are aimed at containing both endogenous and exogenous transmission.

Table 1.4 Characteristics of living organisms.

Cellular structure apparent
Respire and generate energy
Grow and adapt
Metabolise (consume food and convert it into energy)
Maintain homeostasis (keep a stable internal environment despite external environmental change)
Respond to environmental change
Move
Reproduce and transfer genetic material to offspring

Table 1.5   Infections caused by the normal commensal flora: examples.

Escherichia coli: urinary tract infection

Staphylococcus aureus: surgical site infection

Clostridiodes difficile: overgrowth in the large intestine after treatment with broad-spectrum antibiotics

Enterococcus faecalis: urinary tract, wound or bloodstream infection

Streptococcus pneumoniae: pneumonia, otitis media, meningitis, bloodstream infection

Bacteroides fragilis: abscesses, peritonitis

Infection and Colonisation

Understanding the difference between *infection* and *colonisation* is key to interpreting information on microbiology reports. Infection occurs when a pathogen gains access to the host tissues and elicits a host response, giving rise to the signs and symptoms of infection, such as *pyrexia, inflammation* and pus in a wound or the appearance of neutrophils ('pus cells') in urine. Colonisation occurs when pathogens are present but there is no host response and no signs or symptoms of infection.

Infection is very likely to be present if there are large numbers of the same type of pathogen accompanied by large numbers of neutrophils, pain, tenderness and pyrexia. A microbiology report indicating scant growth or 'mixed growth' of a number of different types of micro-organisms with few neutrophils suggests colonisation. Colonisation is clinically significant because the colonised site operates as a reservoir and the micro-organisms can be transferred to a susceptible site such as a wound via hands or fomites. Colonisation often occurs before infection develops.

Bacterial Growth Requirements

Bacteria share the same characteristics of life as higher organisms (see Table 1.5). All bacteria require water but otherwise their growth requirements vary enormously, reflecting the wide variety of environments they inhabit. Gram-negative bacteria have very simple growth requirements, needing only water, simple nutrients and warmth to multiply. Most human pathogens grow and reproduce optimally at 37 °C and thrive in the warm, damp, densely populated hospital environment, explaining why risk of infection, especially from opportunists, is high. A key measure of growth is the doubling time which varies according to environmental conditions. For *E. coli*, doubling time is about 20 minutes in a nutrient-rich environment but 15 hours under less favourable circumstances (Gibson et al. 2018).

Keeping the clinical environment and equipment dry and clean helps eliminate reservoirs and reduces the risk of cross-infection caused by Gram-negative

---

Box 1.5   Risks of Cross-Infection caused by Gram-Negative Opportunists

Gram-negative bacteria have been isolated from damp cleaning equipment in wards and other items (e.g. cleaning cloths, mop heads, wash bowls, infant feeding bottles) where they multiply in large numbers, forming reservoirs that have been associated with outbreaks, and from equipment left immersed in disinfectant solution. Cross-infection should be avoided by using disposables and by drying other equipment after use and storing items dry.

Source: Adapted from Ayliffe et al. (1970).

---

opportunists (Box 1.5). Gram-positive bacteria are generally able to tolerate dry conditions better than Gram-negative bacteria. They can survive in dust, forming reservoirs.

Some species of bacteria, described as fastidious, have very exacting growth requirements. They need specific nutrients and some do not survive for long outside the host or are unable to survive at all (e.g. *Treponema pallidum*).

All bacteria need to respire and generate energy to metabolise. *Aerobic bacteria* utilise oxygen and thrive in wounds close to the skin. Aerobic bacteria are described as *obligate aerobes* if they depend entirely on oxygen to support metabolism (e.g. *M. tuberculosis*). *Obligate anaerobes* are killed in the presence of atmospheric oxygen and use a different source of energy to respire (e.g. *Bacteroides fragilis*, *Clostridium pefringens*, *C. tetani*). They are found in deeper wounds and within abscesses. *Facultative aerobes* use oxygen to support metabolism if it is present but can switch to anaerobic respiration if it is not (e.g. *S. aureus*, *Staphylococcus epidermidis*, *E. coli*). Most human pathogens are aerobic.

Bacteria vary according to the pH optimal for their survival and this influences distribution of the normal flora. An acidic environment favours *S. aureus* which multiples well on skin which is acidic (pH 4). Lactobacilli thrive in the acidic vaginal environment throughout the female reproductive years. Decrease in oestrogen at the menopause reduces vaginal acidity and the lactobacilli tend to be replaced by other micro-organisms. Infection and vaginal discharge may result. The very low pH of gastric secretions (pH 2) destroys many of the bacteria ingested in food but enteric pathogens such as *Salmonella typhi* (causing typhoid) grow and multiply in the alkaline environment of the small intestine (pH 8).

Bacterial Structure

Bacteria are *unicellular* organisms. This means that one cell on its own operates as an independent, viable organism. There is no division of labour between bacterial cells: one cell performs all the functions of living independently of any others.

Before examination in the microbiology laboratory, all cells and tissues must be 'fixed' (killed) and stained with laboratory dyes to make them visible. Neither the light microscope or the electron microscope (which makes it possible to examine specimens at much higher magnification) depicts organisms in their living state. Electron microscopy makes it possible to study the cellular *ultrastructure* (fine, detailed structure) of bacteria and other cells and tissues.

All bacteria are *prokaryotic*. This means that their genetic material (DNA) lies directly in the cell cytoplasm instead of being separated from it by a nuclear membrane. Bacteria contain a single chromosome carrying their genes. Higher organisms are described as *eukaryotic*. Their chromosomes are separated from the cytoplasm by a nuclear membrane and they contain organelles responsible for cellular respiration (mitochondria) and synthesising protein (ribosomes) which are membrane bound. Prokaryotic cells are simpler in structure than the cells higher organisms. Instead of being equipped with discrete organelles, they contain intracellular membranes called *mesosomes* that undertake cellular functions. Figure 1.2 illustrates an 'idealised' bacterial cell demonstrating all the features possible.

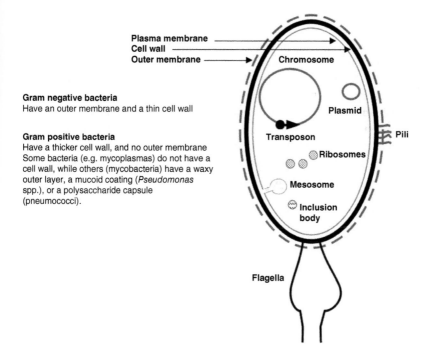

Plasma membrane
Cell wall
Outer membrane
Chromosome

Gram negative bacteria
Have an outer membrane and a thin cell wall

Plasmid

Gram positive bacteria
Have a thicker cell wall, and no outer membrane
Some bacteria (e.g. mycoplasmas) do not have a
cell wall, while others (mycobacteria) have a waxy
outer layer, a mucoid coating (*Pseudomonas*
spp.), or a polysaccharide capsule
(pneumococci).

Transposon
Ribosomes
Pili
Mesosome
Inclusion body

Flagella

Figure 1.2 The 'idealised' bacterial cell.

Bacteria have rigid cell walls giving structural support while protecting the cellular contents. The walls consist of a mesh of polysaccharides and amino acids called peptidoglycans. Historically, bacterial cell walls have been of intense interest because they determine the staining properties of the bacterium (reaction to Gram's dye), many aspects of bacterial behaviour and are the target for antibacterial drugs.

The cell walls of Gram-positive bacteria consist of a very thick peptidoglycan mesh which enables the bacteria to withstand the immune system of the host although they are still susceptible to some enzymes, including lysozyme. Gram-negative bacteria have more complex cell walls consisting of a thin layer of peptidoglycan surrounded by an outer membrane made up of protein, phospholipid and lipopolysaccharide molecules (endotoxins). Endotoxins are highly toxic to eukaryotic organisms and are responsible for many of the signs and symptoms arising when infection occurs. The outer membrane of Gram-negative bacteria enables them to withstand the action of many disinfectants but its relative thinness compared to Gram-positive bacterial cell walls makes them more susceptible to desiccation. The β-lactam ring of the penicillin molecule prevents the synthesis of peptidoglycan, allowing it to destroy the bacterial cell. Eukaryotic organisms do not contain peptidoglycan, explaining why penicillin can be given safely to treat infection. Many other antibiotics also target bacterial cell walls.

The difference between prokaryotic and eukaryotic cells is clinically important because prokaryotic organisms are damaged or destroyed by antimicrobial drugs that do not have the same effect on eukaryotic organisms. Antibiotics operate as 'magic bullets' specifically able to target bacteria without damaging the host in the same way. Some antibiotics prevent the synthesis of bacterial cell walls (e.g. cephalosporins, vancomycin). Others prevent the synthesis of bacterial proteins (e.g. gentamicin, erythromycin) or the formation of bacterial DNA (e.g. trimethoprim, co-trimoxazole).

Some bacteria are equipped with whip-like flagellae. This enables them to be highly motile, e.g. *Salmonella* spp. which cause food poisoning and *Proteus* spp. which are opportunistic and able to cause healthcare-associated infections. Other species are equipped with minute hairs called pili.

Classifying Bacteria
Bacterial Morphology
Bacteria are classified according to their morphological characteristics (shape) (Figure 1.3).

Cocci are round. They form clusters (e.g. *S. aureus*), chains (e.g. *Streptococcus pneumoniae*) or occur in pairs called diplococci (e.g. *N. gonorrhoeae*). *Bacilli* are rod-shaped bacteria occurring singly or in chains (e.g. *E. coli, Pseudomonas, Klebsiella, Proteus, Serratia, Salmonella*). *Vibrios* are curved (e.g. *Vibrio cholerae, Campylobacter*). Spirochaetes are tiny, flexible spirals (e.g. *T. pallidum* [syphilis], *Leptospira* [Weil's disease] and *Borrelia* [Lyme disease].

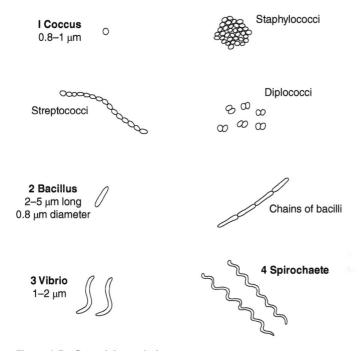

Figure 1.3   Bacterial morphology.

Gram Staining Reaction

Gram staining is the first step taken to identify bacteria in a laboratory specimen (Figure 1.4). Reaction to Gram's dye is determined by the chemical composition of the bacterial cell wall.

Gram-positive bacteria take up and retain Gram's stain, appearing blue. They are generally resistant to desiccation, tolerate dry conditions and are not flagellated or motile. Some species sporulate. They develop a thick layer of peptidoglycan around themselves, protecting the cellular contents against adverse conditions such as desiccation or lack of nutrients. When conditions become less hostile, the spores hatch to release vegetative bacteria able to grow and reproduce. *Bacillus cereus* is a Gram-positive species well known for causing food poisoning associated with Chinese meals. The spores, which are often present in rice, survive boiling. If the rice is then kept at a warm temperature for several hours, the vegetative bacteria emerge and multiply to form a large infective dose. Gentle reheating (to make 'special fried rice') does not destroy them and if ingested, the result is gastrointestinal upset.

Gram-positive bacteria release chemicals called *exotoxins*. Exotoxins are released outside the bacterial cell into the extracellular fluid of the host where they dissolve and are carried throughout tissues. They either destroy host cells or inhibit specific

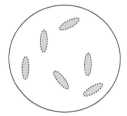

Identify organism of interest

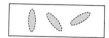

Prepare a smear of the bacteria and then use heat to fix the bacteria to the slide

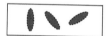

Flood the slide with 0.5% crystal violet and leave for 30 seconds. This will dye the bacteria purple.
Wash the slide with water

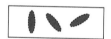

Flood the slide with (1%) Lugol's iodine (also known as Gram's iodine) and leave for 30 seconds.
Wash the slide with water

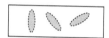

Decolourise with 95–100% ethanol or acetone until colour ceases to run out of the smear
Wash the slide with water

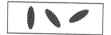

Flood the slide with 0.1% safranin as a counterstain. Wash the slide with water and blot dry
Examine the slide to observe cell morphology and Gram reaction

Gram positive
organisms stain blue or purple.

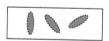

Gram negative
organisms stain pink or red.

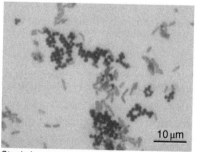

Staphylococcus aureus a Gram positive bacterium in purple, and *Escherichia coli* a Gram negative bacterium in pink

Figure 1.4 The Gram staining reaction.

cellular functions and can have very serious, often lethal effects. The exotoxin released by *C. tetani* is a potent neurotransmitter responsible for the paralysis caused by tetanus. Its release causes the muscles to go into spasm. Tetanus used to be called 'lockjaw' because of its effects on the facial muscles. If paralysis of the respiratory muscles occurs, the result is respiratory arrest, progressing to cardiac arrest and death. Ingestion of the exotoxins released by *S. aureus* causes food intoxication. The signs and symptoms are rapid-onset diarrhoea and vomiting, often within six hours. The illness is often described as 'mild' but can last several days, resulting in dehydration, especially in older people. Food intoxication cannot be prevented by heating food to a high temperature because exotoxins are heat resistant.

Gram-negative bacteria do not retain Gram's stain and appear red under the microscope. They thrive in damp situations, usually have very simple growth requirements, are often flagellated and motile, do not sporulate and many species are intrinsically resistant to antibiotics. *Endotoxins* forming part of cell wall are released when the bacteria die, causing fever and malaise when they escape into the tissue fluids of the host. The symptoms of typhoid (*S. typhi*) and meningitis (*Neisseria meningitidis*) are caused by endotoxin release.

Mycobacterium tuberculosis does not respond well to Gram's stain and is sometimes described as 'acid fast'.

Bacterial Reproduction and Genetics

The way that bacteria reproduce has important clinical implications. All bacteria are able to reproduce asexually by *binary fission*. The parent cell divides into two genetically identical daughter cells, each receiving half the genetic material of the parent (Figure 1.5a). There is no genetic variation and no scope for adaptation to the environment (evolution). The warmth and dampness prevailing in healthcare premises provide ideal conditions for bacterial growth and multiplication. Division can occur every 30 minutes, generating large reservoirs of bacteria, increasing the risk of transmission. If a laboratory specimen is stored at room temperature, any bacteria that it contains multiply rapidly, leading to heavy levels of contamination. The findings of laboratory tests are then more difficult to interpret.

Some species of bacteria are capable of exchanging genetic material, enabling them to adapt to changing environmental conditions. Those best adapted to the environment survive and multiply at the expense of those less well adapted. This process involves the exchange of a circle of extracellular DNA called a *plasmid*. Plasmids are clinically important as they often carry genes conferring resistance to antimicrobial substances (Bennett 2008). Plasmids can replicate and when the bacterial cell, divides each daughter cell will contain a copy of the plasmid. Plasmid transfer between bacteria is possible via four routes (Box 1.6).

Clearly, the progeny arising through plasmid exchange are not genetically identical. Having a gene that enables the bacterium to resist the effects of

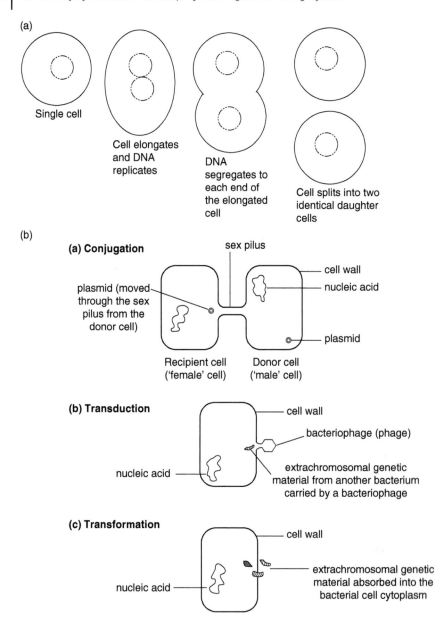

(a)

Single cell

Cell elongates and DNA replicates

DNA segregates to each end of the elongated cell

Cell splits into two identical daughter cells

(b)

(a) Conjugation

sex pilus

cell wall

nucleic acid

plasmid (moved through the sex pilus from the donor cell)

plasmid

Recipient cell ('female' cell)

Donor cell ('male' cell)

(b) Transduction

cell wall

bacteriophage (phage)

nucleic acid

extrachromosomal genetic material from another bacterium carried by a bacteriophage

(c) Transformation

cell wall

extrachromosomal genetic material absorbed into the bacterial cell cytoplasm

nucleic acid

Figure 1.5 (a) Binary fission. (b) Plasmid-mediated bacterial reproduction.

Box 1.6   Mechanisms of Plasmid Transfer

Transformation occurs when some bacteria ('competent bacteria') take up extracellular DNA released into the environment from decomposing or disrupted cells, viral particles or DNA excreted by living cells via their cell walls. This DNA is either carried in the cytoplasm as a plasmid or integrated into the bacterial genome (Thomas and Nielsen 2005).

Conjugation involves the development of a junction between two bacteria, genesis of a pore and a channel called a sex pilus that allows the passage of a plasmid from one cell to the other.

Transduction involves plasmid transfer to a bacterial cell that has become infected with a virus particle called a bacteriophage.

Transposable elements are sequences of DNA able to alter position by moving from a chromosome to a pre-existing plasmid. Once incorporated into the plasmid, they can be transferred to other bacteria through conjugation or transduction. The transposon Tn*1546*, which contains a cluster of genes known as *vanA*, can be transferred between bacteria (Gardete and Tomasz 2014) and has been linked to vancomycin resistance in *S. aureus* (Sievert et al. 2008).

---

antimicrobials will allow it to thrive and multiply by binary fission in an environment where others would be unable to survive. This is the mechanism driving antimicrobial resistance. Genes conferring resistance to the β-lactamase group of antibiotics (e.g. penicillin, cephalosporins, carbapenems) are carried on plasmids. Many bacteria, mainly Gram-negative species, are able to undergo transformation. Conjugation occurs in Gram-negative and Gram-positive bacteria. *S. aureus* is able to acquire resistance to meticillin via a set of genes called MecA transferred by conjugation. It is also possible for plasmid transfer to take place between Gram-negative and Gram-positive species. Gram-negative resistance to carbapenem is plasmid mediated (Codjoe and Donkor 2017).

Mycoplasmas

Mycoplasmas are a genus of small bacteria that lack cell walls. As a result, they are naturally resistant to antimicrobial drugs that exert their effects by disrupting cell wall synthesis. Several species are human pathogens. *Mycoplasma pneumoniae* causes pneumonia; *M. genitalium* is sexually transmitted.

Viruses

Viruses are very small, typically 10–30 nm and visible only with the electron microscope. Each virus particle consists of a nucleic acid core surrounded by a protein coat called a *capsid* which carries receptors that enable the virus to attach

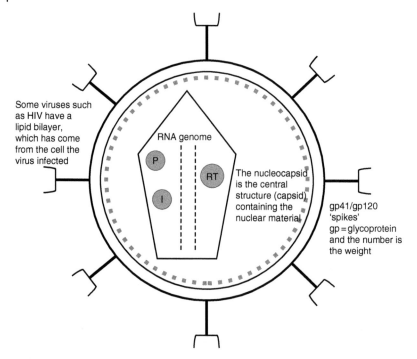

Viruses are much simpler than bacteria or human cells. This is HIV. It can infect CD4+ cells such as T-helper cells because of the fit between the GP41/GP120 on the outside of the virus and CD4 molecules on the cell.
Because of the unique replication of retroviruses such as HIV which involves making a DNA copy of its RNA genome, it has to carry its own enzyme to do this, known as reverse transcriptase (RT). Other important viral enzymes are integrase (I) and protease (P). Each of these is a target of anti-HIV treatment.

Figure 1.6   Structure of a typical virus.

to the host cell (Figure 1.6). Viral nucleic acid consists of either DNA or RNA but never both. Some viruses are described as 'enveloped' because they have an outer lipid (fat) capsule surrounding the protein coat. 'Naked' viruses lack a lipid capsule. The glycopeptide receptors enable the virus to attach to the host cell. Attachment is always at a specific site on the surface.

Viruses cause disease in humans, animals and plants. One group called *bacteriophages* (phages) infect bacteria. Viruses are obligate parasites. They cannot grow and replicate outside living cells and technically are not alive as they lack all the characteristics of living organisms (see Table 1.4) except the ability to reproduce and pass on genetic information to their progeny. There is ongoing debate between biologists and philosophers regarding whether it is correct to regard viruses as living organisms or whether they occupy a grey zone between the animate and inanimate. It is often assumed that because of their simple structure, they represent the first, most primitive form of life but it is more likely that viruses are degenerate organisms that have lost their ability to exist independently during evolution.

Life Cycle of Viruses

An example of the life (or replication) cycle of a virus is shown below, in this case HIV. HIV is a retrovirus, meaning that its genetic material is in the form of RNA which has to be turned into DNA to allow the virus to replicate. Viruses attach themselves to the surface of the host cell at specific receptor sites and enter, leaving the protein coat outside (Figure 1.7). Receptor sites are specific for the virus, and

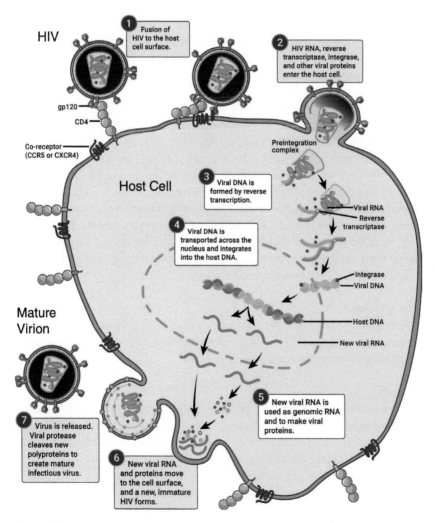

Figure 1.7 Life cycle of a DNA virus.

mean that viruses can only infect cells carrying the receptor that they recognise. They type of cell, tissue or species that a virus can infect is known as its tropism. In the case of HIV, the virus initially attaches itself to CD4 receptors on the surfaces of macrophages lymphocytes and some other cells. Having entered the cell, the viral RNA is converted to DNA by a virus specific enzyme known as reverse transcriptase, and becomes incorporated or integrated into the DNA of the host cell by another viral enzyme known as integrase. It then takes command of its genetic machinery, generating large numbers of new virus proteins. New virus particles are assembled and released into the environment. Most viruses destroy the host cell but as only a few are affected, the host organism recovers. There are exceptions, however. HIV eventually depletes the cells of the host immune system. Viruses able to cause malignancy (e.g. papilloma virus) are also highly destructive.

Treating virus infections with conventional antibiotics is impossible because they lack a cellular structure and are protected inside living cells.

Acute and Dormant Virus Infections

Some virus infections are acute, others cause dormant infections. When the infection is acute, new virus particles either bud out of the host cell membrane or cause it to burst (lyse) and release them. The host cell dies and the infection resolves quickly. Minor respiratory infections such as colds, influenza and varicella (chickenpox) are examples of acute virus infections. When the infection is dormant, the virus remains inactive inside the host cell for months or years. Reactivation occurs under specific circumstances, often when the host becomes unwell. The symptoms of viral infection manifest long after the initial infection. Herpes zoster (shingles) is an example of a dormant virus infection which typically occurs in older people, often if they develop another illness.

Classifying Viruses

Numerous different ways of classifying viruses have been devised over the years. Modern systems are based on the shape of the virus particle. Some of the major groups of clinical importance are presented below.

Adenoviruses

Adenoviruses are DNA viruses able to cause a wide range of common illnesses including colds, sore throats, influenza-like infections, conjunctivitis and gastrointestinal infections. There appears to be more than one mode of spread and portal of entry, including direct contact and the air-borne route. Infections occur most often in young children and those who have close contact with them. Infections are more serious in individuals who are immunosuppressed. The period of infectivity is prolonged. Risk factors include crowded conditions, especially indoors.

Herpesviruses

Herpesviruses are DNA viruses responsible for a number of different types of infection. Herpes simplex types 1 and 2 cause cold sores and genital infections. The varicella zoster virus causes chickenpox, which is an acute, usually mild infection affecting children. The virus can remain dormant in the dorsal horn cells of the nerves after the acute infection is over and become reactivated at a later stage, giving rise to herpes zoster (shingles). Vesicular lesions containing virus particles appear on the skin, mirroring the path of the nerve over its surface. The Epstein–Barr virus is responsible for glandular fever (infectious mononucleosis). *Cytomegalovirus* often results in asymptomatic infections but can cause respiratory or gastrointestinal symptoms.

Caliciviruses

Caliciviruses are RNA viruses responsible for gastroenteritis. The most notorious is norovirus which causes 'winter vomiting'. Outbreaks are very common in community and hospital settings and are very difficult to control.

Other clinically important RNA viruses are shown in Table 1.6.

Prions

Prions are protein particles that do not contain genetic material. They are responsible for a number of serious neurological diseases (Ironside et al. 2017). These conditions have a high public profile but are rare, occasionally causing sporadic infections in the community (Haywood 1997). Examples are Creutzfeld–Jakob disease, bovine spongiform encephalopathy, fatal familial insomnia and kuru. Infection is thought to occur following changes in prion structure. Iatrogenic transmission appears possible, for example during transplant surgery, blood transfusion or if surgical instruments become contaminated with neurological tissue, cerebrospinal fluid or blood.

Prions are resistant to disinfection and sterilization. Special approaches must be taken to contain risks in operating theatres.

Table 1.6   RNA viruses.

Piconaviruses, e.g. rhinovirus, coxsackie virus, hepatitis A
Togavirus, e.g. yellow fever, dengue fever, hepatitis C
Rubella
Orthomyxovirus, e.g. influenza
Calicivirus, e.g. norovirus
Coronavirus, e.g. colds, COVID, SARS
Retrovirus, e.g. HIV, leukaemia viruses

Fungal Infections

Fungi are eukaryotic organisms exhibiting all the characteristics of living organisms (see Table 1.2). They form huge quantities of minute spores spread via the air. Fungi are classified separately from other organisms but have most in common with animals. Their cellular organelles are similar to those of animals and they contain the storage carbohydrate glycogen also found in animals. Over 300 000 species exist and there are undoubtedly many more to be discovered and classified. Most are harmless saprophytes living in soil and water and some are commercially important in cheese and bread making. About 600 species have been associated with human disease and some species are opportunistic (e.g. *Candida* spp., *Aspergillus* spp.) (Caceres et al. 2020). Their similarity to animals makes developing antifungals challenging.

Structurally, fungi fall into two groups: simple forms (yeasts), that reproduce asexually by forming buds, and those with a more complex structure. Complex fungi are made up of microscopic, filamentous *hyphae* which absorb nutrients and water. Collectively hyphae are called a *mycelium*. The visible fruiting bodies of mushrooms and toadstools are large collections of hyphae visible to the naked eye. Fungi are highly invasive because the finger-like hyphae enable them to grow between cells and into organs.

Fungal infections are called mycoses. A *mycosis* can be superficial or systemic. Superficial mycoses are restricted to subcutaneous tissues that contain the protein keratin (the skin and its appendages [nails, hair]) and to the mucous membranes. The deeper tissues are not invaded and if a host response occurs, it is only mild. Nevertheless, superficial mycoses are distressing and because they are often visible to other people, can be a source of embarrassment and lead to stigmatisation. Athlete's foot (*Trichophyton interdigitale*) and ringworm (*Tinea capitis*) are examples of superficial mycoses affecting the skin and appendages. *Candida albicans* is a superficial mycosis responsible for 'thrush' affecting the mucous membranes lining the oral cavity and vagina. Superficial mycoses are usually amenable to topical treatment with creams, ointments and pessaries.

Systemic mycoses affect the internal tissues (Box 1.7). The portal of entry is either via the respiratory or gastrointestinal tract or the skin. The host is usually immunocompromised and the outcome of infection is often a severe illness (Hope et al. 2013). *Aspergillosis fumigatus*, *Candida auris* and *Rhizopus* spp. can give rise to systemic mycoses. *Pneumocystis* spp. are opportunistic but can cause severe lung disease in immunocompromised patients. This mycosis first gained attention during the HIV pandemic in the 1980s when many people became severely ill.

The management of systemic fungal infections is challenging because patients are usually already very ill and few effective antifungal agents are available to treat them. Their development is encouraged by warm, humid conditions. At one time, systemic mycoses were uncommon in temperate climates but the *incidence* is now increasing, probably as an effect of global warming. Advancements in medical

---

Box 1.7 Invasive Fungal Disease

Invasive fungal disease is an important cause of morbidity and mortality amongst critically ill and immunocompromised patients. Construction and renovation activities can cause extensive contamination of the healthcare environment, resulting in clusters of infection. The main culprit is *Aspergillus* spp. Recommendations for decreasing risk include minimising dust likely to be contaminated by spores generated during construction work and preventing dust infiltrating clinical areas by using high-efficiency filtration systems near patients at high risk.

Source: Adpated from Kanamori et al. (2015).

---

science have increased the number of severely immunocompromised patients and this is also considered an important contributory factor to the increasing incidence of invasive fungal disease (de Cássia Orlandi Sardi et al. 2018).

Protozoa

Protozoa are unicellular microscopic animals. Many species exist but most live harmlessly in water and soil. Under adverse conditions, they form thick-walled cysts which can survive for long periods until a return to more favourable conditions. A few species are pathogenic (Table 1.7).

Malaria is a protozoal infection responsible for a major public health problem globally (Box 1.8).

Chlamydiae

Chlamydiae combine the characteristics of bacteria and viruses but can be treated with antibiotics. All are obligate intracellular organisms. Many species exist and a few are important human pathogens responsible for serious public health problems. *C. trachomatis* is the leading cause of blindness in low-income countries. In higher income countries, it is most commonly spread through vaginal, oral and anal sex. Men develop non-specific urethritis. Women develop *salpingitis* which is a leading cause of subfertility. Neonates can develop pneumonia or serious eye infections during passage down an infected birth canal.

Table 1.7 Pathogenic protozoa.

Plasmodium spp. (malaria): biological transmission by insect vector
Trichomonas vaginalis: sexual transmission
Giardia lamblia: food-borne and water-borne transmission
Entamoeba histolytica (amoebic dysentery): food-borne and water-borne transmission
Toxoplasma gondii: transmission in undercooked meat, cat faeces, vertical transmission in the human host

---

Box 1.8   Malaria

According to the World Health Organization (WHO), there are 229 million cases of malaria globally. In 2019, 409 000 deaths were reported, of which nearly 70% were in children. Nearly half the global population is at risk and the most affected nation is Africa. Symptoms vary. Mild infections are hard to diagnose. Severe infections cause acute febrile illness with fever, chills and malaise. The parasites (plasmodia) live and multiple inside erythrocytes and symptoms recur when they burst, releasing the plasmodia into the bloodstream. Long-term effects include anaemia, respiratory distress resulting from metabolic disturbance and cerebral malaria. Developing effective vaccines has been challenging because the plasmodia are protected inside the erythrocytes but the discovery of an effective vaccine was announced by Oxford University in 2021. Malaria is also prevented by public health measures to control the vector: insecticides, use of antimalarial prophylaxis and drainage of swamps where the mosquitoes live.

Numerous drugs are used in malarial chemoprophylaxis, but resistance is widely reported so travellers should be advised to seek the latest information from travel centres. It may be necessary to take several drugs in combination to reduce the possibility of the plasmodia developing resistance. Drug regimens differ between regions according to the levels of risk and existing drug resistance.

Parasites

There are two broad group of parasites: endoparasites which live inside the body and ectoparasites which live on the surface.

Endoparasites
Helminthic (Worm) Infestations
Numerous species can infest humans. Some are microscopic. Others are large and clearly visible to the naked eye but the eggs and early larval stages are visible only under the microscope and specimens are sent to the medical microbiology department for diagnosis. Identification is usually by examining specimens of recently passed faeces ('hot' stools) because any microscopic forms they contain are likely to be alive and active, increasing the chances of diagnosis. There are two groups of helminths: roundworms and flatworms (Table 1.8).

Some helminthic infestations are minor and a nuisance. Others constitute a major public health challenge.

Enterobius vermicularis (threadworm) is the most common helminth in the UK. It usually affects children. The worms infest the large bowel and emerge onto the perineum at night where they lay their eggs. Many people are unaware that they have threadworms but perianal and vaginal itching are common. Scratching followed by swallowing eggs contaminating the fingers perpetuates reinfestation.

Table 1.8   Helminths.

Roundworms

Enterobius vermicularis (threadworm)

Ascaris lumbricoides (roundworm)

Necator spp. (hookworm)

Strongyloides spp.

Flatworms

Taenia spp. (tapeworm)

Adults are less likely to be affected than children because the adult gastric secretions are more acidic and destroy the eggs more effectively. The eggs can survive on surfaces for up to two weeks and are readily transferred to bedclothes, flannels, towels, toys and kitchen utensils. Transmission occurs easily between members of the same household and all must receive treatment.

Mebendazole is the most commonly used medication and is available over the counter. It kills the adult worms within a few days but does not destroy the eggs. Stringent hygiene measures are necessary to eradicate the infestation: washing bedlinen, towels and soft toys, thoroughly vacuum cleaning the house, especially bedrooms, and not eating in bedrooms to avoid swallowing eggs shaken off bedclothes. Thorough hand hygiene and scrubbing nails should be encouraged. Nail biting and thumb sucking should be discouraged. Precautions should continue for six weeks as this is the life cycle of *E. vermicularis*.

Other species of helminths are a leading cause of chronic ill health in warm, moist climates where sanitation is poor. The worms inhabit the intestine, the eggs escape in faeces and are transmitted to other people on contaminated fingers and food. Infestation is very common, especially in children. Light infestations may have few ill effects. More severe infestations interfere with the absorption of food, contributing to undernutrition and anaemia. Helminthic infestation is a major and underappreciated cause of poor educational attainment and economic underdevelopment globally but is preventable.

Ectoparasites

Ectoparasites live outside the host, either on or in the skin (Table 1.9).

Outbreaks of scabies are often reported in hospitals and nursing homes. Infestation is caused by mites.

Scabies is caused by the mite *Sarcoptes scabiei* which is transmitted directly and indirectly by skin contact. The mite burrows into the skin and lays eggs, giving rise to intense itching and a papular rash. Symptoms appear in 4–8 weeks. Scabies causes intense itching which may persist for some time after treatment, can lead to skin infections and can make existing skin conditions (e.g. psoriasis) worse.

Table 1.9 Ectoparasites: examples.

Sarcoptes scabiei	Scabies
Cimex lectularius	Bed bug
Pediculus humanus capitis	Head louse
Pediculus humanus humanus	Body louse
Phthirius pubis	Pubic louse

Transmission requires direct, prolonged skin-to-skin contact, contact on clothing, bedclothing or furnishings. Scabies can spread rapidly in crowded conditions, especially as asymptomatic individuals can be a source of infestation. Eradication involves washing all clothing and bedclothing at 50 °C or higher. Items that cannot be washed should be placed in a bag which should be sealed for three days while the mites perish. Treatment is with 5% permethrin cream or 0.5 malathion lotion available over-the-counter.

'Crusted' (Norwegian) scabies results when large numbers of mites are present and is particularly likely to result in outbreaks in hospitals, nursing homes and prisons which may be hard to control (Vorou et al. 2007). Treatment with ivermectin can be effective.

Head Lice

Head lice (*Pediculus humanus capitis*) are very common. Children and sometimes adults are affected. Transmission occurs when two heads touch and the lice are able to jump. They prefer clean hair because it enables them to move around easily and as they like warmth, they tend to congregate close to the scalp. Lice are difficult to dislodge and cannot be removed by ordinary shampooing. Adult females lay large numbers of eggs close to the base of the hair shafts. The usual symptom, itching, may not develop for several weeks. Lice can be removed by wet combing. Chemical insecticides are not always effective and resistance is developing.

Pubic Lice

Pubic lice (*Phthirius pubis*) infest the coarse body hair and are spread by close contact, including between family members as well as during sexual contact. They die rapidly in the environment and are not spread by clothing or other objects. Treatment is with insecticides, either topically (e.g. malathion) or orally (ivermectin).

Suggested Activities

Exercise 1.1 Self-assessment

1   Complete the following sentence: 'A microbial pathogen is defined as . . .'

2   A reservoir of infection is:
    A Any source of infection inside the patient zone
    B Where the pathogen survives but cannot multiply
    C Where the pathogen lives and multiplies
    D Any source of infection outside the patient zone.

3   List seven ways in which micro-organisms spread.

4   The infectious dose is:
    A The number of organisms required for colonisation to occur
    B The number of organisms required for infection to occur
    C The number of organisms required for cross-infection to occur
    D The number of organisms required for cross-contamination to occur.

5   Under favourable circumstances, most bacteria are able to cause infection.
    True/False

6   Explain the key difference between endogenous infection and exogenous infection.

7   DNA viruses reproduce by binary fission.
    True/False

8   Which of the following cause mycoses?
    A *T. pallidum*
    B *Pneumocystis* spp.
    C *Aspergillus fumigatus*
    D All of the above

9   Which of the following are pathogenic protozoa?
    A *Plasmodium* spp., *Trichomonas vaginalis*, *Entamoeba histolytica*, *T. pallidum*
    B *Plasmodium* spp., *M. genitalium*, *E. histolytica*, *Toxoplasma gondii*
    C *Plasmodium* spp., *Trichomonas vaginalis*, *E. histolytica*, *Toxoplasma gondii*
    D All of the above

10 The commensal flora is always harmless.
    True/False

Exercise 1.2

Choose a pathogen that has caused problems/has the potential to cause problems in your own clinical setting.

- What are the problems/potential problems?
- Apply the chain of infection to suggest solutions.
- Identify lessons for future clinical practice, policy and education in your organisation.

References

Ayliffe, G.A., Collins, B.J., and Pettit, F. (1970). Contamination of infant feeds in a Milton milk kitchen. *Lancet* 1: 559–560. https://doi.org/10.1016/s0140-6736(70)90783-x.

Bennett, P.M. (2008). Plasmid encoded antibiotic resistance: acquisition and transfer of antibiotic resistance genes in bacteria: plasmid-encoded antibiotic resistance. *Br. J. Pharmacol.* 153: S347–S357. https://doi.org/10.1038/sj.bjp.0707607.

Boone, S.A. and Gerba, C.P. (2007). Significance of fomites in the spread of respiratory and enteric viral disease. *Appl. Environ. Microbiol.* 73: 1687–1696. https://doi.org/10.1128/AEM.02051-06.

Caceres, D.H., Mohd Tap, R., Alastruey-Izquierdo, A., and Hagen, F. (2020). Detection and control of fungal outbreaks. *Mycopathologia* 185: 741–745. https://doi.org/10.1007/s11046-020-00494-1.

Casewell, M.W. and Phillips, I. (1978). Epidemiological patterns of klebsiella colonization and infection in an intensive care ward. *J. Hyg.* 80: 295–300. https://doi.org/10.1017/S0022172400053651.

de Cássia Orlandi Sardi, J., Silva, D.R., Soares Mendes-Giannini, M.J., and Rosalen, P.L. (2018). Candida auris: epidemiology, risk factors, virulence, resistance, and therapeutic options. *Microb. Pathog.* 125: 116–121. https://doi.org/10.1016/j.micpath.2018.09.014.

Codjoe, F.S. and Donkor, E.S. (2017). Carbapenem resistance: a review. *Med. Sci.* 6: E1. https://doi.org/10.3390/medsci6010001.

Davies, M.P., Anderson, M., and Hilton, A.C. (2016). The housefly *Musca domestica* as a mechanical vector of *Clostridium difficile. J. Hosp. Infect.* 94: 263–267. https://doi.org/10.1016/j.jhin.2016.08.023.

Drossinos, Y., Weber, T.P., and Stilianakis, N.I. (2021). Droplets and aerosols: an artificial dichotomy in respiratory virus transmission. *Health Sci. Rep.* 4: e275. https://doi.org/10.1002/hsr2.275.

Gardete, S. and Tomasz, A. (2014). Mechanisms of vancomycin resistance in *Staphylococcus aureus. J. Clin. Invest.* 124: 2836–2840. https://doi.org/10.1172/JCI68834.

Gibson, B., Wilson, D.J., Feil, E., and Eyre-Walker, A. (2018). The distribution of bacterial doubling times in the wild. *Proc. R. Soc. B* 285: 20180789. https://doi.org/10.1098/rspb.2018.0789.

Hassard, F., Sharp, J.H., Taft, H. et al. (2017). Critical review on the public health impact of norovirus contamination in shellfish and the environment: a UK perspective. *Food Environ. Virol.* 9: 123–141. https://doi.org/10.1007/s12560-017-9279-3.

Haywood, A.M. (1997). Transmissible spongiform encephalopathies. *N. Engl. J. Med.* 337: 1821–1828. https://doi.org/10.1056/NEJM199712183372508.

Heath, P.T. and Jardine, L.A. (2014). Neonatal infections: group B streptococcus. *BMJ Clin. Evid.* 2014: 0323.

Hope, W., Natarajan, P., and Goodwin, L. (2013). Invasive fungal infections. *Clin. Med.* 13: 507–510. https://doi.org/10.7861/clinmedicine.13-5-507.

Ironside, J.W., Ritchie, D.L., and Head, M.W. (2017). Prion diseases. *Handb. Clin. Neurol.* 145: 393–403. https://doi.org/10.1016/B978-0-12-802395-2.00028-6.

Kanamori, H., Rutala, W.A., Sickbert-Bennett, E.E., and Weber, D.J. (2015). Review of fungal outbreaks and infection prevention in healthcare settings during construction and renovation. *Clin. Infect. Dis.* 61: 433–444. https://doi.org/10.1093/cid/civ297.

Kanamori, H., Rutala, W.A., and Weber, D.J. (2017). The role of patient care items as a fomite in healthcare-associated outbreaks and infection prevention. *Clin. Infect. Dis.* 65: 1412–1419. https://doi.org/10.1093/cid/cix462.

Karimzadeh, S., Bhopal, R., and Nguyen Tien, H. (2021). Review of infective dose, routes of transmission and outcome of COVID-19 caused by the SARS-COV-2: comparison with other respiratory viruses. *Epidemiol. Infect.* 149: e96. https://doi.org/10.1017/S0950268821000790.

Schmid-Hempel, P. and Frank, S.A. (2007). Pathogenesis, virulence, and infective dose. *PLoS Pathog.* 3: e147. https://doi.org/10.1371/journal.ppat.0030147.

Sievert, D.M., Rudrik, J.T., Patel, J.B. et al. (2008). Vancomycin-resistant *Staphylococcus aureus* in the United States, 2002–2006. *Clin. Infect. Dis.* 46: 668–674. https://doi.org/10.1086/527392.

Stamm, W.E. (1978). Stamm highlights device-related infections. *Hosp. Infect. Control* 5: 100.

Tang, J.W., Bahnfleth, W.P., Bluyssen, P.M. et al. (2021). Dismantling myths on the airborne transmission of severe acute respiratory syndrome coronavirus-2 (SARS-CoV-2). *J. Hosp. Infect.* 110: 89–96. https://doi.org/10.1016/j.jhin.2020.12.022.

Thomas, C.M. and Nielsen, K.M. (2005). Mechanisms of, and barriers to, horizontal gene transfer between bacteria. *Nat. Rev. Microbiol.* 3: 711–721. https://doi.org/10.1038/nrmicro1234.

Vorou, R., Remoudaki, H.D., and Maltezou, H.C. (2007). Nosocomial scabies. *J. Hosp. Infect.* 65: 9–14. https://doi.org/10.1016/j.jhin.2006.08.012.

Wells, W.F. (1934). On air-borne infection: study ii. droplets and droplet nuclei. *Am. J. Epidemiol.* 20: 611–618. https://doi.org/10.1093/oxfordjournals.aje.a118097.

Wong, G., Liu, W., Liu, Y. et al. (2015). MERS, SARS, and Ebola: the role of super-spreaders in infectious disease. *Cell Host Microbe* 18: 398–401. https://doi.org/10.1016/j.chom.2015.09.013.

2

Applying the Principles of Evidence-based Practice to Infection Prevention and Control

The Evidence-based Medicine Movement

The modern age of evidence-based medicine (EBM) arose through the work of Archie Cochrane and David Sackett in the 1960s and 1970s. At that time, many healthcare interventions were based on treatments that had not been demonstrated to be effective through scientific study. Instead, junior nurses and doctors copied the practice of senior staff and applied the same treatments and rituals. EBM was conceived to encourage the uptake of healthcare interventions of known effectiveness based on empirical evidence obtained through research. The aims of EBM were to avoid wasting time and resources and avoid the harm that can arise through the use of untested treatments.

The move towards EBM resulted in the Cochrane Collaboration and Cochrane systematic reviews. These synthesise the evidence underpinning clinical interventions intended to improve patient care. Their goal is to use the best evidence available to support practice, while taking into consideration the needs of the individual patient. EBM is based on a hierarchy called the Levels of Evidence (Figure 2.1). The hierarchy was developed to classify evidence obtained through quantitative research, predominantly through randomised controlled trials (RCTs) which traditionally have been considered as the 'gold standard' empirical approach to research. The use of similar hierarchies for quantitative evidence is controversial and not universally accepted (Aromataris and Munn 2020).

Evidence generated through research high up the hierarchy is by convention considered more robust than evidence of research lower down because it is less subject to bias. *Bias* is defined as the systematic influence of factors other than those under investigation that might affect the outcomes of the study. It should be reduced as far as possible because it undermines the validity of the findings – the extent to which they can be regarded as a genuine reflection of reality.

Infection Prevention and Control in Healthcare Settings,
First Edition. Edward Purssell and Dinah Gould.
© 2023 John Wiley & Sons Ltd. Published 2023 by John Wiley & Sons Ltd.

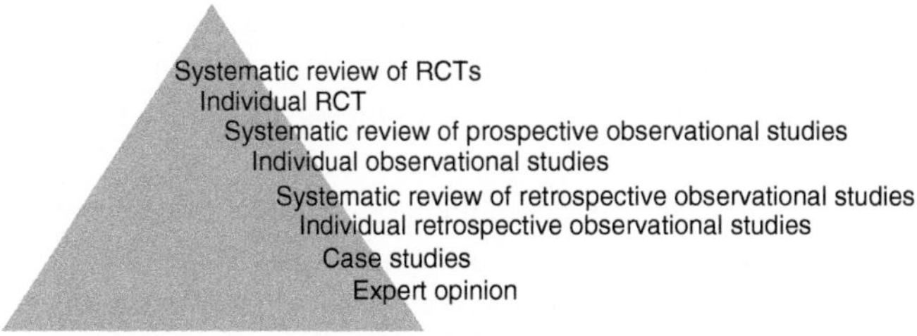

Systematic review of RCTs
Individual RCT
Systematic review of prospective observational studies
Individual observational studies
Systematic review of retrospective observational studies
Individual retrospective observational studies
Case studies
Expert opinion

At each level a systematic review is a higher level of evidence than an individual study.
Expert opinion is not really a level of evidence, but rather an interpretation of evidence.
Prospective studies are a higher level of evidence than retrospective studies because data
collection can be planned.
Observational evidence that can be upgraded using GRADE may provide stronger evidence than
downgraded RCT evidence.

There is no direct equivalent for qualitative studies.

Figure 2.1   Levels of evidence.

Research Paradigms

Research paradigms represent shared beliefs concerning the way that research is
understood. Proponents of the same school of thought hold the same ontological
(philosophical) beliefs relating to research, see the world in a particular way
('worldview') and interpret its findings (epistemology) accordingly (Kuhn 1970).

In broad terms, two types of research paradigm have evolved: positivism and
interpretivism. According to the proponents of positivism, it is possible to generalise the findings of one study to other situations and circumstances. Positivism is
the paradigm employed by life scientists and utilises quantitative methodologies.
Quantitative research is primarily concerned with numbers and taking data from
a sample and making inferences about a population based on that sample.

According to the interpretivist school of thought, it is not appropriate to
generalise the findings from one study to other situations and circumstances.
These researchers study human behaviour which they consider likely to change
according to situational and environmental factors. Members of the interpretivist
school of thought are social scientists and their research adopts qualitative methodologies that are context specific. The aim is not to generalise to other situations
and settings but to understand a phenomenon and generate theory.

Application to Infection Prevention and Control

Infection prevention is a multidisciplinary endeavour. Knowledge about
micro-organisms and their behaviour is derived from the life sciences by microbiologists and epidemiologists. Such knowledge on its own does not, however,

explain why guidelines to prevent infection are implemented better in some settings and by some health workers than others and it is here that the expertise of social scientists, founded on interpretivism and employing qualitative methodologies, is invaluable.

Much contemporary research addressing challenges in infection prevention does not depend on a single paradigm or set of assumptions. Instead, an eclectic approach is adopted by research teams whose members have different expertise in order to obtain complementary insights about the phenomenon under scrutiny, combining quantitative and qualitative methodologies. A large mixed-methods research project might seek to establish not just whether a treatment is effective in a clinical trial but also why it is or is not effective by adopting qualitative approaches (e.g. interviews, focus groups).

Interventions and Observational Research

Research studies are often described as interventional or observational.

- Intervention studies, such as randomised or quasi-randomised studies, are designed to test the truth of an assumption (hypothesis); although using traditional methods, this is usually done indirectly by testing the results against a null hypothesis. They always involve quantitative methods and employ manipulation. The intervention is the action taken (e.g. administering a new antibiotic) and the aim of the study is to determine whether the treatment achieves the desired outcome (resolution of infection). This is an example of a simple intervention in which the impact of a single action is evaluated. Interventions can also be complex. A bundle of actions intended to increase adherence to hand hygiene that involves providing alcohol handrub at every bedside, staff education with reminders and performance feedback would constitute a complex intervention. Sometimes trials evaluate a number of different interventions and might involve two or more treatment groups ('arms'). A trial might be set up with one arm evaluating the impact of the bundle described above and a second arm consisting of education only, as well as a control group receiving no intervention. A complex bundled intervention is inevitably more expensive and takes more time to organise than a single intervention and a complex package of care is more expensive than a single one. Consequently, a complex trial might evaluate the relative merits of each of the components of the bundle in separate arms compared to a control.
- Observational studies draw inferences from a sample to a population without manipulation (e.g. surveys, cohort studies, case–control studies). They are often used when conducting a trial would be impossible because of ethical concerns or

would not be feasible (e.g. prohibitive cost). Observational studies are lower down the hierarchy of evidence because the lack of control increases the risk of bias but such studies should not be dismissed as generating low-quality evidence. The risk of bias arising from a poorly controlled trial can be greater than the risk of bias associated with a well-conducted observational study (Black 1996).

Many infection prevention precautions have been in place for years and are firmly entrenched in practice. Deliberately withholding them in a control group would not be sanctioned by an ethics committee and would not be acceptable to health workers or patient support organisations. For example, to evaluate a hand hygiene campaign, the new approach or intervention would be compared to usual hand hygiene practice rather than having a control group where the practice is withheld entirely (no hand hygiene). Alternatively, a methodology lower down the hierarchy of evidence could be used, such as observing two different wards.

Today, it is appreciated that different disciplines value sources of evidence differently and address different types of research question. The Cochrane Collaboration has responded by developing protocols for synthesising a wider range of research studies and a number of other organisations have proposed their own methodologies (e.g. Campbell Collaboration for social sciences and Joanna Briggs Institute for qualitative and mixed-methods research). There are also circumstances in which a research design high up the conventional hierarchy would be superfluous to requirements because the research question requires a different approach. RCTs are not designed to explore the reasons why health workers do not adhere to hand hygiene protocols or to explore public anxiety about a new, highly infectious pathogen. Qualitative methodologies are more appropriate to address these issues.

Critical Appraisal

Some clinicians engage in research as part of their usual work. For others, their main research responsibility is to ensure that clinical practice is based on the best research evidence available and that the findings are appropriate to their organisation or specific clinical setting. The ability to critically appraise research findings is essential when making these decisions.

Undertaking critical appraisal requires the ability to assess the trustworthiness, value and relevance of research to practice in a particular context. A range of critical appraisal tools are available to guide evaluation (Table 2.1). The Critical Appraisal Skills Programme (CASP) is among the most widely used (Brice 2021).

Key questions to consider when using CASP to decide whether to implement the findings of research locally are:

Table 2.1   Critical appraisal tools: examples.

Critical Appraisal Skills Programme (CASP) – wide range of tools:
https://casp-uk.net/casp-tools-checklists
Joanna Briggs Institute – another wide range of tools:
https://jbi.global/critical-appraisal-tools
Newcastle Ottawa Scale – for assessing the quality of non-randomised studies:
https://www.ohri.ca//programs/clinical_epidemiology/oxford.Asp tool

- What are the study findings?
- Can we believe them?
- Would the study findings be helpful to support local practice?

The following sections provide an overview of the main research methodologies that clinicians need to know about when critically appraising research.

Quantitative Research Methods

Classic Randomised Controlled Trials

The classic double-blind RCT was originally developed to test the effectiveness of new drugs and is designed to establish whether the medication is directly responsible for bringing about its desired outcome (e.g. reduce inflammation, resolve infection). This is achieved by ruling out the possibility that the outcome has been influenced by some other variable that has not been measured (effect of bias). 'Double blind' means that neither the patient or the research team responsible for administering the drug or analysing the data knows whether the patient has received the real drug or a placebo that looks exactly like it. The aim is to avoid patients or clinicians being influenced by awareness of group allocation. It is possible, for example, that the pain associated with inflammation might resolve because a patient knows that they have received an antibiotic and expects to feel better.

Patients in the population to be tested are randomly allocated to the intervention or control group using a computer program. The purpose of randomisation is to ensure that every patient recruited has an equal chance of receiving the drug or placebo. Randomisation is intended to avoid bias by distributing characteristics of the patients (e.g. age, gender) that might influence the outcome of treatment between the groups. If this has been done correctly, it should allow any difference in outcome between the intervention and test group to be attributed to the treatment.

The association between the treatment and outcome is determined by undertaking statistical tests. The dose of the drug, the period of time over which it is to

---

Box 2.1   Ability of ward leadership to enhance nurses' adherence to hand hygiene guidelines

---

Aim: evaluate the impact of a campaign to increase nurses' adherence to hand hygiene

Underpinning theory: sound ward leadership is associated with effective implementation of change in clinical settings

Intervention: leadership programme to enable ward leaders to manage change designed to promote a hand hygiene campaign

Control: usual hand hygiene protocol with no other intervention

Sample: 67 wards in three hospitals randomised to the two groups; 10 785 hand hygiene opportunities documented for 2733 nurses

Results:
- Test wards: hand hygiene adherence increased from 20% to 53%
- Control wards: hand hygiene adherence increased from 23% to 46%

Source: Adapted from Huis et al. (2013).

---

be administered, the outcomes that will be taken to indicate success (e.g. resolution of the symptoms of infection, negative bacteriology test) and how they will be measured are stated in a research protocol drawn up before the trial commences. Box 2.1 presents a complex intervention study evaluating the impact of a hand hygiene campaign.

Sources of Bias in Randomised Controlled Trials

The robustness of an RCT depends on its ability to minimise all possible sources of bias. In practice, this may not be possible.

Selection Bias

Selection bias occurs if randomisation is impaired. Some people in the population eligible to be included might refuse. A ward manager might not allow staff to participate in a study evaluating the impact of alcohol handrub coupled with special training because they suspect that their staff will not perform well.

Performance (Confounding) Bias

Performance (confounding) bias occurs when people in a test group receive extra attention (e.g. greater interaction with health workers, more diagnostic tests) that could result in better outcomes compared to the control group. Receiving a new alcohol handrub and being shown how to use it during extra visits by the infection prevention team could operate as a source of performance bias.

Attrition Bias

Attrition bias occurs when differences arise between test and control groups (e.g. patients dying or deciding to withdraw). Ward closures could result in attrition from the above hand hygiene study. Risk of attrition bias increases over time and is highest when data collection is protracted.

Measurement Bias

Measurement bias occurs when data are not collected in the same way for the test and control group participants and is often the result of inability to achieve blinding. Many infection prevention interventions involve training or the introduction of a new policy or guideline. Health workers inevitably become aware that change is being implemented and are very likely to alter their behaviour. Measurement bias is also possible if the study outcome is not measured in exactly the same way for all participants. In a large hand hygiene trial, responsibility for audit might be devolved to ward managers who might monitor hand hygiene adherence differently even if they have received training by the research team.

Contamination Bias

Contamination bias occurs when control group participants receive the intervention by mistake or become alerted to it by accident. Health workers might discuss a training intervention with colleagues allocated to a control group, prompting them to change behaviour.

Adapting Trials for Use in the Real World

Randomised controlled trials have been adapted to test the effectiveness of the types of complex interventions frequently evaluated in public health, including infection prevention. Because RCTs are very highly controlled, they often do not reflect clinical practice well. Thus RCTs are said to test *efficacy* and answer the question 'can something work under highly controlled (often ideal) circumstances?' rather than *effectiveness*, which answers the question 'does something work in real life?'.

In the real world, it is usually impossible to attain the degree of control that is achievable in a drug trial. In addition to bias, other events and changes in practice occurring throughout the life of such trials have the capacity to influence the findings. Interventions intended to increase hand hygiene adherence are open to the influence of other factors affecting hand hygiene performance: local shortages of alcohol handrub; an outbreak of norovirus in the community (health workers might increase hand hygiene to reduce personal risk of infection); or a new government directive on hand hygiene. Interventions to improve infection prevention are highly susceptible to the influence of seasonal and secular trends.

- *Seasonal* trends recur and are often cyclical. They are very likely to influence infection rates and are often associated with behaviour, although not always in ways that are easy to predict. Respiratory virus infections increase in winter when people spend more time indoors. The associated increase in hospital admissions ('winter pressures') increases health workers' workload and could in turn reduce the amount of time available to perform frequent and thorough hand hygiene. Conversely, concern about developing respiratory infection might increase adherence to hand hygiene protocols.
- *Secular* trends are any trends not attributable to seasonal or cyclical changes. They are often long-term, one-off events (e.g. new policy, changes in public health, changes in treatment). The visit of an accreditation panel might boost hand hygiene adherence in the short term. A new policy to decrease the unnecessary use of non-sterile disposable gloves might influence hand hygiene adherence.

Other Types of Randomised Controlled Trials

The classic RCT has been adapted for use in public health in an attempt to overcome the above challenges. Different research designs have been developed. There are advantages and disadvantages associated with each, depending on the nature of the intervention, the setting and the rigour with which it is possible to conduct the study.

Cross-over Randomised Controlled Trials

Cross-over RCTs evaluate the impact of one or more interventions, enabling all participants to receive treatment with each acting as their own control (Box 2.2). Participants are randomised into two or more groups, depending on the number of interventions being evaluated, and each group receives each intervention in turn. In this type of study, it is the sequence in which each group receives a particular intervention and acts as a control that is randomly assigned. The advantage of cross-over study designs is that all participants receive a potentially beneficial new intervention, a situation welcomed by patients and ethics committees but at the expense of rigour. The study groups receive the intervention at different times, making it difficult to compare outcomes between groups, especially in infection-related studies subject to the influence of seasonal and secular trends. A 'washout period' is often needed when crossing between intervention and control to allow the effects of treatment to wear off.

Cross-over designs are not feasible when the effect of an intervention is irreversible (e.g. a new policy, staff training).

Box 2.2   Example of a cross-over research design

Aim: establish the ability of alcohol handrub with training to increase hand hygiene adherence and reduce infection rates in intensive care units.

Study design: cross-over RCT over 2 years with cross-over between test and control groups after 12 months.

Sample: two critical care units in a Canadian hospital.

Intervention: alcohol handrub with training.

Outcome measures: hand hygiene adherence, infection rates.

Results: hand hygiene increased adherence in both groups for all health workers:

Group 1: 37–68%
Group 2: 38–69%

Infection rates: unchanged.

Source: Adapted from Rupp et al. (2008).

Cluster Randomised Controlled Trials

Cluster randomised controlled trials (CRCTs) are large, expensive studies which involve randomising whole organisations (e.g. wards, hospitals, primary care centres) into test and control groups (clusters), not the individuals in them (Box 2.3). CRCTs overcome the risk of contamination between participants allocated to the different arms of the trial. The drawback is that they are unable to overcome common factors shared throughout a cluster that might influence outcomes. For example, organisational culture has a well-known influence on the quality of healthcare (Davies et al. 2000). It is very likely that any new infection prevention guideline evaluated in a CRCT will be implemented more effectively in a 'good' ward or hospital.

Step-Wedge Cluster Randomised Controlled Trials

Step-wedge cluster randomised controlled trials are used to evaluate the effectiveness and safety of interventions intended for routine use (e.g. vaccines), particularly but not exclusively in low-income countries. Baseline data are collected for the whole population which is then subdivided into units (e.g. 'wards' in a constituency, villages, towns). Participants in one of the units are randomised into control and test groups and the impact of the intervention is evaluated. If all is well, the control participants also receive treatment and the procedure is repeated until participants in all the units have been included in the trial and received the intervention.

Box 2.3   Example of a cluster randomised controlled trial

Aim: investigate the effectiveness of a campaign to promote hand hygiene adherence in long-term care facilities (LTCFs) in Hong Kong.

Study design: CRCT in six LTCFs randomised to receive/not receive the hand hygiene intervention with follow-up seven months later.

Outcome measures: uptake of alcohol handrub uptake.

Results:
Test LTCFs
Hand hygiene
Baseline 25.8%, follow-up 33.3%
Control LTCFs

Hand hygiene: no change

Source: Adapted from Yeung et al. (2011).

Step-wedge CRCTs are major studies which require very good organisation although they are usually manageable as the sample for each unit is often small. The switch from control to test group occurs at different time points, allowing difficulties to be resolved as they arise rather than occurring together. This type of study design is considered ethical (all participants benefit from the intervention), encouraging governments to take part. A disadvantage is that groups receive the intervention at different times and are affected differently by seasonal and secular trends. Box 2.4 describes a CRCT in a school in Kenya. It was impossible to blind participants to group allocation and as record keeping in the schools was poor (e.g. no records of time missed from school, examination results), data loss was inevitable.

Box 2.4   Example of a step-wedge cluster randomised controlled trial

Aim: determine the health and educational benefits of a school-based deworming programme in western Kenya.

Intervention: antihelminthic (worming) medication administered at school with health education (e.g. lectures, posters).

Sample: 25 schools randomised into three groups, each receiving the intervention at a different time (order of intervention randomised) over 12 months.

Outcome measures: school attendance, examination performance.

Results: school attendance improved, examination performance did not change.

Source: Adapted from Davey et al. (2015).

Non-randomised Controlled Trials

Non-randomised controlled trials (quasi-experimental studies) estimate the impact of an intervention without random allocation of participants to test and control groups. They are often used to evaluate standard practice when randomisation is not possible (Box 2.5) and are relatively low down the hierarchy of evidence because there is considerable risk of bias, which research teams usually try to minimise by ensuring that test and control participants are as similar as possible.

Uncontrolled Before-and-After Studies

Uncontrolled before-and-after studies (UCBAs) adopt a pre- and post-test data collection procedure. Baseline data collected for the chosen outcome measures are obtained, the intervention is put in place, then postintervention data are collected. Follow-up may take place once or be repeated over a period of weeks or months, and data are compared before and after the intervention. There is no control group. UCBAs are far down the hierarchy of evidence because external validity is low and it is impossible to rule out the influence of confounding variables. Nevertheless, UCBAs are very frequently reported in infection prevention and some have had a powerful influence on policy and practice (Box 2.6).

Box 2.5 Example of a non-randomised controlled trial

Aim: to establish the impact of filtering facepiece class 2 (FFP2) masks compared to surgical masks on the risk of SARS-CoV-2 acquisition among healthcare workers in Switzerland

Study design: prospective multicentre study

Sample: 3259 participants from nine healthcare institutions

Intervention: particpants were asked about their usually worn mask type when caring for COVID-19 patients when not performing aerosol-generating procedures. They were not randomised or allocated a mask type.

Outcome measures: self-reported SARS-CoV-2-positive nasopharyngeal PCR/rapid antigen tests and SARS-CoV-2 seroconversion

Results: FFP2 use was associated with a non-statistically significant reduction in:

1) having a positive swab – adjusted hazard ratio: 0.8 (95% CI 0.6–1.0)
2) seroconversion – adjusted odds ratio: 0.7, 95% CI 0.5–1.0)

Source: Haller et al. (2022).

Box 2.6   Example of an uncontrolled before-and-after study

Aim: evaluate the impact of a bundled intervention to promote hand hygiene adherence and reduce rates of healthcare-associated infection.

Bundle components: alcohol handrub placed at every bedside, staff training, reminders, audit with performance feedback, organisational support.

Study design: UCBA over four years with repeated postintervention data collection.

Outcome measures: hand hygiene frequency, overall rates of healthcare-associated infection, MRSA rates.

Sample: all health workers in one university teaching hospital.

Results:
Hand hygiene adherence increased: 47.6–66.8%
Overall rates of healthcare-associated infection declined: 16.9–9.9%
MRSA rates declined: 2.16–0.93%.

Source: Adapted from Pittet et al. (2000).

Observational Studies

Interrupted Time Series Studies

Interrupted time series studies (ITSs) are the most robust study designs available to assess the impact of an intervention when randomisation is not feasible. With an ITS, it is possible to document trends in the data over time on repeated, predetermined occasions, with comparison before and after a change occurred. The change can be a deliberate intervention or a natural event. ITSs are particularly valuable in infection prevention because it is possible to take into account the impact of seasonal and secular changes. Data collection can be prospective or retrospective or a combination of both (Box 2.7).

A second advantage when using an ITS is that it is often possible to make use of the large amounts of infection-related data routinely collected by public health bodies and health provider organisations (e.g. national statistics collected for MRSA, hospital hand hygiene audit data). The data are expressed graphically and the impact of change is identified by measuring the slope of the graph (Figure 2.2). The disadvantage of ITSs is that analysis can be very complicated. Access to expert statistical expertise is essential to interpret the findings.

Cohort Studies

Cohort studies (longitudinal studies) are used to explore the incidence, cause and prognosis of conditions, often new diseases, and to examine the association

---

Box 2.7   Example of an interrupted time series study

Aim: determine whether terminal cleaning of surfaces with bleach in isolation rooms could reduce the high incidence of *Clostridioides difficile* infection identified by a local infection prevention team during routine surveillance.

Study design: ITS with retrospective preintervention data analysis and prospective follow-up over 14 months in three hospitals.

Result: 48% reduction in *C. diff* rates post intervention.

Source: Adapted from Hacek et al. (2010).

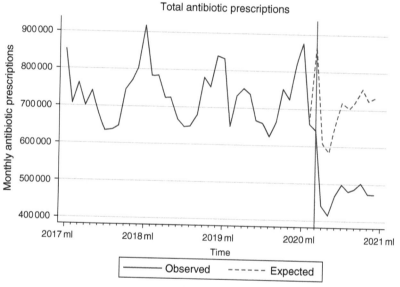

Figure 2.2   Antibiotic prescriptions before and after COVID-19. The dotted line shows what would have been expected based on previous years, the solid line what actually occurred. *Source:* https://academic.oup.com/ofid/article/8/11/ofab533/6414697

between exposure and outcomes (Box 2.8). There is no manipulation. Data collection can be retrospective or prospective, often by examining routinely collected data (e.g. hospital records). If there is reliance on data not obtained for the specific purpose, there is a risk of missing data that affect the study conclusions. For this reason, prospective data are preferred over retrospectively collected data.

Cohort studies can be expensive if they take place over a long period and are prone to bias, especially confounding bias (e.g. knowing they are taking part in a study might encourage participants to change their behaviour).

Box 2.8 Example of a cohort study

Aim: explore the relationship between age and mortality from COVID-19 infection among inpatients.

Study design: retrospective cohort study analysing electronic case records of the first 450 patients with positive PCR COVID-19 tests admitted to one hospital.

Outcome measures: disease severity, mortality.

Results: 60% of patients >80 years died compared to 28% patients <80 years.

Source: Adapted from Brill et al. (2020).

Case–control Studies

Case–control studies compare exposures in those with and without the condition of interest. People with the outcome (cases) are identified and then similar people without the outcome (controls) are compared, the aim being to find out what the cases did or were exposed to that the controls were not. Because the outcome has already occurred to the cases, these studies are by definition retrospective. They are also useful in outbreak conditions because they can be done very quickly, where the outcome is rare and a very large cohort would be needed to identify enough cases, or when the outcome takes a long time to occur (Box 2.9).

Case Study Series

Case study series are by convention classified as quantitative studies, although this is arguable as they describe patients in their natural setting and numbers are often very small. They are used to describe new, unusual diseases or cases of a

---

Box 2.9 Example of a case–control study

Aim: to evaluate the effectiveness of personal protective measures against severe acute respiratory disease coronavirus 2 (SARS-CoV-2) infection.

Study design: comparison of 211 contacts of COVID-19 patients who later tested positive (the cases) and 839 contacts who did not test positive (controls).

Result: wearing masks all the time reduced the risk of infection compared with not wearing masks, while wearing a mask sometimes during contact did not lower infection risk. Maintaining at least 1 m distance from a person with COVID-19, having close contact for less than 15 minutes, and frequent handwashing reduced the risk of infection.

Source: Adapted from Doung-ngern et al. (2020).

Box 2.10   Example of a case study series

Four cases of *Rhizopus microsporus* mycosis were documented in the same neonatal unit, with three mortalities. Investigation failed to identify any source of environmental contamination. Cross-infection was considered unlikely as the neonates were not on the unit at the same time. Searches of the literature revealed that cases of *R. microsporus* pulmonary infection had been reported among sawmill workers who had inhaled fungal spores. This information helped to narrow the investigation and the outbreak was eventually traced to wooden tongue depressors used to make splints for intravenous cannulae on the unit as traditional ones were too large for the neonates. They were issued by the manufacturer without being sterilised and stored in an open box. No new cases emerged when they were removed.

Source: Adapted from Mitchell et al. (1996).

---

condition presenting under unexpected circumstances and differ from cohort studies because there is no comparison between groups (Box 2.10). Selection bias is high and external validity (generalisability to other populations) is very low. Data collection is retrospective or prospective.

Surveys

Surveys collect data from a predefined group of respondents to obtain data on one or more topics of interest (Box 2.11). Data collection is usually by questionnaire and is often online although interviews are sometimes conducted either by

---

Box 2.11   Example of a cross-sectional survey

Aim: explore teaching arrangements for aseptic technique among pre-registration student nurses.

Study design: cross-sectional survey.

Sample: all universities teaching pre-registration student nurses in the UK (national sample).

Methods: structured telephone interviews conducted with a representative nurse educator in each university.

Results: response rate was 70% (n = 49/70). Aseptic technique was taught throughout the programme, mainly applied to wound care. The focus was on how to conduct a procedure applying aseptic technique rather than the underpinning principles.

Source: Adapted from Hawker et al. (2020).

---

telephone or more rarely face to face. As well as for research purposes, surveys are widely used commercially (e.g. to assess household spending habits) and by organisations (e.g. political opinion polls). They may be conducted as 'one-off' events (cross-sectional surveys) or on repeated occasions with the same sample to obtain longitudinal data. Unless a representative sample is obtained or all the individuals eligible to be included in a population take part, surveys lack external validity.

Qualitative Research Methods

In contrast to quantitative research, where the aim is to generalise from a sample to a population by testing a theory based on a hypothesis, qualitative research is usually context specific. Instead of testing theories or hypotheses, the aim is to generate theory (Forman et al. 2008). A range of qualitative methodologies exist (Table 2.2). In large studies, qualitative methodologies are often combined with quantitative methods (e.g. open-ended questions in surveys).

The main methods of data collection include:

- in-depth interviews
- focus groups
- observation (non-participant, participant)
- analysis of existing documentary material and narratives (e.g. minutes of meetings, official records).

The success of infection prevention depends heavily on adherence to protocols and guidelines and is often suboptimal. Employing qualitative methodologies can help to explain why health workers or patients do not always comply and can suggest avenues for improvement.

Phenomenology

Phenomenology takes an issue of interest and seeks to understand participants' subjective 'lived experiences' of it to understand individual experiences (Cristancho et al. 2018). This approach has been used to obtain an understanding

Table 2.2 Qualitative research methodologies.

Phenomenology
Ethnography
Grounded theory

of health workers' anxieties and gaps in expertise when providing care for patients suffering from emerging infectious conditions and to suggest ways of improving support when future outbreaks occur (Lee et al. 2020).

Ethnography

Ethnography seeks to understand people in the context of their culture, social organisation and shared values (Cristancho et al. 2018). Ethnographic studies are gaining importance in infection prevention. They have been used to identify barriers to adherence to infection prevention guidelines and to explore patient perceptions of different infection prevention practices and barriers to implementation (Knobloch et al. 2017).

Grounded Theory

Grounded theory seeks to identify participants' experiences and develop theory to explain social relationships and behaviours. The distinctive approaches characteristic of studies adopting grounded theory are as follows.

- *Theoretical sampling*: data already obtained are coded and analysed as the study progresses and used to make decisions about further sources of information. Data collection is said to be 'controlled by emergent theory'.
- *Theoretical saturation*: the decision to stop sampling is taken when no new codes are emerging.
- *Constant comparative method* (Glaser and Strauss 2010): as data are coded, they are compared with previous information in the same and different codes. Two or more concepts pertaining to the same phenomenon are grouped into categories which are used to generate theory.

Grounded theory has been used to explain how nurses learn to use new technology to improve hand hygiene adherence (Granqvist et al. 2022).

Human Factors and Ergonomics

Human factors and ergonomics (HFE) is a method of enquiry used to examine the design of individual work system components and the way they interact with each other, taking into account human capabilities and characteristics. The goal is to achieve optimum safety and performance (Gurses et al. 2012, 2020). HFE experts are trained to design and adapt work systems, identify barriers and enablers to adherence to guidelines and protocols, maximise individual and team performance and minimise risk (Harrison et al. 2007). There is increasing interest in the application of HFE to infection prevention. It was used to redesign workflow in paediatric outpatient services during the COVID-19 pandemic. Different methods of communication between families and health workers were explored and the results were used to facilitate service improvements that will be valuable in future outbreak situations (Gurses et al. 2020).

Synthesising Literature

Most clinicians develop critical appraisal skills during undergraduate preparation but it is rarely practical for them to undertake a full-scale systematic review and usually unnecessary as reviews already exist for a vast number of topics. Systematic reviewing is a lengthy, time-consuming process demanding specialist expertise. Such reviews are supposed to include all available evidence, much of which is often unpublished ('grey' literature) and busy clinicians rarely have the time or skills to locate it.

Systematic Reviews

Systematic reviews are positioned very high up the hierarchy of evidence because they adopt an agreed, highly organised, methodical approach to obtaining and assessing all the best evidence available on a specific topic. Different methods of undertaking systematic reviews have been described but the most widely used approach for quantitative studies is that developed by the Cochrane Collaboration.

Meta-analysis

Meta-analysis is a particular form of systematic reviewing. It combines the statistical results of more than one study to provide an overall weighted average ('pooled' result). Meta-analysis is more sophisticated than simply taking the average result of the individual studies because it weights them according to the relative contribution that they should make to the final, overall result; a sample of 1000 participants would be weighted more heavily than a study with only 100 participants, for example.

The quality of a systematic review or meta-analysis depends on whether or not it is possible to draw meaningful comparisons between studies addressing the topic of interest.

Heading Heterogeneity

Studies are described as heterogeneous if they are not the same. Three types of heterogeneity exist.

- *Clinical diversity*: differences in types of patients or treatments in the different studies available.
- *Methodological diversity*: differences in the methods used to undertake the studies.
- *Statistical heterogeneity*: differences between studies in terms of the effect the intervention has exerted.

It is usually not sensible to combine the findings of very dissimilar studies, especially when the results will be used to generate clinical recommendations. Whether or not to include studies with a high degree of heterogeneity in a review is a matter of judgement.

Box 2.12 presents an example of a Cochrane systematic review in which the individual studies were compared but meta-analysis was not considered meaningful because all three types of heterogeneity were marked.

Important topics are likely to attract the attention of more than one research team undertaking a systematic review and it is necessary to appraise and compare the quality of each (Smith et al. 2011). Of 20 systematic reviews evaluating interventions to assess the effectiveness of hand hygiene, the one presented in Box 2.12 above was considered to have the lowest risk of bias (Price et al. 2018).

Box 2.12   Example of a Cochrane systematic review

Aims: assess the effectiveness of strategies to increase adherence to recommendations for hand hygiene and determine whether increased hand hygiene adherence can reduce rates of healthcare-associated infection.

Method: systematic review adopting Cochrane methodology.

Selection criteria for included studies: randomised trials, non-randomised trials, controlled before-after studies and interrupted time series studies that evaluated any intervention to improve hand hygiene adherence.

Results: 26 studies were included. Implementing a bundled intervention based on the use of alcohol handrub resulted in a modest increase in hand hygiene adherence but it was not possible to detect any impact on infection rates. There was risk of bias in all the included studies.

Source: Adapted from Gould et al. (2017).

Synthesising the Findings of Qualitative Research

Synthesising the findings of qualitative research and marrying together the findings of quantitative and qualitative studies are emerging methodologies. Numerous methods have been described and are accompanied by their own critical appraisal tools. Specialist information about these mixed-methods approaches is available from the Joanna Briggs Institute (Aromataris and Munn 2020).

Guideline Development

Clinical practice is widely informed by recommendations and guidelines. These are not legally binding and may or may not apply in a specific clinical situation (Table 2.3).

A range of organisations develop guidelines (Table 2.4).

Table 2.3 Definitions of policies, protocols, recommendations and guidelines.

A *policy* is usually an organisational decision that shows how it functions or how something should be done. It is a formal statement of a principle that should be followed by everyone covered by the policy.

A *protocol* specifies a particular sequence of activities that allow healthcare workers to respond consistently in clinical practice.

A *guideline* is an evidence-based *recommendation* for health and care. It usually sets out the care and services suitable for most people who have a particular condition or need, and people in particular circumstances or settings.

Sources: Anonymous (1993), NICE (2021), Wrensch (2020).

Table 2.4 Infection prevention guidelines.

International	
World Health Organization	
National	
National Institute for Health and Care Excellence	UK
Centers for Disease Prevention and Control	US
Department of Health	UK (epic3)
Professional bodies	
Association for Professionals in Infection Control	US
Society for Hospital Epidemiology for America	US
Infection Prevention Society	UK

Grading of Recommendations, Assessment, Development and Evaluation

The Grading of Recommendations, Assessment, Development and Evaluation (GRADE) system is widely used to turn evidence into recommendations through a transparent process that involves appraising research evidence whilst taking additional key factors into account (Schünemann et al. 2013).

Use of GRADE begins with an assessment of the quality of the body of evidence. Unlike traditional hierarchies that are fixed, GRADE allows for a body of high-quality observational evidence to form a higher level of evidence than a body of weaker quality observational evidence (Box 2.13). It is important to remember that GRADE is distinct from critical appraisal with tools such as CASP, as it is applied to the whole body of evidence used to make a decision, not to individual studies.

Box 2.13   Assessing the body of evidence using GRADE

Begin by looking at the studies. RCT evidence starts at a high level but can be downgraded; observational evidence starts at a lower level but can be upgraded.

Type of evidence	Criteria
Evidence from RCTs receives high initial rating but is reduced in the event of:	Study limitations (risk of bias)
	Inconsistency of results
	Indirectness of evidence
	Imprecision
	Publication bias
Evidence from observational evidence receives low initial rating but is increased in the event of:	Large magnitude of an effect
	Dose–response gradient
	Effect of plausible residual confounding from observational studies may be working to reduce the demonstrated effect or increase the effect, if no effect was observed

Qualitative evidence does not have a hierarchy in the same way; all study types start equal.

Qualitative evidence factors to consider include (Lewin et al. 2018):	Methodological limitations of the individual qualitative studies contributing to a review finding
	The coherence of the review finding
	The adequacy of data supporting a review finding
	The relevance of the data from the primary studies supporting a review finding to the context (perspective or population, phenomenon of interest and/or setting) specified in the review question

Expert opinion is not considered to be a level of evidence, but rather an interpretation of evidence.

Having assessed the quality of the evidence, GRADE incorporates other factors that are used to make decisions. These factors are incorporated into Evidence to Decision Frameworks, and include:

- the certainty of the evidence
- the balance of benefits and harms associated with uptake
- outcome importance: the value placed by stakeholders on the main outcomes
- use of resources
- equity
- acceptability
- feasibility.

Integrating these across the entire body of evidence generates five types and strengths of recommendation.

- *Strong recommendation for an intervention*: confidence that most individuals would want the recommended course of action and only a small proportion would not.
- *Strong recommendation against an intervention*: confidence that most individuals would not want the recommended course of action and only a small proportion would.
- *Weak recommendation for an intervention*: most individuals would want the suggested course of action, but many would not.
- *Weak recommendation against an intervention*: most individuals would not want the suggested course of action, but many would.
- *No recommendation.*

These recommendations are based on whether the desirable effects of the intervention outweigh its undesirable effects (Schünemann et al. 2013). Assessment is reached by a guideline development team which is usually multidisciplinary, and which must include representatives of those among whom the recommendations are to be implemented.

Using GRADE, it is possible to make a strong recommendation for an intervention in the absence of high-quality evidence from an RCT if the other factors support that recommendation. For example, a strong case can be made for promoting hand hygiene because it is aesthetically desirable, low risk, the potential benefits are great, the outcome is important, the costs relatively modest, it is generally acceptable to those concerned and feasible to implement, with few potential harms associated with it.

Where direct evidence for an intervention is lacking evidence, it may be possible to make a Good Practice Point (GPP). These are short pieces of advice which may not have an evidence base but which are seen as good clinical practice (SIGN) or for which there is indirect evidence. Numerous infection prevention precautions could be seen as GPPs; for example, it is good practice to use different coloured cloths for different cleaning purposes.

The Challenge of Infection Prevention Research

Undertaking well-designed research studies to support infection prevention policy and practice is challenging. For many clinical studies, the primary outcome measure is easily decided; for example, a trial to determine the effectiveness of a new analgesic would take decrease in reported pain as the primary outcome. Secondary outcomes might include impact on mobility or quality of life assessed by validated scales completed by participants. For studies evaluating the impact of infection prevention interventions, the obvious primary outcome measure is decrease in infection rates but seasonal and secular trends can have such a powerful influence that they can undermine the validity of research where infection rate is taken as the primary outcome. A further complication is that many patients become colonised rather than infected or infection can be mild and asymptomatic unless confirmed by laboratory investigation, which in a large study could become prohibitively expensive. Proxy indicators are often taken as primary outcome measures in such studies.

To evaluate the impact of hand hygiene campaigns, the primary outcome measure is very often change in hand hygiene frequency without any attempt to document infections (Gould et al. 2017). This leaves the most important question unanswered: whether or not the intervention can break the chain of infection. Many infection prevention guidelines and recommendations are supported by evidence from poorly controlled studies or are pragmatic and supported only by the consensus opinion of experts. Table 2.4 illustrates the level of evidence underpinning recommendations in official guidelines.

There are numerous challenges in using evidence to inform practice, including finding and understanding individual studies, assessing the body of evidence, and then applying it to a particular area of practice. The most important aspect of this process is being aware of uncertainty and incorporating this into any decision.

Suggested Activities

Exercise 2.1 Self-assessment

1   Complete the sentence 'Intervention studies are positioned high up the hierarchy of evidence because . . .'

2   In quantitative research a hypothesis tests the truth of an assumption.
True/False

3   Undertaking critical appraisal means:
A   Undertaking a full systematic review
B   Assessing the trustworthiness, value and relevance of a research study to practice in a particular context
C   Assessing the relevance of a research study to practice
D   Criticising research.

4   External validity means that the findings of a study are generalisable to other patient groups and populations in similar settings.
True/False

5   Look at Box 2.1. What sort of trial is being conducted?

6   Briefly explain the difference between seasonal and secular trends.

7   The findings of cross-over randomised controlled trials are subject to the effects of seasonal and secular trends.
True/False

8   The findings of uncontrolled before-and-after studies are high up the hierarchy of evidence because their findings influence clinical policy and practice.
True/False

9   Interrupted times series studies:
A   Can be undertaken with retrospective data
B   Can be undertaken with prospective data
C   Can be undertaken with routinely collected data
D   All of the above.

10   The acronym GRADE stands for:

Exercise 2.2

Obtain the paper by Rupp et al. (2008) from the chapter reference list (open access is available). Read the paper without first looking at the abstract and write notes.

A Use your notes to write a structured abstract for the paper in 500 words under the headings: background; aims; methods; analysis; main study findings; study limitations; conclusions. Compare your abstract to the one supplied in the paper.

B The intervention in the above study increased hand hygiene adherence but, contrary to expectations, did not decrease infection rates. Why might this have occurred? (The materials and methods section of the paper gives a strong hint although the authors do not comment on it in their discussion.)

Exercise 2.3

Go online and retrieve one of the sets of guidelines presented in Table 2.4 (all are open access). Look at the recommendations for a topic of clinical importance in your workplace. What type of evidence underpins the recommendations presented? Is the supporting research mostly from RCTs, from study designs further down the hierarchy of evidence or supported by expert opinion?

References

Anonymous (1993). Protocols: guidance for good practice: the use of standardised protocols in patient care is becoming widespread. They offer a posit he adjunct to nurses, but can be misused by managers to effect changes in staffing skill mix. This article offers guidance for nurses on the essential criteria a protocol must achieve before being considered acceptable. *Nurs. Stand.* 8: 29–29. https://doi.org/10.7748/ns.8.8.29.s49.

Aromataris, E. and Munn, Z. (ed.) (2020). *JBI Manual for Evidence Synthesis*. JBI https://doi.org/10.46658/JBIMES-20-01.

Black, N. (1996). Why we need observational studies to evaluate the effectiveness of health care. *BMJ* 312: 1215–1218. https://doi.org/10.1136/bmj.312.7040.1215.

Brice, R. (2021). CASP CHECKLISTS. CASP – Critical Appraisal Skills Programme. https://casp-uk.net/casp-tools-checklists

Brill, S.E., Jarvis, H.C., Ozcan, E. et al. (2020). COVID-19: a retrospective cohort study with focus on the over-80s and hospital-onset disease. *BMC Med.* 18: 194. https://doi.org/10.1186/s12916-020-01665-z.

Cristancho, S., Goldszmidt, M., Lingard, L., and Watling, C. (2018). Qualitative research essentials for medical education. *Singapore Med. J.* 59: 622–627. https://doi.org/10.11622/smedj.2018093.

Davey, C., Aiken, A.M., Hayes, R.J., and Hargreaves, J.R. (2015). Re-analysis of health and educational impacts of a school-based deworming programme in western Kenya: a statistical replication of a cluster quasi-randomized stepped-wedge trial. *Int. J. Epidemiol.* 44: 1581–1592. https://doi.org/10.1093/ije/dyv128.

Davies, H.T., Nutley, S.M., and Mannion, R. (2000). Organisational culture and quality of health care. *Qual. Health Care* 9: 111–119. https://doi.org/10.1136/qhc.9.2.111.

Doung-ngern, P., Suphanchaimat, R., Panjangampatthana, A. et al. (2020). Case–control study of use of personal protective measures and risk for SARS-CoV 2 infection, Thailand. *Emerg. Infect. Dis.* 26: 2607–2616. https://doi.org/10.3201/eid2611.203003.

Forman, J., Creswell, J.W., Damschroder, L. et al. (2008). Qualitative research methods: key features and insights gained from use in infection prevention research. *Am. J. Infect. Control* 36: 764–771. https://doi.org/10.1016/j.ajic.2008.03.010.

Glaser, B.G. and Strauss, A.L. (2010). *The Discovery of Grounded Theory: Strategies for Qualitative Research*, 5e. New Brunswick: Aldine Transaction.

Gould, D.J., Moralejo, D., Drey, N. et al. (2017). Interventions to improve hand hygiene compliance in patient care. *Cochrane Database Syst. Rev.* 9: CD005186. https://doi.org/10.1002/14651858.CD005186.pub4.

Granqvist, K., Ahlstrom, L., Karlsson, J. et al. (2022). Learning to interact with new technology: health care workers' experiences of using a monitoring system for assessing hand hygiene – a grounded theory study. *Am. J. Infect. Control* 50: 651–656. https://doi.org/10.1016/j.ajic.2021.09.023.

Gurses, A.P., Ozok, A.A., and Pronovost, P.J. (2012). Time to accelerate integration of human factors and ergonomics in patient safety. *BMJ Qual. Saf.* 21: 347–351. https://doi.org/10.1136/bmjqs-2011-000421.

Gurses, A.P., Tschudy, M.M., McGrath-Morrow, S. et al. (2020). Overcoming COVID-19: what can human factors and ergonomics offer? *J. Patient Safety Risk Manage.* 25: 49–54. https://doi.org/10.1177/2516043520917764.

Hacek, D.M., Ogle, A.M., Fisher, A. et al. (2010). Significant impact of terminal room cleaning with bleach on reducing nosocomial *Clostridium difficile*. *Am. J. Infect. Control* 38: 350–353. https://doi.org/10.1016/j.ajic.2009.11.003.

Haller, S., Güsewell, S., Egger, T. et al. (2022). Impact of respirator versus surgical masks on SARS-CoV-2 acquisition in healthcare workers: a prospective multicentre cohort. *Antimicrob. Resist. Infect. Control* 11: 27. https://doi.org/10.1186/s13756-022-01070-6.

Harrison, M.I., Koppel, R., and Bar-Lev, S. (2007). Unintended consequences of Information Technologies in Health Care – an interactive sociotechnical analysis. *J. Am. Med. Inform. Assoc.* 14: 542–549. https://doi.org/10.1197/jamia.M2384.

Hawker, C., Courtenay, M., Wigglesworth, N., and Gould, D. (2020). National cross-sectional survey to explore preparation to undertake aseptic technique in pre-registration nursing curricula in the United Kingdom. *Nurse Educ. Today* 90: 104415. https://doi.org/10.1016/j.nedt.2020.104415.

Huis, A., Schoonhoven, L., Grol, R. et al. (2013). Impact of a team and leaders-directed strategy to improve nurses' adherence to hand hygiene guidelines: a cluster randomised trial. *Int. J. Nurs. Stud.* 50: 464–474. https://doi.org/10.1016/j.ijnurstu.2012.08.004.

Knobloch, M.J., Thomas, K.V., Patterson, E. et al. (2017). Implementation in the midst of complexity: using ethnography to study health care-associated infection prevention and control. *Am. J. Infect. Control* 45: 1058–1063. https://doi.org/10.1016/j.ajic.2017.06.024.

Kuhn, T. (1970). Logic of discovery or psychology of research. In: *Criticism and the Growth of Knowledge: Proceedings of the International Colloquium in the Philosophy of Science, London, 1965* (ed. I. Lakatos and A. Musgrave). Cambridge: Cambridge University Press https://doi.org/10.1017/CBO9781139171434.

Lee, J.Y., Hong, J.H., and Park, E.Y. (2020). Beyond the fear: nurses' experiences caring for patients with Middle East respiratory syndrome: a phenomenological study. *J. Clin. Nurs.* 29: 3349–3362. https://doi.org/10.1111/jocn.15366.

Lewin, S., Bohren, M., Rashidian, A. et al. (2018). Applying GRADE-CERQual to qualitative evidence synthesis findings – paper 2: how to make an overall CERQual assessment of confidence and create a Summary of Qualitative Findings table. *Implementation Sci.* 13: 10. https://doi.org/10.1186/s13012-017-0689-2.

Mitchell, S.J., Gray, J., Morgan, M.E. et al. (1996). Nosocomial infection with *Rhizopus microsporus* in preterm infants: association with wooden tongue depressors. *Lancet* 348: 441–443. https://doi.org/10.1016/s0140-6736(96)05059-3.

NICE 2021. NICE guidelines. www.nice.org.uk/about/what-we-do/our-programmes/nice-guidance/nice-guidelines

Pittet, D., Hugonnet, S., Harbarth, S. et al. (2000). Effectiveness of a hospital-wide programme to improve compliance with hand hygiene. *Lancet* 356: 1307–1312. https://doi.org/10.1016/S0140-6736(00)02814-2.

Price, L., MacDonald, J., Gozdzielewska, L. et al. (2018). Interventions to improve healthcare workers' hand hygiene compliance: a systematic review of systematic reviews. *Infect. Control Hosp. Epidemiol.* 39: 1449–1456. https://doi.org/10.1017/ice.2018.262.

Rupp, M.E., Fitzgerald, T., Puumala, S. et al. (2008). Prospective, controlled, cross-over trial of alcohol-based hand gel in critical care units. *Infect. Control Hosp. Epidemiol.* 29: 8–15. doi: 10.1086/524333.

Schünemann, H., Brożek, J., Guyatt, G., Oxman, A. (2013). GRADE handbook. https://gdt.gradepro.org/app/handbook/handbook.html

Smith, V., Devane, D., Begley, C.M., and Clarke, M. (2011). Methodology in conducting a systematic review of systematic reviews of healthcare interventions. *BMC Med. Res. Methodol.* 11: 15. https://doi.org/10.1186/1471-2288-11-15.

Wrensch, J.-L. (2020). The difference between a policy, procedure, standard and guideline. https://www.michalsons.com/blog/the-difference-between-a-policy-procedure-standard-and-a-guideline/42265

Yeung, W.K., Tam, W.S.W., and Wong, T.W. (2011). Clustered randomized controlled trial of a hand hygiene intervention involving pocket-sized containers of alcohol-based hand rub for the control of infections in long-term care facilities. *Infect. Control Hosp. Epidemiol.* 32: 67–76. https://doi.org/10.1086/657636.

3

Immunity: Response of the Body to Infection

Introduction to Immunology

Immunology is the study of how the body protects itself from invasion by foreign substances (e.g. potential pathogens, pollen, dust) and malignant or damaged cells. Immunity is a state of resistance to harmful agents. It depends on the ability of the cells of the immune system to respond to antigens present on the surfaces of foreign cells. An antigen is defined as any substance able to stimulate an immune response, and any one antigen may contain many different antigenic epitopes which are the smaller parts of an antigen actually recognised by the immune system. Bacteria and viruses carry many antigens on their surfaces, some better at provoking an immune response than others.

Overall, the immune response takes place in a number of overlapping steps.

1) Foreign substances, micro-organisms, or their toxins are detected.
2) Their presence is communicated to the parts of the immune system responsible for neutralising and destroying them.
3) The immune attack is launched.
4) Once the harmful agent has been eliminated and the immune response is no longer required, it is suppressed.

To operate effectively it is necessary for the immune system to:

- differentiate between 'self' and 'non-self' molecules and eliminate those that are 'not-self' without reacting to 'self' molecules. If a response to a persons own body does occur, it is referred to as 'autoimmunity'
- prevent damage from the pathogen without causing excessive harm to the individual. Most immune responses cause some local and occasionally systemic damage, but this must not be excessive
- mount the right kind of immune response. For example, bacterial and viral infections require different types of immune response

Infection Prevention and Control in Healthcare Settings,
First Edition. Edward Purssell and Dinah Gould.
© 2023 John Wiley & Sons Ltd. Published 2023 by John Wiley & Sons Ltd.

- take place at the right location. Many of the cells of the immune system are present in the blood and lymphatic systems but most infections occur in the tissues. The blood-borne and lymph-borne cells must reach the appropriate site. Migration occurs in response to chemicals called *chemoattractants* released in the damaged tissues many of which are inflammatory
- take place rapidly enough to prevent excessive damage.

The immune system is highly complex and many of its actions are closely inter-related. Not surprisingly, mistakes in functioning are possible: autoimmunity occurs when the immune system reacts to the individual's own cells. Type 1 diabetes mellitus, rheumatoid arthritis, systemic lupus erythematosus, inflammatory bowel disease, multiple sclerosis and Guillain–Barré syndrome are all examples of autoimmune diseases.

Allergy (Hypersensitivity)

Approximately 10% of the population experience exaggerated hypersensitive (allergic) reactions to otherwise harmless materials (e.g. pollen, dust, fur, nuts, shellfish) which act as antigens. Allergic reactions are triggered when too much immunoglobulin E (IgE) is produced, which binds to the surface of mast cells and other inflammatory cells. On subsequent exposure to the same antigen, they release inflammatory substances such as histamine and bradykinin causing local or systemic inflammation. If this occurs locally it is referred to as an allergy, if it occurs systemically it is anaphylaxis. Many allergic reactions involve the respiratory tract because potential allergens are often inhaled and a large number of mast cells are present in the lungs. Mild allergic reactions are very common (e.g. hay fever resulting from exposure to pollen). Before nitrile and neoprene gloves were introduced, health workers often developed allergy to latex. Severe allergic reactions can be life-threatening (Box 3.1).

Lymphoid Tissues

The lymphoid tissues are concentrated at sites of the body particularly susceptible to microbial invasion (Table 3.1).

The lymphoid tissues are interconnected by a network of vessels making up the lymphatic system. The cells of the immune system develop in the bone marrow and migrate to the lymphoid tissue when mature. When microbial invasion occurs, the lymph nodes swell and may become tender.

Immune System Function

The immune system offers three sequential layers of protection:

- anatomical and physical barriers to avoid invasion
- innate immunity
- adaptive or acquired immunity.

Box 3.1 Anaphylaxis

Anaphylaxis is a severe, systemic allergic reaction caused by the rapid release of vasoactive amines (e.g. histamine, serotonin). These substances cause inflammation, increase the permeability of capillary walls and cause vasodilation, leading to oedema, shock, respiratory failure and cardiac arrest. The incidence of anaphylaxis is increasing and it is estimated that 0.3% of the general population in the UK experiences an episode annually. The signs and symptoms include urticarial rash with wheals; swelling of the lips, eyes and tongue; respiratory distress; stridor; wheezing; tachycardia and hypotension. Guidelines for emergency treatment are available from the Resuscitation Council (Resuscitation Council UK 2021). Specific guidelines for settings where vaccines are administered were developed during the COVID-19 pandemic.

If a patient collapses and anaphylaxis is suspected, the emergency services must be alerted. Key emergency actions are:

- maintaining the airway
- administering oxygen if available
- administering basic life support if necessary
- administering adrenaline (epinephrine) as soon as possible to combat shock by reversing peripheral vasodilation, reducing oedema and encouraging bronchodilation.

Table 3.1 Sites of lymphoid tissue.

Liver
Spleen
Tonsils
Adenoids
Peyer's patches in the gastrointestinal mucosa
Appendix
Lymph nodes

Anatomical and Physical Barriers to Invasion

Intact Skin and Mucous Membranes

Intact skin and mucous membranes are the body's chief defences against infection. Skin is acidic (pH 4) because sebaceous secretions create an 'acid mantle'. This supports a population of micro-organisms, mainly bacteria, that are able to keep pathogens at bay. Infection supervenes when the skin is broken or becomes excessively moist which supports microbial growth. For example, dampness beneath the breasts or between the toes frequently leads to infection, especially if hygiene is poor.

Gastrointestinal Tract

Many of the pathogens present in food are destroyed in the stomach because of the very low pH (2) of gastric acid. Patients taking proton pump inhibitors and H2 receptor blocking drugs are at risk of infection because they prevent the secretion of hydrochloric acid by the gastric mucosa. Further down the GI tract, the high pH (8–9) of secretions in the small intestine destroys most pathogens but not those responsible for typhoid and cholera.

Respiratory Tract

The respiratory tract is protected by the coughing and sneezing reflexes. Within the nose, the nasal conchae increase the surface area of the mucosae and cause inspired air to eddy, trapping small particles as it travels over them. Lymphoid tissues in the tonsils operate as further defences. The entire respiratory tree, except for the alveoli, is lined with mucus-secreting epithelium. The mucus traps foreign substances and is carried upwards to the pharynx by the action of the cilia and swallowed. Smoking paralyses ciliary action, explaining why people who smoke heavily are at particular risk of lower respiratory tract infections.

Female Genital Tract

The adult vagina contains lactobacilli which metabolise glycogen present in cervical secretions, forming lactic acid. The pH of the healthy adult vagina is approximately pH 4.5, inhibiting the growth of other micro-organisms. After the menopause, cervical secretions are scant because oestrogen production is low and vaginal pH rises, increasing the risk of infection. Taking antibiotics also increases the risk of developing vaginal infections such as *Candida* spp. ('thrush') because they suppress the normal bacterial vaginal flora.

Urinary Tract

In health, the bladder is kept free of micro-organisms. The epithelial cells lining its internal surface resist bacterial adhesion; any bacteria gaining access via the narrow urethra are diluted as the bladder fills and are flushed out during micturition.

Antimicrobial Secretions

Lysozyme is an enzyme secreted by macrophages and is present in many body fluids (e.g. tears, saliva). It destroys bacteria by attacking their cell walls but has no action against those protected by a thick extracellular mucous coat.

Innate Immunity

Innate immunity is the body's first line of defence against invading pathogens and occurs swiftly. It is not specific to each individual antigen, and it is essentially functional from birth. Components of the innate immune system include:

- phagocytic cells
- antigen presenting cells
- inflammatory substances
- complement proteins
- extracellular antimicrobial chemicals.

The cells of the innate immune system include:

- neutrophils
- macrophages and monocytes
- mast cells
- dendritic cells
- eosinophils
- natural killer cells.

These cells recognise antigens on the surfaces of micro-organisms according to their molecular patterns. These arrangements of molecules on the micro-organism are known as pathogen-associated molecular patterns (PAMPS) (Kobayashi et al. 2018). PAMPS are identified by complementary pattern recognition receptors on the cells of the body's innate immune system. Neutrophils and macrophages remove pathogens directly by *phagocytosis* (Figure 3.1). The stages of phagocytosis are as follows.

- *Opsonization*: a ligand (particle or group of molecules) attaches to the surface of the phagocyte, stimulating contraction of the proteins within its cytoplasm.
- *Endocytosis*: the pathogen is engulfed by the phagocyte.
- Formation of a *vacuole* created by the phagocytic membrane around the pathogen.
- Fusion of the vacuole with an organelle in the cytoplasm of the phagocyte called a *lysosome*. Lysosomes contain hydrolytic enzymes (e.g. catalase and myeloperoxidase).
- *Release* of the enzymes into the vacuole, destroying the pathogen.

Some cells of the innate immune system (e.g. dendritic cells, macrophages) enhance the immune response by promoting adaptive immunity. These are described as antigen-presenting cells (APCs). APCs recognise antigens on the surfaces of foreign cells and molecules and 'present' them to T-lymphocytes which are part of the acquired immune system.

Neutrophils

Neutrophils develop from stem cells in the bone marrow but migrate to the bloodstream and other tissues where they become active. They comprise 50–70% of the total phagocytic count (Summers et al. 2010). Neutrophils take approximately seven days to appear in the circulation but mature cells survive for only 6–8 hours (Dancey et al. 1976).

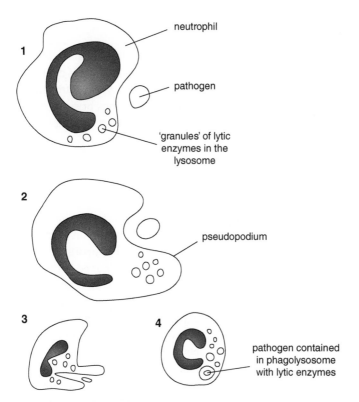

Figure 3.1 Phagocytosis.

Organelles in the neutrophil cytoplasm called lysosomes contain enzymes destructive to pathogens and the neutrophil membrane carries receptors for antibodies and complement proteins. Neutrophils migrate to the traumatised tissues about an hour after the inflammatory response has been initiated. Migration is stimulated by the release of leucocyte-releasing factors which increase the activity of leucopoietic (leucocyte-producing) tissue in the bone marrow. Neutrophils entering the bloodstream are transported along the edges of the capillaries to the site of injury (mural flow) and enter the tissues by squeezing through tiny apertures between the capillary cells, a phenomenon called *diapedesis*. Migration to the injured area takes under two minutes and is caused by chemical attraction (chemotaxis).

Neutrophils identify substances acting as *opsonins* on the surface of the pathogen (Kobayashi et al. 2018). Opsonins are 'chemical tags' carrying receptors enabling the neutrophils to recognise and attach to antigens. Opsonisation enhances phagocytosis. Antibodies and the proteins of the complement cascade operate as opsonins. Patients with low neutrophil counts (neutropenia) are at high risk of infection (Box 3.2).

Box 3.2   Neutropenia

Neutropenia is one of the most common immune deficiencies and occurs mainly in patients undergoing chemotherapy. In cancer, neutropenia is defined as a neutrophil count of 0.5×10^9 per litre or less. Patients with neutropenia and a temperature greater than 38 °C or displaying other signs or symptoms associated with sepsis should be assessed rapidly and receive empirical antibiotic therapy.

Source: Adapted from National Institute for Health and Care Excellence (2012).

Macrophages and Monocytes

Macrophages develop in the bone marrow and enter the bloodstream as immature monocytes. Once they have matured and migrated to the tissues, they are known as macrophages. They are long-lived phagocytic cells particularly important in the later stages of infection, scavenging foreign cells and molecules filtered in the lymphoid tissues. Macrophages play a key role in the destruction of intracellular pathogens (e.g. *Mycobacterium tuberculosis*). Once engulfed by neutrophils, these pathogens are able to withstand the destructive action of their enzymes and continue to grow and multiply. Macrophages phagocytose neutrophils containing intracellular pathogens and destroy them. They also activate the adaptive immune system.

Distinct lineages of macrophages have been identified, with function depending on their location (Gordon and Plüddemann 2017). Langerhans cells are macrophages in the epidermis able to migrate to the lymph nodes and are thought to play a key role in immunosurveillance.

Mast Cells

Mast cells circulate in the bloodstream and congregate in connective tissue. They are activated by injury to the tissues and the complement proteins C3a and C5a, releasing molecules that increase the permeability of the capillaries (e.g. histamine, leucotrienes, prostaglandins) and molecules that attract neutrophils. Mast cells also play roles in the allergic and anaphylactic responses.

Dendritic Cells

Dendritic cells take up antigens in the tissues and carry them to the lymph nodes where they are most likely to encounter and be dealt with by macrophages or T-helper cells, thus helping to launch the adaptive immune response.

Natural Killer Cells

Natural killer cells comprise 5–20% of circulating lymphocytes. They respond to many different types of pathological challenge very rapidly. They attach to the surfaces of host cells infected with viruses and release a protein called *perforin* which creates pores in the membrane, setting in train a sequence that culminates in cellular destruction. NK cells also recognise cells in the early stages of neoplastic change and destroy them.

Eosinophils

Eosinophils are leucocytes activated by the proteins of the complement cascade. They attack parasites (e.g. protozoa, helminths) too large to be phagocytosed. Instead, they are destroyed by the action of enzymes produced by eosinophils.

Complement Proteins

Complement comprises a group of about 30 proteins present in inactive form in body fluids (Dunkelberger and Song 2010). Activation of the first complement in the sequence occurs when it is exposed to antigens and by the 'labelling' actions of opsonins and antibodies. When the complement cascade is triggered, each activated complement protein activates the next one in the sequence (Figure 3.2).

Once activated, complement proteins play a role in the inflammatory response; they increase permeability of the capillary walls, attract phagocytes, act as opsonisers and destroy bacteria by perforating their cell walls. The attachment of complement to an antigen–antibody complex results in its destruction (complement fixation). Several complement proteins have additional functions important in the overall immune response, illustrating the highly complex nature of immunity. C3b is a potent opsoniser. C3a stimulates macrophages to release bactericidal agents and enhances mast cell activity. C5b is a chemotactic attractor for neutrophils and macrophages (Merle et al. 2015).

Extracellular Antimicrobial Chemicals

A number of extracellular antimicrobial chemicals contribute to the innate immune response. They include:

- interferons
- lactoferrin
- acute phase proteins.

Interferons are released by cells infected with viruses. They limit the spread of viruses throughout the tissues and stimulate the immune response against malignant cells. Clinically, interferons are used to treat some cancers but cause severe side-effects including influenza-like symptoms and bone marrow suppression. *Lactoferrin* circulates in the bloodstream and is present in breast milk, saliva, tears and nasal secretions. Its antimicrobial properties are most marked in infants. *Acute phase proteins* are synthesised in the liver and appear in the bloodstream in the early stages of infection. A number have been identified, including C-reactive

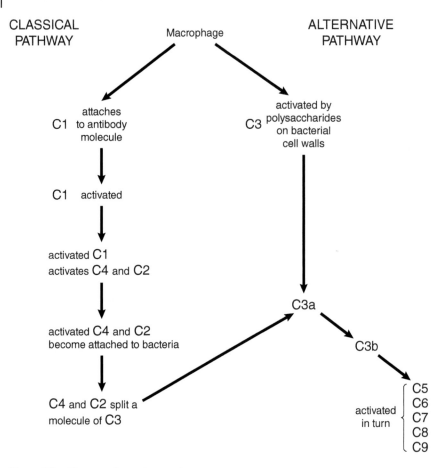

Figure 3.2 The complement cascade.

protein (CRP) which is important clinically as it used to diagnose infection and as a general marker of inflammation (Sproston and Ashworth 2018).

The inflammatory response and pyrexia are both considered to form part of the innate immune. Therefore, although sometimes considered harmful these are actually important responses to infection. Fever, as opposed to hyperthermia is hardly ever harmful, although inflammation may be if excessive or if it occurs in particular parts of the body.

Inflammatory Response

Inflammation is the response of the tissues to trauma. It takes place in response to physical damage (e.g. cuts, extremes of temperature), chemical damage and pathogenic invasion. The classic hallmarks of inflammation are:

- erythema (redness)
- swelling
- heat
- pain
- loss of function; the extent depends on the site and magnitude of injury.

When injury is sustained, the capillary walls in the surrounding tissues dilate and become more permeable in response to the release of locally acting hormones (e.g. bradykinin, histamine, prostaglandins). Oedema is caused by plasma leaking through the capillary walls into the intercellular spaces and contributes to the pain of inflammation by exerting pressure on adjacent nerve endings. The increased blood supply explains the erythema and sensation of heat associated with inflammation. Inflammation is beneficial: any microbial toxins present are diluted and increased numbers of phagocytic cells are carried to the site.

Fever (Pyrexia)

Fever, or pyrexia occurs in response to infection in all vertebrates. It is thought to play a beneficial role, possibly by increasing metabolic rate to eliminate bacteria and their toxins from the tissues quickly, and may also heighten the immune response. Although not usually harmful, and in many ways fever may be beneficial, there are some potential disadvantages. For example

- *Negative nitrogen balance*: for every 1 °C rise in temperature, the adult pulse rises by approximately 10 beats per minute and the rate of respiration by seven inspirations per minute.
- *Depletion of glycogen stores* leading to nitrogen wastage as protein is catabolised to generate energy.
- *Rigors*: uncontrollable violent shivering, frequently coinciding with the release of bacterial toxins into the bloodstream.
- *Febrile seizures* (convulsions) may occur in young children (six months to five years of age) and individuals with a history of epilepsy. Although transient, convulsions are frightening and can be dangerous as they may lead to trauma, aspiration of secretions or asphyxia.
- *Delirium*: this is most often seen in young children, older people and patients with marked pyrexia. It causes disorientation and restlessness, complicating the management of infectious patients in isolation.

Although fever may be treated symptomatically to reduce discomfort or excessive energy requirements, it should not be routinely treated.

Temperature Regulation and Infection

Temperature is controlled by the hypothalamus. Increase in body temperature is a systemic effect of the inflammatory response when prostaglandins and proteins called *pyrogens* released by the leucocytes induce fever. The temperature-regulating centre operates in the same way as a thermostat. Human core temperature is usually maintained at about 37 °C although normal temperature varies between people and at different sites. Deviations detected by receptor cells in the skin and tissues are relayed to the hypothalamus along the afferent nerves (Figure 3.3).

If temperature falls below the set point of 37 ° C, heat-conserving or -generating mechanisms are initiated. A rise above the set point triggers heat loss (Table 3.2).

When infection supvervenes, antigens on the surface of the pathogens 'reset' the thermostat to a higher set point by stimulating neutrophils and other cells of the immune system to release substances which can cause fever, known as pyrogens. Temperature is maintained at this new level until the foreign particles have been removed and the pyrogens are no longer present. Vasoconstriction and shivering are accompanied by increased metabolic rate. The patient feels cold and huddles up irrespective of the number of bedclothes provided.

The magnitude of fever depends on the pathogen and its interaction with the individual. Individuals have varying normal temperatures, and similarly varying

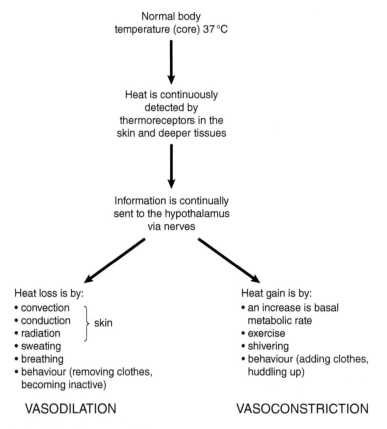

Figure 3.3 Thermoregulation.

Table 3.2 Mechanisms of thermoregulation.

Heat loss	Heat conservation
Skin capillaries dilate, increasing heat loss through: • convection • conduction • radiation • the evaporation of sweat	Skin capillaries constrict, decreasing heat loss through: • convection • conduction • radiation
	Shivering (involuntary muscular activity) and non-shivering thermogenesis
Behavioural activities, e.g. removing clothes, stretching out, reducing activity	Behavioural activities, e.g. huddling up, putting on extra clothes

---

Box 3.3 Care of Patients with Pyrexia

Monitor temperature, pulse and respiratory rate
Monitor fluid balance
Ensure adequate nutrition
Ensure adequate rest
Provide supportive care including help with hygiene
Change bedclothing as it becomes damp
Observe for signs of disorientation and febrile seizures in children under five

As the fever develops:
Provide extra bedclothes
Obtain specimens for laboratory diagnosis

Because fever is a regulated rise in temperature, external cooling will not reduce the temperature. Sometimes when cooled in this way, people shiver. This is known as a rigor, and is the body aiming to increase its temperature. Administration of antipyretic drugs, such as paracetamol (acetaminophen) or ibuprofen, will reduce the temperature, although their use in this way is controversial.

---

responses to infection. Mild infections may have little or no effect but others (e.g. *Salmonella enterica* serovar *typhi* causing typhoid) induce very high pyrexia (39–40 °C). Vasodilation and perspiration are stimulated once the infection begins to subside, promoting heat loss and making the patient feel hot and sticky (Box 3.3).

Some infections are associated with characteristic changes in body temperature pointing to diagnosis. In patients with brucellosis ('undulating fever'), temperature gradually rises and then resolves over a period of about 10 days before the cycle repeats. It is of the utmost importance to differentiate fever, which is regulated within the body, from hyperthermia which is not (Ogoina 2011).

Adaptive or Acquired Immunity

Pathogens occasionally escape the action of the innate immune system because they either evade phagocytosis or are not inactivated by the complement proteins. The body has evolved additional ways of destroying them through the action of the adaptive immune system. Adaptive immunity takes longer to develop (10–14 days) than the innate immune response because it provides a specific response to each individual antigen. Considering the very large number of antigens to which an individual will be exposed throughout their life, it is easy to see why this process may take a little time. This is in contrast to the innate immune system which is not antigen specific and so can respond much more quickly. This is sometimes referred to as the specific immune system because of its antigen specificity, or the acquired immune system because immunity is 'acquired' through exposure to a specific antigen. Two broad types of acquired immunity exist, using different types of lymphocytes:

- B-lymphocytes which produce antibodies (humoral immunity)
- T-lymphocytes which attack infected cells and malignant cells (cell-mediated immunity) and co-ordinate the immune response (T-cell 'help').

Both recognise and bind to antigens on the surface of foreign cells and inactivate or remove them.

B-Lymphocytes and Humoral Immunity

B-lymphocytes (which can mature into antibody-producing plasma cells) are produced in the bone marrow and move into the tissues when mature. Numbers are highest in the lymphoid tissues where foreign materials are filtered from body fluids ('humors'). B-lymphocytes bind to antigens on the surface of pathogens and neutralise them (Figure 3.4). Binding takes place between antigen-binding sites on the surface of the B-lymphocyte and a region of the pathogen called the antigenic determinant or *epitope* that has a complementary shape. The two fit together like a key fitting into a lock. An individual antigen will contain many epitopes.

Key features of humoral immunity are:

- antigen specificity
- clonal selection
- clonal expansion
- clonal suppression and the formation of memory cells
- release of antibodies.

Antigen Specificity

B-lymphocytes are able to recognise and respond to at least 10^8 different antigenic epitopes. Consequently, every different antigen the body encounters is recognised independently of all the others. It is not possible for every B-lymphocyte to carry all the receptors necessary to recognise all the thousands of antigenic epitopes it might

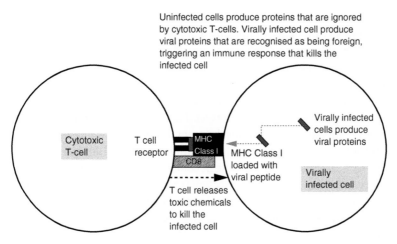

Uninfected cells produce proteins that are ignored by cytotoxic T-cells. Virally infected cell produce viral proteins that are recognised as being foreign, triggering an immune response that kills the infected cell

Figure 3.4 Binding between a B-lymphocyte and an antigen, and the B-cell receiving T-cell help.

encounter because there would be insufficient physical space on the surface of the cell and not enough DNA to code for them. Instead, each B-lymphocyte carries receptor molecules of a unique structure and specificity to allow it to recognise a few of similar configuration (shape).

Clonal Selection

There are thousands of different types of B-lymphocytes. Each responds to the same few antigenic epitopes. Those responding to the same epitopes are called a *clone*. The body contains thousands of different clones 'selected' because they match antigenic epitopes the best. A large bacterial cell carrying numerous different antigenic epitopes would select several different clones of B-lymphocytes.

Clonal Expansion

Clonal expansion involves the rapid replication of thousands of identical B-lymphocytes in response to the arrival and binding of antigens. An immune response begins with a very small number of cells that recognise a specific antigenic epitope. Through a repeated process of positive selection of those which bind the antigen best, clonal expansion, change through mutation, and more positive selection, the immune system is able to generate large numbers of antigen specific cells. It is the length of time that this process takes that accounts for the relative slowness of the primary immune response. Future responses are quicker due the immunological memory.

Immunological Memory

A key feature of the acquired immune system is immunological memory. Unlike the innate immune system which starts anew each time an infection occurs, the acquired immune system has long-lived memory cells specific for each antigen.

These memory cells are able to respond more quickly to an infection on the second and subsequent exposure. For example, memory B cells are able to produce antibody more quickly than was originally the case, and they are able to produce different types of antibody that are of higher avidity and affinity which are measures of the biding strength of antibodies. Similar memory cells are generated from T-cell population. The more rapid response to infection is shown in Figure 3.5. This is the rationale for vaccination. By presenting the antigen if a form that does not cause disease this stimulates the development of a primary immune response. When the real (or wild-type) organism is encountered the immune system recognises that it has been exposed to the antigen before. The faster, stronger immune response is set in train and the risk of infection is averted. Although it is not know for sure how long immunological memory lasts, epidemiological data would suggest that in some cases it may be life-long, partially explaining why it is rare to get diseases such as chicken pox and measles more than once.

Antibodies (Immunoglobulins)

Immunoglobulins (Igs) are proteins carried on the surface of B-lymphocytes, and then secreted into body fluids. Approximately 10^5 immunoglobulins are present on the surface of each lymphocyte. Binding to the specific antigen occurs between the immunoglobulin and a corresponding antigenic determinant or epitope (see Figure 3.5). Immunoglobulin molecules are Y-shaped and consist of two distinct parts connected by a hinged region (Figure 3.6).

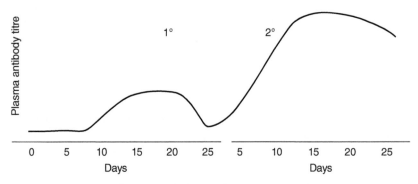

Figure 3.5 The primary and secondary immune responses. *Primary immune response (1°).* Day 0 Vaccination: exposure to an inactive or weakened strain of antigen. Days 10–20 Release of antibodies in response to the antigens in the vaccine and creation of memory cells. Day 25 Return to low plasma antibody levels. Memory cells persist. *Secondary immune response (2°).* Before Day 5 Exposure to the antigen results in steep increase in antibodies released from the memory cells persisting from the primary response. Days 10–20 The antibody titre is much higher than during the primary response. A sizeable and successful immune response is mounted. Day 25 The antibody level gradually wanes but remains relatively high for months or years.

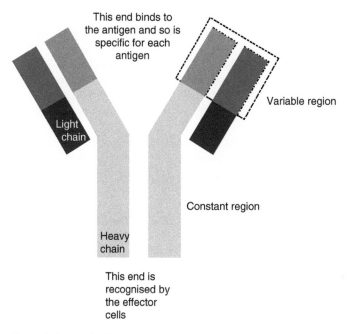

This end binds to the antigen and so is specific for each antigen

Variable region

Light chain

Constant region

Heavy chain

This end is recognised by the effector cells

Figure 3.6   Antibody molecule.

- The Fab region of the antibody is the antigen binding site.
- The Fc (crystalline fragment) of the antibody interacts with the other cells of the immune system when the antibody is secreted, controlling the immune response when binding occurs.

Binding of the antigen and antibody is the signal for clonal expansion. Once a B-lymphocyte binds to its antigenic determinant epitope on the micro-organism, it secretes further antibodies into the blood and body fluids at a rate of thousands per second. Immunoglobulins bind to their matching antigenic determinant epitope causing agglutination (clumping) and the resulting aggregates are more readily phagocytosed.

Once binding has occurred, the antibody:

- functions as an opsonin, labelling antigens and targeting them for phagocytosis
- enhances the cytotoxic action of the NK cells and eosinophils
- triggers the complement cascade, generating C3a and C3b to contribute to the inflammatory response.

Five classes of immunoglobulin have been identified (Table 3.3).

Table 3.3   The classes of immunoglobulins.

Ig type	Role in the immune response
IgA	The main antibody in external secretions and on mucous membranes; also present in breast milk. Acts as an early defence against pathogens by coating them to prevent them adhering to epithelial cells
IgD	Part of the B-cell receptor
IgE	Attached to cells, including mast cells and is an important inflammatory mediator. Triggers the allergic response and active against parasites
IgG	The main circulating antibody, important in the secondary immune response by initiating phagocytosis and neutralising bacterial toxins. Crosses the placenta in third trimester
IgM	The first antibody produced in response to pathogenic invasion, playing a key role in the primary immune response by facilitating phagocytosis. Sometimes used as a marker of recent infection

IgM is the first antibody produced by the B-lymphocytes. After a few days, different classes of antibodies are released, usually IgG. IgM is a large molecule able to bind to a large number of antigens. IgG molecules are much smaller and able to enter the tissues more effectively. IgG can also be produced in far greater amounts.

Cell-Mediated Immunity

Cell-mediated immunity is a function of the T-cells. They develop in the bone marrow and migrate to the thymus gland behind the sternum, where they mature. T-cells produce messenger molecules called *cytokines* (e.g. interferon). These activate many of the other cells of the immune response.

Cell-mediated immunity is stimulated when an antigen binds to a receptor site on the surface of a T-cell. The cell-mediated immune response:

- offers protection against viral and fungal infections and parasites
- offers protection against intracellular invasion by bacteria able to survive phagocytosis (e.g. *M. tuberculosis*)
- maintains the inflammatory response when chronic infection occurs (e.g. tuberculosis, leprosy)
- monitors the presence of foreign cells, detects malignant cells and plays a role in transplant rejection
- regulates the adaptive immune response.

T-cells release chemicals called *lymphokines* which activate macrophages, enhancing phagocytosis and stimulating the activity of other cells vital for the immune response.

Types of T-Cell

T-cells multiply rapidly after they have been exposed to an antigen and undergo differentiation. Numerous subsets have been identified. Sometimes these are referred to by their cluster of differentiation (or CD number). This refers to the presence of particular molecules on the cell surface.

- T-cytotoxic cells (CD8+ cells) recognise peptides (protein fragments) presented to them by proteins of the major histocompatibility complex (MHC) on the surfaces of cells infected with viruses and those that have undergone neoplastic change. Viruses take over the genetic machinery of the host cell, stimulate it to make virus proteins and alter the MHC proteins on the cell surfaces. Neoplastic change also alters the surface MHC proteins. T-cytotoxic cells release interferon and perforin which destroy foreign cells. MHC Class I molecules are found on all nucleated cells of the body, and present proteins that are being produced inside of the cell, on the outside of the cell. Normally these would be 'self' proteins, which are recognised and ignored by cytotoxic T-cells. Virally infected cells however will produce viral proteins that are presented by MHC Class I molecules in the same way. These are recognised by cytotoxic T-cells as being foreign causing the T-cell to kill the infected cells. This is shown in Figure.
- T-helper cells (CD4+ cells) launch and regulate the immune response. They stimulate the B- and other T-lymphocytes to mature. This function is executed only after they have themselves been activated. Cells that can act as antigen presenting cells (APC cells) such as dendritic cells, macrophages, and many others possess another type of MHC proteins known as MHC Class II. In contrast to MHC I, these do not present proteins made within the cell, but rather proteins taken up by the cell. Antigen presenting cells take up foreign proteins and after breaking them down the literally 'present' the antigen held by MHC Class II proteins to T-helper cells, thus activating them. Other activation signals include cytokines from other cells of the immune system.
- T-suppressor cells deactivate the immune response by 'switching off' the action of the T-helper cells. They help prevent autoimmunity (Geginat et al. 2014).

Variations in the Immune Response and the Prevention of Autoimmunity

The activity of the immune system is genetically regulated. Some children are born with congenital or genetic deficiencies of the immune system and are highly susceptible to infection. Inherited lymphocytopenia (a low level of lymphocytes in the blood) and agammaglobulinaemia (the absence or deficiency of gammaglobulin in the blood) are X-linked genetic disorders. Affected children seldom survive infancy. People with chronic granulomatous disease are highly susceptible to opportunistic infections because they have defective phagocytic enzymes unable to kill and digest bacteria. If one twin of a monozygotic (identical) pair develops tuberculosis, the other is more likely to do so at some stage in their life than other siblings who do not share all the same genes but whose degree of exposure is the same.

Some ethnic groups appear susceptible to particular infections (e.g. tuberculosis, COVID-19). Other infections are species specific; norovirus appears to infect the human host only. In order to prevent autoimmunity, many immune responses require two separate signals to become activated, and if both are not present apoptosis or programmed cell death may occur. Cells of the acquired immune system are also monitored for autoimmune tendencies throughout their development, and any that are likely to cause autoimmunity are removed.

Immunity throughout the Lifespan

Immunity may be depressed during ill health and other changes throughout the life of the individual and is influenced by a range of factors.

- *Age*: infection is more common at the extremes of life. Infants acquire IgG via the placenta and IgA via breast milk. Although their effects do not persist for long, these antibodies offer valuable protection while the adaptive system is immature. Ability to mount an inflammatory response and to form new antibodies declines in the very elderly.
- *Drugs*: steroids depress the inflammatory response and inhibit antibody formation. Antimicrobials disrupt the normal body flora, encouraging superinfection by extraneous micro-organisms. Replacement of the normal bowel flora can result in superinfection with *Clostridioides difficile*. Replacement of the normal vaginal flora can result in superinfection with *Candida* spp.
- *Radiotherapy and chemotherapy* depress the leucocyte count if the bone marrow or lymphatic tissues are affected. Patients with reduced neutrophil count (neutropenia) are highly susceptible to infection.
- *Metabolic disorders* including diabetes and malignancy reduce the immune response.
- *Malnutrition*: obesity reduces the ability to heal because adipose tissue has a poor blood supply. Undernutrition interferes with all aspects of the immune response, as demonstrated by the devastating effects of measles in parts of the world with diminished food supplies. In malnourished patients, the capacity of the gastrointestinal mucosa to act as a barrier against pathogens is impaired.
- *Immobility* contributes to increased susceptibility to infection because it inhibits the drainage of respiratory secretions, induces urinary stasis and increases

the risk of pressure ulcers, which breach the normally intact cutaneous barrier and allow the entry of skin commensals not usually able to cause infection.

- *Psychological stress* appears to depress the immune response.
- Specific and acquired immunity depend on the antigens to which an individual has been exposed, either naturally or through immunisation.

Types of Immunity

Immunity is either active or passive.

Active Immunity

Active immunity is acquired throughout the lifespan. Different types exist.

- *Natural active immunity*: antibodies develop in response to exposure to an antigen.
- *Artificial active immunity*: antibodies are produced in response to vaccination.

Passive Immunity

Passive immunity results when preformed antibodies are received and lasts only as long as they remain in the body. Different types exist.

- *Natural passive immunity*: IgG is received from the mother across the placenta and IgA via breast milk, giving immunity for the first few months while the baby's immune system is immature.
- *Artificial passive immunity* is induced by immunising an individual exposed to a pathogen against which they have no existing immunity. Recipients are injected with antibodies obtained from individuals who have high levels of antibodies because they have either recently been infected or immunised. Immunity is rapidly induced but is short-lived, waning as the antibodies are gradually lost. Artificial passive immunity is used to provide temporary protection against hepatitis B after needlestick injury, and for some children who are immunosuppressed and who do not have immunity to chickenpox.

Artificial Active Immunity: Vaccination

Vaccination is the process of giving a vaccine. Immunisation results either as a result of receiving a vaccine or through natural exposure.

Vaccines are biological agents able to generate an immune response, giving protection against infection on future exposure to a pathogen while causing minimal adverse effects (Pollard and Bijker 2021). Most vaccines stimulate antibody production, but some also stimulate cell-mediated responses. For example, the bacillus Calmette–Guérin (BCG) vaccine for tuberculosis induces cell-mediated immunity. Two types of protection are offered: protection of the individual and protection for the population as whole, sometimes referred to as herd immunity. This occurs when a sufficient proportion of the population are protected, preventing widespread transmission of the micro-organism. Crucially it does not mean that no one will become ill.

Most vaccines provide medium to long-term immunity. The main exception is the influenza vaccine. Type A influenza, which is most often responsible for epidemics, carries two main antigens, haemagglutinin and neuramidase, which mutate slowly (antigenic drift) and sometimes suddenly (antigenic shift). Antigenic drift occurs slowly all the time but antigenic shift occurs rapidly; the last time was in 2009 when H1N1 entered the human population. Constant change means that a new vaccine is required for type A influenza every year. The World Health Organization (WHO) analyses the predominant strains each year and advises changes necessary to the vaccine formulation. Most vaccines give protection after two or three injections but some (e.g. measles, mumps, rubella [MMR]) achieve a high antibody level after a single dose.

The first vaccine was developed by Jenner in 1796. He observed that milkmaids who had developed cowpox rarely contracted the similar but much more serious smallpox. Jenner prepared a rudimentary vaccine from the cowpox virus able to induce immunity in people not previously exposed to either infection. This was a major advance in public health as at the time, smallpox was a major cause of mortality. Smallpox vaccination was highly successful and in 1980 the WHO declared that smallpox had been eradicated. It is hoped that polio may one day also be eradicated from the world.

Types of Vaccines

Modern vaccines are prepared from the agent causing the disease, its products or a synthetic substitute treated with heat or chemicals (e.g. formaldehyde) to induce immunity without causing the disease itself. Different types of vaccines have been developed (Table 3.4).

The *valency* of a vaccine is the number of antigens that it contains. The influenza vaccine is either trivalent or quadrivalent, containing three or four antigens respectively. The MMR vaccine is trivalent; it contains a single strain of each of the three viruses it offers protection against. There are a variety of pneumococcal vaccines, with the polysaccharide vaccine containing 23 different types of pneumococcus (known as serotypes because they appear different to the immune system), while conjugate vaccines may contain 7, 10, 13, and in newer versions even more serotypes. Factors affecting the development of new vaccines and their introduction are influenced by changing patterns of disease within the community. Traditionally, it took years to develop new vaccines but a number of vaccines for COVID-19 were developed rapidly during the pandemic in 2020–2021.

Table 3.4 Types of vaccines.

Type of vaccine	Examples
Live attenuated vaccines contain an altered or weakened version of the organism. These can replicate in the body and usually provide high levels of immunity persisting for a long period of time	Tuberculosis (BCG)
	Oral polio vaccine (OPV)
	Measles, mumps, rubella (MMR)
	Shingles (herpes zoster)
	Rotavirus
	Nasal influenza
Inactivated vaccines contain whole organisms that have been inactivated and are unable to replicate.	Whole-cell pertussis (wP)
	Inactivated polio virus (IPV)
	Influenza (not nasal influenza)
Subunit (purified antigen) vaccines contain individual antigens from the organism	Acellular pertussis (aP)
	Hepatitis B (HepB)
	Human papiloma virus (HPV)
Polysaccharide vaccines contain parts of the polysaccharide capsule found on the outside of some bacteria. These provide T-cell-independent immunity by stimulating B cells directly, which is more limited in strength and duration, with little immunological memory. These vaccines have limited effect in children under two years	Pneumococcal polysaccharide vaccine (PPV23)
	Meningococcal quadrivalent (ACWY)
Polysaccharide conjugate vaccines contain parts of the polysaccharide capsule found on the outside of some bacteria attached (conjugated) to a protein carrier. This turns a T-cell-independent immune response into a dependent response, overcoming many of the limitations of pure polysaccharide vaccines	*Haemophilus influenzae* type b (Hib)
	Pneumococcal conjugate (PCV-7, PCV-10, PCV-13)
	Meningococcal B, C & quadrivalent (ACWY)
Toxoid vaccines comprise inactivated toxins. They are used where the illness is caused by a toxin produced by an organism rather than the organism itself	Tetanus toxoid (TT)
	Diphtheria toxoid
Viral vector vaccines. The genes for key antigens are inserted into a harmless vector. When the vector multiplies, the genes replicate	COVID-19
mRNA vaccines. Messenger RNA (mRNA) for key antigens is injected. The RNA is translated into protein which stimulates immunity. It is important to note that these do not affect cellular DNA	COVID -19
DNA vaccines. These are similar to mRNA vaccines but use DNA	None presently available

Technical challenges still limit the development of vaccines for many serious infections. It is difficult to develop vaccines for pathogens that can survive intra-cellularly (e.g. *Neisseria gonorrhoeae*). HIV mutates so rapidly that an effective vaccine has never been developed.

Herd Immunity

Herd immunity is resistance to an infectious disease exhibited by the population as a whole. If a high percentage are immunised (or have acquired immunity natu-rally), the risk of transmission to those who are susceptible is reduced because exposure is less likely. However, this does not mean that no one will ever catch the disease, only that widespread community transmission should not occur. The pro-portion of people needed to be successfully immunised in order to achieve herd immunity varies and is dependent upon how transmissible the organism is. For very transmissible organisms such as measles, the proportion needed to achieve herd immunity is around 95%. Before vaccination was introduced, outbreaks of measles and pertussis (whooping cough) occurred cyclically every few years. In between, cases occurred sporadically throughout the population. A large number of infections occurring simultaneously was possible only when a cohort of chil-dren lacking previous exposure were infected. Once all had been infected, the outbreak waned until the number of susceptible children increased again.

In community health terms, sporadic infection is significant as epidemics are possible as long as some individuals lacking immunity are present in a popula-tion. Conditions favouring outbreaks occur when susceptible people are clustered together geographically or socially (May and Silverman 2003). The aim of immu-nisation programmes is to induce acquired immunity in all the people in a popula-tion susceptible to an infection to prevent outbreaks. The proportion of people required to be successfully immunised for herd immunity to exist can be as high as 95% for highly infectious diseases such as measles.

Standard Immunisation Programmes

Vaccination schedules differ between countries for epidemiological, organisa-tional and economic reasons. Key issues in their design include the ability to deliver the vaccine, including the need to space doses and maintain the supply chain. The childhood immunisation programmes against infectious disease were introduced in the UK in the 1940s and are regularly reviewed and updated; for example, vaccination against pneumococcal disease was introduced in 2006 and against the human papilloma virus in 2008. In the UK, the Department of Health recommends a schedule of immunisation commencing in early childhood and responsibility for vaccination falls to the primary care services. These details are contained within the Green Book (UK Health Security Agency 2021), while the equivalent in the United States is the Pink Book (Centers for Disease Control and Prevention 2021).

Vaccines need to be given as early as possible to maximise protection but not so early that the infant is unable to develop effective immunity because of the immaturity of their immune system. Generally, vaccines given before 12 months of age do not result in long-term immunity and booster vaccinations are required unless the pathogen is likely to cause less severe disease in adults (e.g. rotavirus). MMR is given after maternal antibodies for measles have declined to avoid interference between this maternal antibody and the vaccine (Zinkernagel 2001). Few vaccines are thought to work in the neonatal period, two exceptions being the BCG for tuberculosis and that against hepatitis B.

Health promotion and administering vaccines are an important aspects of the work of health professionals employed in primary care. Uptake can be increased by promoting public awareness, especially in relation to adverse reactions and safety. Parents sometimes worry that vaccines might overwhelm their child's immune system but this is not a valid concern. If each vaccine contained 100 antigens each with 10 epitopes, infants could still respond to approximately 10 000 vaccines at one time point (Offit et al. 2002). Parents can be reassured that anaphylaxis following vaccination is rare and that the risk is far outweighed by the risk of infectious disease.

Severe adverse effects of vaccines are very unusual. The link between the MMR and autism has been discredited.

Primary care staff should include vaccination history whenever children are assessed and for other groups where vaccines are recommended. The UK Green Book immunisation against infectious disease emphasises the importance of recommending vaccination even if individuals are older than the scheduled age (UK Health Security Agency 2021). There are only a few contraindications for vaccination (Table 3.5).

Health workers responsible for giving immunisations must be trained to recognise and manage anaphylaxis. They should also be familiar with the storage of vaccines (Box 3.4).

Vaccinations for 'At-risk' Populations

Some people require additional vaccinations because they are at particularly high risk of infection. Children with impaired immunity can be immunised against varicella although this vaccine does not form part of the routine immunisation schedule in the UK. Travellers are offered vaccination for hepatitis A if they visit areas where hygiene is poor. Vaccinations against yellow fever and typhoid are offered to people travelling to countries where these diseases are endemic.

Table 3.5 Contradictions against routine vaccination.

All vaccines

History of anaphylaxis after receiving a vaccine or its components, although alternatives may be available

Febrile illness, although this probably does not affect the immunogenicity, it may appear to be a side-effect of the vaccine

Active infection

Live vaccines

Pregnant women, the theoretical risk for the unborn baby needs to be weighed against the protection the vaccine offers. In general live vaccines are not given however

People who are immunosuppressed

Cancer patients receiving chemotherapy or radiotherapy

Box 3.4   Storing Vaccines
• The recommended temperature for polio vaccine is 0–4 °C. All other vaccines should be stored at 2–8 °C.
• The temperature of the refrigerator should be monitored and recorded regularly.
• Written procedures should be developed and adopted if the refrigerator breaks down.
• The refrigerator should be defrosted regularly, placing the vaccines in another refrigerator or coolbox.
• Reconstituted vaccine should be used within the period recommended by the manufacturer. Partially used vials should be destroyed at the end of the clinic session.
• Stocks should be rotated so the oldest batch of numbered vaccines is used first.
• Vaccines should be removed from the refrigerator and reconstituted only when they are about to be administered.
Source: Adapted from Purssell (2015).

Vaccine Hesitancy

As long as vaccines have existed, there have been concerns about their safety. The 'life cycle' of vaccine scepticism tends to follow a pattern.

- People are worried about an infectious disease.
- A vaccine is developed and concern is reduced.
- As the risks of the disease are forgotten, adverse reactions begin to attract attention, often exacerbated by the media. For example, young health professionals

and young parents, never having witnessed the effects of pertussis on a small baby, may be heavily influenced by media stories documenting adverse effects.

- Confidence in the vaccination programme declines.
- Vaccination uptake decreases, followed by resurgence of the disease.

Vaccine hesitancy is sometimes a feature of belonging to a specific group, often associated with religious or other beliefs. Members often live in the same area or attend the same social and other events, enabling the infection to spread readily (May and Silverman 2003).

Sepsis

Sepsis is described by the World Health Organization (n.d.) as the most serious complication related to infection, particularly in low- and middle-income countries. It is a potentially life-threatening condition occurring when the inflammatory response causes extensive tissue damage by activating the coagulation and complement cascades. A recent definition of sepsis is: 'a life-threatening organ dysfunction caused by a dysregulated host response to infection' (Singer et al. 2016). It is prevented by fundamental infection prevention and control strategies.

Sepsis is possible as the result of minor injuries in otherwise healthy people (World Health Organization n.d.) but some groups are at particular risk.

- Older age groups
- Very young children
- Immunocompromised patients
- Patients with diabetes
- Patients with chronic liver or kidney disease
- Previous treatment with antimicrobials or steroids
- Patients with indwelling invasive devices

In severe cases, sepsis progresses to septic shock: a dramatic fall in blood pressure resulting in lack of tissue perfusion and multiple organ failure (Gotts and Matthay 2016). Six types of organ dysfunction have been described (Table 3.6).

Recovery from mild sepsis is possible, especially if patients receive antimicrobial treatment and drugs to combat the effects of shock (e.g. epinephrine) promptly, but mortality is very high, especially for older people, those who are immunocompromised or receiving treatment for cancer (Vincent et al. 2019). Patients who survive sepsis frequently experience long-term physical and mental health problems (e.g. post-traumatic stress disorder, cognitive problems, chronic pain, organ dysfunction) and are at higher risk if they develop infection again.

Table 3.6   Organ dysfunction associated with sepsis and septic shock.

- Neurological and altered mental status: lethargy, confusion, or delirium
- Pulmonary dysfunction manifesting as increased respiratory rate (tachypnoea) associated with abnormal arterial blood gases (usually respiratory alkalosis with hypoxaemia and hypercarbia)
- Myocardial depression with decreased ventricular ejection
- Reduced circulating volume resulting from capillary leakage leading to reduced renal function and oliguria
- Haematological disorders resulting in either disseminated intravascular coagulation (DIC) with cyanosis, that can progress to gangrene, or blood loss. These apparently paradoxical findings result from the balance between the clotting and fibrinolytic systems, with the result depending upon which dominates
- Liver damage probably resulting from poor hepatic perfusion

Source: Hotchkiss et al. (2016).

It is estimated that 49 million people develop sepsis every year with 11 million deaths (Rudd et al. 2020). There are 123 000 cases in England annually and 37 000 deaths. Nurses in close patient contact are well placed to recognise the early signs of sepsis:

- increased respiration rate
- low oxygen saturation
- low systolic blood pressure
- bradycardia
- disorientation or impaired consciousness in previously lucid patients.

In UK hospitals, the National Early Warning Score (NEWS) (Royal College of Physicians 2017) is used to standardise assessment and response to acute illness, including sepsis. There are equivalent systems for children, which are more complicated because they are different for each age group. Training to identify and report early warning signs can improve patient outcomes (Torsvik et al. 2016).

Suggested Activities

Exercise 3.1 Self-assessment

1   How is an antigen defined?

2   Which of the following contain lymphoid tissue?
   A Appendix
   B Trachea

C Liver

D Body fluids

3 Which of the following cells are phagocytic?

A T-helper cells

B Mast cells

C Plasma cells

D Macrophages

4 The innate and adaptive immune systems function independently of one another. True/False

5 Complete the following sentence: 'The classic signs of inflammation are . . .'

6 Complete the following sentence: 'Pyrexia is part of the innate immune response because . . .'

7 Which of the following are key features of humoral immunity?

A Clonal expansion

B Formation of memory cells

C Phagocytosis

D All of the above

8 Give an example of each of the following:

A Natural active immunity

B Artificial active immunity

C Natural passive immunity

D Artificial passive immunity

9 The vaccine for influenza type A is effective for life. True/False

10 How many antigens are contained in a divalent vaccine?

Exercise 3.2

Vaccination is an important part of the overall infection control and prevention strategy. There are two main vaccination strategies – universal vaccines offered to everyone, and those which are targeted at a specific groups. Examining the vaccination schedule for your country or region, see which vaccines are offered and to which groups. In particular, note the timings (including the number of doses and gaps between doses), and any contraindications.

Exercise 3.3

Vaccination coverage is rarely 100%. What barriers to vaccination are there and why do some people choose not to be vaccinated? What can be done to improve this? See if you can find any local guidance about improving vaccination uptake.

Exercise 3.4

Access the reference by Torsvik et al. (2016). Read the paper and address the following questions.
  A What type of study was conducted?
  B What are the study findings?
  C Are they trustworthy?
  D Would the findings be helpful to support local practice elsewhere?

References

Centers for Disease Control and Prevention (2021). Epidemiology and Prevention of Vaccine-Preventable Diseases. www.cdc.gov/vaccines/pubs/pinkbook/index.html.

Dancey, J.T., Deubelbeiss, K.A., Harker, L.A., and Finch, C.A. (1976). Neutrophil kinetics in man. *J. Clin. Invest.* 58: 705–715. https://doi.org/10.1172/JCI108517.

Dunkelberger, J.R. and Song, W.-C. (2010). Complement and its role in innate and adaptive immune responses. *Cell Res.* 20: 34–50. https://doi.org/10.1038/cr.2009.139.

Geginat, J., Paroni, M., Maglie, S. et al. (2014). Plasticity of human CD4 T cell subsets. *Front. Immunol.* 5: 630. https://doi.org/10.3389/fimmu.2014.00630.

Gordon, S. and Plüddemann, A. (2017). Tissue macrophages: heterogeneity and functions. *BMC Biol.* 15: 53. https://doi.org/10.1186/s12915-017-0392-4.

Gotts, J.E. and Matthay, M.A. (2016). Sepsis: pathophysiology and clinical management. *BMJ* 353: i585. https://doi.org/10.1136/bmj.i1585.

Hotchkiss, R.S., Moldawer, L.L., Opal, S.M. et al. (2016). Sepsis and septic shock. *Nat. Rev. Dis. Primers.* 2: 16045. https://doi.org/10.1038/nrdp.2016.45.

Kobayashi, S.D., Malachowa, N., and DeLeo, F.R. (2018). Neutrophils and bacterial immune evasion. *J. Innate Immun.* 10: 432–441. https://doi.org/10.1159/000487756.

May, T. and Silverman, R.D. (2003). 'Clustering of exemptions' as a collective action threat to herd immunity. *Vaccine* 21: 1048–1051. https://doi.org/10.1016/S0264-410X(02)00627-8.

Merle, N.S., Church, S.E., Fremeaux-Bacchi, V., and Roumenina, L.T. (2015). Complement system part I: molecular mechanisms of activation and regulation. *Front. Immunol.* 6: 262. https://doi.org/10.3389/fimmu.2015.00262.

National Institute for Health and Care Excellence (2012). Neutropenic sepsis: prevention and management in people with cancer. www.nice.org.uk/guidance/cg151.

Offit, P.A., Quarles, J., Gerber, M.A. et al. (2002). Addressing parents' concerns: do multiple vaccines overwhelm or weaken the infant's immune system? *Pediatrics* 109: 124–129. https://doi.org/10.1542/peds.109.1.124.

Ogoina, D. (2011). Fever, fever patterns and diseases called 'fever' – a review. *J. Infect. Public Health* 4: 108–124. https://doi.org/10.1016/j.jiph.2011.05.002.

Pollard, A.J. and Bijker, E.M. (2021). A guide to vaccinology: from basic principles to new developments. *Nat. Rev. Immunol.* 21: 83–100. https://doi.org/10.1038/s41577-020-00479-7.

Purssell, E. (2015). Reviewing the importance of the cold chain in the distribution of vaccines. *Br. J. Community Nurs.* 20: 481–486. https://doi.org/10.12968/bjcn.2015.20.10.481.

Resuscitation Council UK (2021). Guidance: Anaphylaxis. www.resus.org.uk/library/additional-guidance/guidance-anaphylaxis.

Royal College of Physicians 2017. National Early Warning Score (NEWS). www.rcplondon.ac.uk/projects/outputs/national-early-warning-score-news-2.

Rudd, K.E., Johnson, S.C., Agesa, K.M. et al. (2020). Global, regional, and national sepsis incidence and mortality, 1990–2017: analysis for the Global Burden of Disease Study. *Lancet* 395: 200–211. https://doi.org/10.1016/S0140-6736(19)32989-7.

Singer, M., Deutschman, C.S., Seymour, C.W. et al. (2016). The third international consensus definitions for sepsis and septic shock (Sepsis-3). *JAMA* 315: 801. https://doi.org/10.1001/jama.2016.0287.

Sproston, N.R. and Ashworth, J.J. (2018). Role of C-reactive protein at sites of inflammation and infection. *Front. Immunol.* 9: 754. https://doi.org/10.3389/fimmu.2018.00754.

Summers, C., Rankin, S.M., Condliffe, A.M. et al. (2010). Neutrophil kinetics in health and disease. *Trends Immunol.* 31: 318–324. https://doi.org/10.1016/j.it.2010.05.006.

Torsvik, M., Gustad, L.T., Mehl, A. et al. (2016). Early identification of sepsis in hospital inpatients by ward nurses increases 30-day survival. *Crit. Care* 20: 244. https://doi.org/10.1186/s13054-016-1423-1.

UK Health Security Agency 2021. Immunisation against infectious disease. www.gov.uk/government/collections/immunisation-against-infectious-disease-the-green-book

Vincent, J.-L., Jones, G., David, S. et al. (2019). Frequency and mortality of septic shock in Europe and North America: a systematic review and meta-analysis. *Crit. Care* 23: 196. https://doi.org/10.1186/s13054-019-2478-6.

World Health Organization n.d. Sepsis. www.who.int/news-room/fact-sheets/detail/sepsis.

Zinkernagel, R.M. (2001). Maternal antibodies, childhood infections, and autoimmune diseases. *N. Engl. J. Med.* 345: 1331–1335. https://doi.org/10.1056/NEJMra012493.

4

The Microbiology Laboratory

Medical Microbiology Services

In the UK, most acute hospitals have their own medical microbiology laboratory. These often provide services for smaller institutions such as nursing homes and general practices. In other countries such as the US, large centralised laboratories provide a commercial service to a range of health providers. In high-income countries, the public health services provide additional, more specialist services to identify organisms only occasionally encountered in clinical care (e.g. those responsible for food-borne and water-borne infection).

Introduction to the Microbiology Laboratory

The functions of the microbiology laboratory are to:

- diagnose infections and give advice about the most effective antimicrobial treatment for individual patients
- investigate clusters of infection
- undertake routine surveillance
- identify antimicrobial-resistant organisms and inform antimicrobial policy.

Laboratory staff work closely with the infection prevention team but all clinicians need to understand the work of the medical microbiology laboratory in order to:

- provide information to patients about diagnostic tests
- obtain specimens: success depends on good practice when the patient is prepared for the test, the specimen is obtained and correct storage and handling
- interpret the findings of laboratory reports.

Infection Prevention and Control in Healthcare Settings,
First Edition. Edward Purssell and Dinah Gould.
© 2023 John Wiley & Sons Ltd. Published 2023 by John Wiley & Sons Ltd.

Diagnostic Laboratory Services

Diagnostic tests fall into two broad categories.

- *Phenotypic* tests based on microbial behaviour (e.g. growth under different conditions, sensitivity to antimicrobials). The most commonly used phenotypic tests are microscopy, culture and sensitivity. Many organisms are hard to grow in laboratory culture and diagnosis can be challenging.
- *Molecular* tests which identify parts of the organism or immune responses to it. Examples are polymerase chain reaction (PCR) tests, antigen detection and serology. Molecular testing, including the use of near-patient testing based on PCR tests, is increasingly undertaken routinely.

Key differences between the two types of tests are the requirement for the organism to be grown in the laboratory in the case of culture-based tests, but not necessary for the PCR which requires only that the genome is in the specimen. This is important when collecting and handling specimens, as some organisms die or become non-viable quickly after collection and so need to be sent to the laboratory immediately if they are to be cultured. This is less important for PCR and similar tests. Also, tests that seek to identify the organism are somewhat different to those which look for the immune response to the organism, since the latter requires sufficient time and immune response for this to be identified. Those who are significantly immune suppressed may not, for example, produce high levels of immunoglobulin. This poses a particular issue for children born to HIV-positive mothers, as they will be born with maternal HIV antibodies which do not necessarily reflect the baby's HIV status. Serological (antibody) tests are not useful in these children who should be tested for the virus directly (World Health Organization 2021a).

Direct Examination

Microbiology laboratories most often deal with specimens of urine, sputum, faeces and wounds. The first step towards diagnosis is examination of the specimen with the naked eye, constituting the microscopy component of microscopy, culture and sensitivity testing (MC&S). Microscopic examination is followed by Gram staining (see Chapter 1). These procedures are often used to make a provisional diagnosis when patients are acutely ill and it is necessary to commence treatment as soon as possible. More precise identification requires culturing (growing) the bacteria in an appropriate medium. If the specimen was obtained from a site where other organisms are present (e.g. skin, faeces), techniques are used to isolate those likely to be causing the infection by using a culture medium that supports particular organisms or suppresses the growth of others.

Biochemical and serological tests may also be necessary to confirm diagnosis. Sensitivity tests are undertaken to determine the most effective antimicrobial.

This is achieved by exposing the organisms to a range of different antimicrobials to determine which inhibit growth.

When examination and testing are complete, a laboratory report is compiled and sent to the clinical team (Figure 4.1). This includes important information about the patient, including their current condition, significant previous history and recent antimicrobial therapy. This is important as it will help the microbiologists select appropriate tests and antimicrobials for sensitivity testing.

Patient name: Violet Dew					
Date of Birth: 28/06/2001			**Hospital number: H123456**		
Patient details including previous antimicrobial therapy: Cloudy, dark offensive urine for 3 days. Catheter in situ 7 days. Antimicrobials: none					
Specimen type: Urine (indwelling urinary catheter) Test ordered: MC&S (microscopy, culture, and sensitivity) Date: 28/12/21					
Organism	**Quantifier**	**Level**	**Coded text**	**Free text**	
E. coli	+++	Authorised			
Enterococcus spp.	+	Authorised			

E. coli - antibiotic	**Result**
Trimethorprin	Sensitive
Ampicillin	Resistant
Nitrofurantoin	Sensitive
Cefpodoxime	Sensitive

Enterococcus spp. - antibiotic	**Result**
Ampicillin	Resistant
Nitrofurantoin	Sensitive

Microscopy:
E. coli: 10^6 cfu/L
Enterococcus spp.: $<10^6$ cfu/L
WBC: 10^7/L
RBC: Not seen
Casts: Not seen

Figure 4.1 A microbiology report.

Table 4.1 Examples of alert organisms.

Bacillus anthracis
Bordetella pertussis
Legionella spp.
Campylobacter spp.
Escherichia coli (toxin-producing strains, e.g. *E. coli* O157)
Meticillin-resistant *Staphylococcus aureus*
Clostridioides difficile

The laboratory report identifies the organisms identified although the amount of detail varies depending on the information required in a particular clinical situation. The laboratory report identifies organisms found and whether or not the organisms are susceptible or resistant to selected antimicrobials.

Laboratory reports carrying urgent findings are flagged for immediate attention. Alert organism reports convey information about the early isolation of new or unusual bacteria to enable the infection prevention team to act quickly to prevent transmission (e.g. arrange patient isolation) (Table 4.1).

Initial Examination

Information about the nature of the infection can be obtained through initial inspection (e.g. odour, appearance). A foul-smelling, purulent specimen suggests the presence of anaerobic bacteria (e.g. *Bacteroides*). Urine or cerebrospinal fluid that looks cloudy is likely to contain large numbers of neutrophils indicative of infection. Mucus or blood in a stool suggests dysentery. Many roundworms and the segments of tapeworms are visible macroscopically (without magnification).

Microscopic Examination

The different microscopic techniques are presented below.

Wet Films

A drop of fluid from the specimen is placed on a microscope slide beneath a cover slip and examined at low power under light microscopy (×400). The following are examined in wet film.

- *Body fluids*: they may contain 'pus' cells (neutrophils) or whole organisms (e.g. *Trichomonas vaginalis* in vaginal discharge).
- *Faeces* may contain ova or the cysts of parasites.
- *Scrapings* from hair, skin or nails may reveal signs of fungal infection.

Dry Films

Dry films give detailed information about the infection. A higher magnification is usually necessary (×1000) and stains are used to aid identification. A thin film obtained from the specimen is placed on a microscope slide, the material is 'fixed' (killed) by passing it through a flame and Gram staining is undertaken. In some laboratories, Gram staining is now automated rather than undertaken by hand. Many other routine laboratory procedures are now automated, improving patient care by increasing the efficiency of microbiological testing, reducing costs and increasing precision.

Special Microscopy Techniques

Special techniques are necessary to identify specific bacteria that do not respond well to Gram's stain.

- The acid-fast (Ziehl–Neelsen [ZN]) technique is used to identify *Mycobacterium* spp. which have thick cell walls impermeable to the dyes used in Gram staining.
- Dark ground microscopy is used to identify spirochaetes which react poorly to traditional stains but are visible at high magnification against a darkened background. Wet films from a recently collected specimen are examined because spirochaetes die rapidly outside the host tissues.

Identifying Bacteria

Many related bacteria appear identical under the microscope. Diagnosis involves growing them in special media and laboratory testing.

Cultures

Broth is a solution of nutrients used grow specific bacteria likely to be present in small numbers in the sample. Solid media are used more often. They are made by mixing nutrients with agar which is poured into petri dishes. The agar solidifies and colonies of the organisms in the sample form over the surface (Figure 4.2). A variety of culture media are used, including peptones, meat and yeast extracts. Blood agar is very commonly used in clinical laboratories.

The concentration of different chemicals added to the medium changes its properties to encourage the growth of a particular organism while suppressing others to help identify the pathogen. For example, MacConkey's medium contains a small amount of lactose and a pH indicator. Bacteria able to grow on MacConkey agar and ferment lactose generate acid which turns the pH indicator red. There is no colour change with species unable to ferment lactose.

(a)

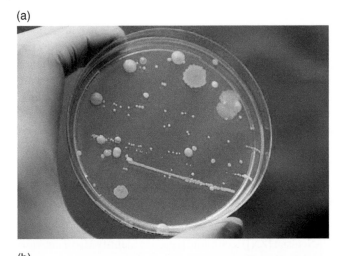

(b)

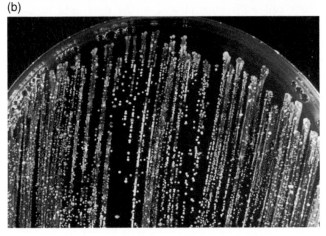

Figure 4.2 (a,b) Culture media and bacterial colonies. *Source:* (a) luchschenF / Adobe Stock.

After the culture medium has been inoculated (Figure 4.3), the specimen is incubated.

Most bacteria able to cause human infection thrive best at 37 °C and give rise to visible colonies on the surface of the agar within 24–48 hours (see Figure 4.3). Cultures are stored and re-examined over several weeks. If the specimen is likely to contain anaerobes (e.g. wound swab), a part of the specimen is cultured in a container free of oxygen (anaerobic jar). *Mycobacterium tuberculosis* grows slowly and is difficult to identify using a culture and difficult to treat as most antimicrobials exert their effects by preventing or reducing growth. Under these

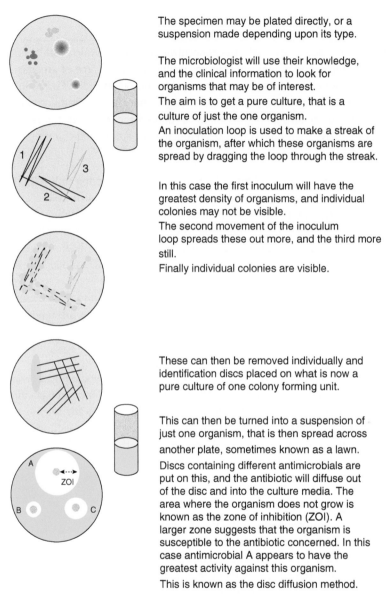

The specimen may be plated directly, or a suspension made depending upon its type.

The microbiologist will use their knowledge, and the clinical information to look for organisms that may be of interest.
The aim is to get a pure culture, that is a culture of just the one organism.
An inoculation loop is used to make a streak of the organism, after which these organisms are spread by dragging the loop through the streak.

In this case the first inoculum will have the greatest density of organisms, and individual colonies may not be visible.
The second movement of the inoculum loop spreads these out more, and the third more still.
Finally individual colonies are visible.

These can then be removed individually and identification discs placed on what is now a pure culture of one colony forming unit.

This can then be turned into a suspension of just one organism, that is then spread across another plate, sometimes known as a lawn.
Discs containing different antimicrobials are put on this, and the antibiotic will diffuse out of the disc and into the culture media. The area where the organism does not grow is known as the zone of inhibition (ZOI). A larger zone suggests that the organism is susceptible to the antibiotic concerned. In this case antimicrobial A appears to have the greatest activity against this organism.
This is known as the disc diffusion method.

Figure 4.3 Technique used to inoculate culture media.

circumstances, molecular methods which do not rely on the ability to grow the organism are preferred.

Colonies become visible over the surface of solid culture media. Each cell divides repeatedly until a clump becomes visible to the naked eye. Each bacterial

---

Box 4.1 Colony-forming Units

A CFU is the unit used to estimate the concentration of viable microbial cells present in a sample. The number of colonies visible on the surface of an agar plate is multiplied by a dilution factor to provide the number of CFU/ml. In theory, one cell could give rise to a colony through binary fission. Traditionally, the number of CFUs on an agar plate used to be counted and recorded manually. This labour-intensive method has now been replaced by automated counting.

---

cell leading to the growth of a colony is known as a colony-forming unit (CFU). All the organisms in the colony are the same type (Box 4.1). The size, colour and shape of a colony depend on the type of bacteria and provide information about the species. *Pseudomonas aeruginosa* produces characteristic green colonies. *Serratia marcescens* gives rise to red colonies. Haemolytic bacteria (e.g. *Streptococcus pyogenes*) release enzymes that destroy erythrocytes in blood agar so each colony becomes surrounded by a clear halo.

One of the challenges associated with this method is isolating individual organisms. Occasionally when microbial growth is excessive, the findings are reported as 'mixed growth'.

Biochemical Tests

The identity of many species of bacteria is confirmed with biochemical tests employing commercially prepared kits. Most detect the presence of specific enzymes by revealing a visible, readily detectable change, usually the release of gas or altered pH, by activating an indicator incorporated into the medium. For example, different species of *Shigella* are differentiated by their ability to ferment carbohydrates to release gas. Biochemical tests do not overcome the need to grow the organism in the laboratory.

Antimicrobial Sensitivity Tests

Appropriate prescribing depends on the use of sensitivity tests to identify which antimicrobial drugs destroy or deactivate the pathogen. The bacteria are inoculated onto solid media, a paper disc impregnated with different antimicrobials is placed over them and the culture is incubated. If the bacteria are sensitive to a particular antimicrobial, the agar remains clear of growth.

Typing Bacteria

Typing is a technique used to enable the infection prevention team to reduce the risks of transmission when clusters of infection occur. If all the cases identified are caused by the same strain, the implication is that the organisms are from a common source. A variety of different typing methods are available. Some employ molecular techniques. Others distinguish between related strains belonging to the same species by establishing their susceptibility to bacteriophages or whether they have identical surface antigens. Phage typing is used to identify different strains of MRSA.

Serological Tests

Serological testing is undertaken with samples of blood and other body fluids to identify the immune response to organisms based on the presence of antibodies. This approach does not usually diagnose a current infection as the antibodies may be present from previous infections and because enough time needs to occur before antibodies are produced in sufficient numbers to be detected. If antigens on the surface of the pathogen and the antibodies belong to the same species, the antibody binds to the antigens, causing visible clumping (agglutination).

Serological tests are particularly useful to identify pathogens that grow slowly and for viruses. The amount and type of antibody present can be used to determine whether a patient is in the acute or convalescent stages of infection or whether they have previously been immunised. High levels of IgM may be indicative of a recent infection because it is the first antibody to be released when the body responds to a pathogen. Findings can be difficult to interpret for patients who are immunocompromised because they do not manufacture antibodies very well. The results of serological testing are usually available within 10–14 days.

Serology is frequently used in epidemiological work (seroprevalence) to identify the number of people in a population who have been infected and numbers still susceptible, especially for infections not usually identified during routine surveillance.

Other Technologies Used in Diagnostics
MALDI-ToF

MALDI-ToF (matrix-assisted laser desorption/ionisation time of flight mass spectrometry) is frequently used to identify bacteria by analysing the chemical compounds they contain and matching them against an existing database of micro-organisms. The chemicals matched include proteins, peptones, sugars and nucleic acids. MALDI-ToF generates results within a few hours, is highly reliable and inexpensive because few consumables are used (Singhal et al. 2015). Drawbacks are that it is unable to distinguish between different antimicrobial strains present in the same specimen.

Molecular Diagnostics

Molecular diagnostics is a rapidly advancing technology used to diagnose and monitor the progress of different types of disease, including infections, cancers and inherited conditions, opening the way for personalised medicine. Tests detect the presence of specific proteins, DNA or RNA in a sample of tissue, blood or another body fluid. Commercial test kits are available to identify a number of infections including *Chlamydia*, HIV, tuberculosis and specific strains of some pathogens including SARS-Cov-2. The organisms do not have to be cultured so the procedure is safe and the results are available quickly.

Electrophoresis

Electrophoresis involves transferring DNA obtained from an organism onto a flat gel surface and splicing it into fragments by an enzyme called *restriction endonuclease*. An electric current is applied, causing the fragments to separate across the surface according to electric change and size. The fragments are stained to aid visualisation. This approach is used to identify different species of bacteria present in chronic wounds and body fluids.

Polymerase Chain Reaction Tests

Polymerase chain reaction tests are molecular tests very widely used in diagnostics to identify specific infections. PCR testing is rapid, highly sensitive, highly specific and inexpensive. The technology works by rapidly 'photocopying' large numbers of copies of the specific sequence of microbial DNA present until very large numbers are available to be detected. Consequently, only a small sample is required. Initial fears that generating multiple copies of the microbial genome might lead to increased risk of infection have not been realised (Wu et al. 2017).

Crucially, PCR identifies a specific gene and is appropriate only when the presence of an organism carrying it is suspected. PCR testing is particularly valuable for organisms such as mycobacteria that grow slowly and for viruses including HIV and norovirus. It is possible to use PCR tests to identify DNA sequences responsible for antimicrobial resistance. PCR testing is reliable and accurate providing staff have received training and that patients obtaining their own specimens have received clear instructions.

Near Patient Testing

Point-of-care (POC) tests are based on PCR tests and are portable, so they can be undertaken at the location where healthcare is delivered (e.g. primary care, outpatient clinics, domiciliary care, accident departments). Patients can perform the test themselves providing clear instructions are given. The results are available rapidly, enabling treatment to begin straight away, and there may be considerable cost savings (Davis et al. 2017). POC tests are particularly useful when dealing with patients who access healthcare sporadically or when patients need the results quickly for some other reason. For example, those with COVID-19 needed to know that they were infected at once to enable them to isolate and inform contacts of their infectious status (Box 4.2). POC testing is cheaper than traditional laboratory testing and the findings can be highly reliable (McIntosh et al. 2018).

Box 4.2   The REACT Study

The Real-time Assessment of Transmission (REACT) study (Imperial College London 2021) investigated how the SARS-CoV-2 virus was spreading across England during the 2020–2021 COVID-19 pandemic. It assessed the sero-prevalence of COVID antibodies in successive random samples of the population invited to undertake self-administered swab tests. The study also analysed the genetic code of a proportion of those testing positive and helped identify the spread of variants of concern.

Whole-genome Sequencing

Epidemiology has been revolutionised by whole-genome sequencing (WGS). Using this technique, it is possible to determine the whole genetic sequence of a micro-organism. WGS is now widely used to identify routes of transmission during outbreaks and is rapidly replacing conventional typing because it is more accurate (Parcell et al. 2021). It has become the standard typing technique for a range of bacteria in reference laboratories including *Escherichia coli*, *Shigella* spp., *Listeria* spp., *Campylobacter* spp., *Staphylococcus aureus* and *Mycobacterium* spp. The technology is portable and was used to sequence the genome of the Ebola virus endemic in West Africa (Quick et al. 2016). In the UK, WGS is used in routine surveillance for *Streptococcus pneumoniae*. Throughout the COVID-19 pandemic, it was used to determine whether infections were hospital or community acquired, set up intrahospital contact tracing and identify cases that might otherwise have been undetected.

Identifying Viruses

Samples intended to identify viruses must transported to the laboratory in media containing antibiotics to inhibit bacterial growth. Four diagnostic approaches are available.

- Culture
- Electron microscopy
- Serological tests
- Molecular approaches

Culturing Viruses

Viruses do not survive outside living tissues. In the laboratory, some but not all can be grown in tissue cultures: sheets of cells suspended on plastic or glass bathed in nutrient media. The presence of a specific virus is indicated by the characteristic way that it changes the shape of the cells.

Electron Microscopy

Viruses subjected to special staining techniques can be identified by their characteristic size and shape under the high magnification of the electron microscope. This method is limited because virus particles are minute and can be overlooked unless they are present in large numbers. A negative result should not be taken as definitive evidence that they are not present.

Serological Tests in Virology

The most commonly used serological test in virology is the enzyme-linked immunosorbent assay (ELISA). It has been used extensively in HIV testing and for hepatitis and Lyme disease. ELISA is used for screening donated blood and tracking outbreaks.

Identifying Fungi

Fungi can be detected in stained films during the routine examination of sputum, swabs and vaginal secretions. Most species grow in the same types of media as those used to culture bacteria.

A few species of fungi grow quickly on agar plates (e.g. *Candida* spp.) but most take much longer to grow. When fungal infection is suspected, special cultures are set up and examined at intervals of 2–3 weeks. A medium containing antibiotics to inhibit bacterial growth, usually Sabouraud glucose agar, is used. Identification is based on the characteristic appearance of the fungus on the surface of the agar and microscopy.

Obtaining Specimens for Microbiological Examination

The success of diagnostic testing depends on good practice when the patient is prepared, when the specimen is obtained and the way it is stored and handled in transit to the laboratory. Clinicians play a key role ensuring that specimens are obtained correctly and reach the laboratory in optimal condition. The procedure used to collect them must protect the health and safety of the patient, the health worker obtaining the specimen and all those handling it. In the UK, Public Health England (now the UK Health Security Agency) provides standards for good practice when obtaining and handling microbiological specimens. All specimens must be transported in the appropriate container placed within a special self-sealing bag with two compartments. One compartment holds the specimen container, the other holds the laboratory request form. Leak-proof boxes should be used during transport.

Effective Technique when Obtaining Specimens

Principles of best practice are shown in Box 4.3.

Box 4.3   Principles of Best Practice when Obtaining Specimens for Microbiological Examination

- Obtain informed consent by explaining the procedure to the patient and secure informed verbal consent.
- Use appropriate personal protective equipment (PPE).
- Employ an effective sampling technique: the specimen must contain micro-organisms from the site being investigated (e.g. saliva must not be obtained as a substitute for sputum).
- Obtain sufficient material for clinical examination (e.g. rectal swabs must not replace a specimen of faeces because there will be insufficient material for culture).
- Use the appropriate specimen container (viruses do not survive in bacterial transport media).
- Label the specimen and request card correctly: particular care is necessary when patients on the same ward have similar names. Use unique identification, for example, bar code or hospital number.
- Provide adequate data on the request form: clinical signs and details of antimicrobial therapy.
- Ensure that the specimen reaches the laboratory as soon as possible, at the correct temperature. Wherever possible, specimens should be obtained immediately before collection. If necessary, the specimen can be stored until collection in a refrigerator at 4 °C. Stool specimens obtained to detect the presence of parasites and vaginal swabs obtained when *Trichomonas vaginalis* infestation is suspected should not be refrigerated because the low temperature makes the organisms sluggish and harder to detect.
- Record the time, date and nature of specimen obtained in the patient's notes.
- Advice for dealing with spillages is provided by the Health and Safety Executive.

Source: Adapted from Health and Safety Executive (2003).

Types of Specimens

Urine Specimens

Urine specimens should as free of contamination as possible. In health, urine is sterile but is easily contaminated when the specimen is obtained by contact with the perineum or the hands. Gram-negative bacteria contaminating a specimen multiply rapidly, especially if it is stored without refrigeration, leading to a false-positive result or a result that is difficult to interpret.

Collecting a 5–10 ml midstream urine specimen reduces the risk of error. Uncircumcised males should be requested or helped to withdraw the foreskin. The urethral meatus is cleansed with soap and water and the middle portion of the flow is collected in a sterile receptacle. Collecting an uncontaminated urine specimen from females is not straightforward, especially if the patient is bed-bound or too disorientated to co-operate. The patient should pass urine with the labia separated, catching the middle part of the stream in a sterile container.

For patients who are catheterised, a syringe is used to aspirate freshly passed urine from the sampling port on the drainage bag tubing, adopting aseptic technique. The drainage apparatus and catheter should never be disconnected to obtain a specimen because of the risk of introducing infection. Urine from the drainage bag will not give satisfactory results because it will be contaminated from environmental sources.

Obtaining uncontaminated urine specimens from infants is challenging. The baby may be held over a sterile container to obtain a 'clean catch' specimen. The least satisfactory method is a bagged' sample in which a plastic bag is applied to the perineum. In an emergency a specimen can be obtained by suprapubic bladder aspiration.

All urine specimens should be examined within three hours of collection, before any contaminating bacteria not responsible for the infection have had time to multiply to avoid distorting the results.

In the laboratory, the specimen is inoculated onto nutrient agar and placed in an incubator overnight. The colonies are counted and the number of bacteria present in 1 ml of the urine is calculated the next day. Counts of 10^5 or more organisms per ml indicate the presence of infection, especially if neutrophils are present. A lower bacterial count suggests contamination rather than infection.

Wound Specimens

Wound infection is usually suspected if the signs of clinical infection are apparent: inflammation, pyrexia and purulent exudate. Skin is colonised by large numbers of potentially pathogenic organisms and chronic wounds (e.g. pressure ulcers, leg ulcers) are likely to be very heavily colonised, so interpreting the findings of microbiological investigation is not straightforward and specimens should only be obtained if there is good reason to suspect that infection is present. Swabs taken from the surface of the wound are likely to yield poor results if stored too long before reaching the laboratory as they will dry out and the bacteria will no longer be viable. Wound swabs are usually supplied with special transport media to prevent drying out.

If possible, pus should be aspirated from the wound or it might be possible to obtain a small piece of excised tissue. If swabbing is the only practical method, two or three specimens are better than one; the first can be stained for microscopy and the others used to inoculate the culture medium. Two agar plates are inoculated – one to grow aerobes, the other to grow anaerobes.

Stool Specimens

Stool specimens are obtained to identify enteric bacteria and viruses and to iden-tify parasites. Protozoa and the eggs of parasitic worms are microscopic but the adult forms of many worms are visible to the naked eye. If their presence is sus-pected, the specimen should be examined as soon as possible; the ova of parasites survive desiccation and cold, but worms and protozoa become sluggish on cooling and are more difficult to detect. Rectal swabs should not be sent to the laboratory instead of stool specimens because there is insufficient material for culture. Stools contain millions of bacteria and interpreting the results can be very difficult. Another limitation is that food-borne disease caused by toxins cannot be detected by examining faeces. If *Clostridioides difficile* is suspected, a special test to identify the toxin responsible is performed.

Sputum Specimens

The lower airways and their secretions are free of micro-organisms in health. The oral and nasal cavities are heavily colonised by micro-organisms able to cause infection if they reach the lower airways. Consequently, diagnosing pneumonia is not straightforward and is based on a combination of clinical examination, x-ray findings and microscopy and culture of the sputum. Specimens should contain material recently discharged from the bronchial tree and sent to the laboratory as quickly as possible to avoid overgrowth by Gram-negative contaminants. At least 5–10 ml are required for microscopy and culture and this may be difficult if patients are unable to expectorate. It may be necessary to enlist the help of the physiotherapist. Early-morning collection is best because secretions pool in the respiratory tract when the patient is supine and are likely to contain larger num-bers of micro-organisms. In the intensive care unit, sputum specimens can be obtained by tracheobronchial suction or bronchoalveolar lavage (washing a seg-ment of the lung with sterile saline via a bronchoscope).

Throat Swabs

The tongue is depressed with a wooden spatula and the tip is passed over the tonsils, the posterior pharyngeal wall and any other areas that appear inflamed or where exudate is visible (Figure 4.4). A good source of illumination is required to avoid contaminating the swab by contact with the oral mucosa. Patients usually find this procedure unpleasant and should be warned in advance about the gag reflex. Children may be more co-operative if parental assistance is enlisted.

Nasal Swabs

Nasal swabs are taken with the patient's head tilted, rotating the swab to ensure that as much secretion as possible is obtained. For infants and very young

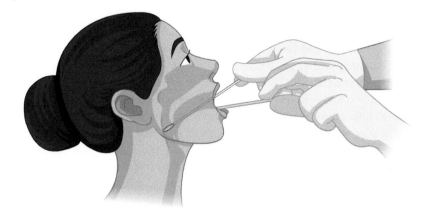

Figure 4.4 Obtaining a throat swab.

children, a fine wire swab-holder can be used instead of a wooden swab-stick. Care is necessary to avoid damaging the delicate epithelium. When healthy people are screened to exclude staphylococcal carriage, the tip of the swab is moistened with sterile water because the nasal mucosae are usually dry in healthy people.

Pernasal Swabs
Pernasal swabs are used to confirm a presumptive diagnosis of pertussis (whooping cough). *Bordetella pertussis* is most readily recovered from the posterior nasopharynx, especially if the specimen is obtained immediately after coughing. The tip of the swab is connected to a fine, flexible wire so that it can be introduced without contamination (Figure 4.5).

Eye Swabs
Eye swabs tend give poor results because lysozyme (enzyme in tears) destroys bacteria. It is possible to obtain scrapings from the conjunctivae with a plastic loop to test for chlamydial infection. Special training is required.

Blood Cultures
Blood cultures should be obtained from peripheral lines unless a central line is suspected as the source of infection. Strict aseptic technique must be adopted to avoid contamination from the skin of the patient or clinician. Two bottles containing broth are inoculated – one for aerobic bacteria, the other for anaerobes. It is advisable to obtain more than one set of specimens to maximise the chance of identifying the cause of infection because the number of organisms circulating in the bloodstream is likely to be small (less than 1000 per ml). Patients likely to have

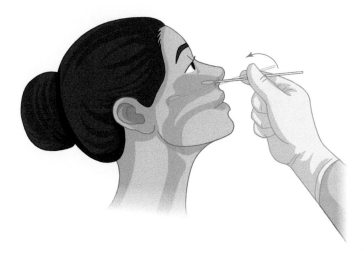

Figure 4.5 Obtaining a pernasal swab.

bloodsteam infections are critically ill, so the specimens must be dispatched at once. Laboratories provide an incubator to receive blood cultures outside usual working hours.

Blood cultures are incubated for at least seven days and monitored for signs of growth every day. Microscopy and Gram staining are undertaken as soon as growth appears to ensure that the patient is receiving appropriate antimicrobials.

Specimens of Cerebrospinal Fluid

Cerebrospinal fluid (CSF) is obtained when meningitis is suspected. It is obtained by spinal tap using strict aseptic technique to avoid contamination and transported to the laboratory at once because the patient is likely to be very ill and also to optimise the survival of meningococci which do not remain viable outside the tissues for long.

Vaginal and Cervical Swabs

Most pathogens recoverable from the female genital tract survive poorly in the environment and contamination is less problematic than with other specimens. Special transport media (Stuart's or Amies' medium) are used. Storage at room temperature enables the laboratory staff to identify *Trichomonas vaginalis* as it is highly motile at this temperature, aiding detection. *Neisseria gonorrhoeae* survives poorly outside the tissues. Diagnosis is easier if specimens are examined as soon as they have been obtained. Most genitourinary medicine (GUM) clinics have satellite laboratories where specimens are examined as soon as they have been obtained.

Environmental Sampling

Environmental sampling is only undertaken under specific circumstances (e.g. to identify possible reservoirs of infection when an outbreak occurs). Routine sampling is pointless as the environment is contaminated with large numbers of organisms that are mostly harmless.

Safe Transport of Specimens

It is essential to prevent leakage during transit. Procedures that comply with health and safety legislation are necessary to protect all staff (Box 4.4).

Box 4.4 Transporting Specimens Safely

Specimens must be transported in leak-proof boxes with the request card carried separately from the specimen container in a special pocket. The outside of the container must be free of contamination with blood or any other body fluid and must not be overfilled otherwise fermentation may occur, especially with faeces, leading to the accumulation of gas and a build-up of pressure that could dislodge a tightly fitting lid. Staff handling specimens need to be aware of the hazards attached to spillage, wear overalls and undertake hand hygiene before and afterwards.

All specimens contain potentially infectious material and present a hazard during transport. To reduce the risks to handlers, the use of leak-proof boxes and agreed protocols for dealing with spillages is recommended (Health and Safety Executive n.d.; World Health Organization 2021b). Biohazard labels are used to indicate to handlers and laboratory staff that a specimen may contain particularly hazardous pathogens (e.g. viruses responsible for haemorrhagic fevers, blood-borne viruses).

Because much of the testing for Covid-19 has been carried out in homes and non-healthcare locations, a significant number of tests have been returned by the postal system. The same principles of packaging apply; that is, there should be three layers:

1) primary packaging – sealed plastic bag
2) secondary packaging – sealed plastic bag
3) outer packaging – cardboard box suitably closed which must have a minimum dimension of 100 mm × 100 mm).

Source: Adapted from Department for Transport (2020).

Interpreting Laboratory Results

The results of microbiological findings must be combined with clinical interpretation. The ability of the laboratory staff to provide useful therapeutic information depends on the clinical details provided on the request form. It is particularly important to include details of any recent antimicrobial treatment the patient may have received as this will increase the risk of antimicrobial resistance. Some of the organisms isolated might be contaminants or part of the normal flora from a site where they do not cause infection. Diagnosis should also take into consideration the signs and symptoms of infection. For example, *Staphylococcus epidermidis* identified in a blood culture would probably be a contaminant in an apyrexial patient.

Quality Control and Quality Assurance in the Microbiology Laboratory

Quality control is essential to ensure the precision and accuracy of microbiology laboratory reporting and prevent error. Quality assurance in microbiology laboratories comprises all the processes used to ensure that the quality of laboratory procedures is guaranteed and that it is possible to verify the results of testing (e.g. culture media must be tested for sterility and performance).

Standards for Microbiology Investigations (SIMs) indicate when microbiological investigations should take place and outline the laboratory methods that underpin quality assurance. In the UK, SIMs are drawn up by consultation between clinicians with input from professional organisations and patients. SIMs documentation consists of algorithms and procedures covering all stages of microbiological testing from specimen collection to laboratory analysis and reporting to standardise diagnostic processes between different laboratories. Across Europe, the European Committee on Antimicrobial Susceptibility Testing (EUCAST) standardises and works towards a pan-European and international consensus and harmonisation of technical matters regarding antimicrobial susceptibility testing (The European Committee on Antimicrobial Susceptibility Testing - EUCAST 2021).

Suggested Activities

Exercise 4.1 Self-assessment

1   The main functions of the medical microbiology department are to:
    A   Diagnose infections
    B   Investigate clusters of infection
    C   Undertake routine surveillance

D Identify antimicrobial-resistant organisms

E All the above.

2 Phenotypic tests involve microscopy, culture and sensitivity testing. True/False

3 List five micro-organisms that would be considered 'alert organisms' in the clinical setting where you work.

4 All the bacterial cells in the same CFU originate from the same original bacterial cell. True/False

5 Complete the following sentence: 'Point of care testing improves the patient experience because . . .'

6 Which of the following are free of micro-organisms in health? Blood, sputum, lower airways, urine, upper airways, urinary drainage bags, large bowel, cerebrospinal fluid.

7 Is it good practice to monitor the clinical environment routinely for microbial contamination? Explain your answer.

8 Look at the laboratory report illustrated in Figure 4.1. Does the patient have a urinary infection? Why do you think this?

9 Describe good practice when obtaining a wound specimen.

10 Which of the following should *not* be placed in ward specimen refrigerators: urine; stool specimens; sputum; vaginal swabs; blood specimens; cerebrospinal fluid? Explain why.

Exercise 4.2

Review specimen taking and storage in your clinical setting. What types of specimens are most commonly obtained? Can you identify any ways of improving practice based on what you have read in this chapter?

Exercise 4.3

Look at a laboratory report recently returned to your clinical setting and interpret the findings. Would you rate the amount and quality of the information provided for laboratory staff as good, adequate or poor? Based on your knowledge of the patient, what additional information might have been provided?

References

Davis, S., Allen, A.J., O'Leary, R. et al. (2017). Diagnostic accuracy and cost analysis of the Alere™ i influenza A&B near-patient test using throat swabs. *J. Hosp. Infect.* 97: 301–309. https://doi.org/10.1016/j.jhin.2017.05.017.

Department for Transport (2020). Packaging and transport requirements for patient samples – UN3373. www.gov.uk/government/publications/packaging-and-transport-requirements-for-patient-samples-un3373/packaging-and-transport-requirements-for-patient-samples-un3373

Health and Safety Executive (2003). *Safe Working and the Prevention of Infection in Clinical Laboratories and Similar Facilities.* Sudbury: HSE Books.

Health and Safety Executive (n.d.) Transportation of infectious substances – blood-borne viruses (BBV). www.hse.gov.uk/biosafety/blood-borne-viruses/transportation-of-infectious-substances.htm

Imperial College London (2021). Real-time Assessment of Community Transmission findings. www.imperial.ac.uk/medicine/research-and-impact/groups/react-study/real-time-assessment-of-community-transmission-findings

McIntosh, B.W., Vasek, J., Taylor, M. et al. (2018). Accuracy of bedside point of care testing in critical emergency department patients. *Am. J. Emerg. Med.* 36: 567–570. https://doi.org/10.1016/j.ajem.2017.09.018.

Parcell, B.J., Gillespie, S.H., Pettigrew, K.A., and Holden, M.T.G. (2021). Clinical perspectives in integrating whole-genome sequencing into the investigation of healthcare and public health outbreaks – hype or help? *J. Hosp. Infect.* 109: 1–9. https://doi.org/10.1016/j.jhin.2020.11.001.

Quick, J., Loman, N.J., Duraffour, S. et al. (2016). Real-time, portable genome sequencing for Ebola surveillance. *Nature* 530: 228–232. https://doi.org/10.1038/nature16996.

Singhal, N., Kumar, M., Kanaujia, P.K., and Virdi, J.S. (2015). MALDI-TOF mass spectrometry: an emerging technology for microbial identification and diagnosis. *Front. Microbiol.* 6: 791. https://doi.org/10.3389/fmicb.2015.00791.

The European Committee on Antimicrobial Susceptibility Testing – EUCAST 2021. www.eucast.org

World Health Organization (2021a). Consolidated guidelines on HIV prevention, testing, treatment, service delivery and monitoring: recommendations for a public health approach. www.who.int/publications-detail-redirect/9789240031593

World Health Organization (2021b). Guidance on regulations for the transport of infectious substances 2021–2022. www.who.int/publications-detail-redirect/9789240019720

Wu, P.J., Jeyaratnam, D., Tosas, O. et al. (2017). Point-of-care universal screening for meticillin-resistant *Staphylococcus aureus*: a cluster-randomized cross-over trial. *J. Hosp. Infect.* 95: 245–252. https://doi.org/10.1016/j.jhin.2016.08.017.

5

Antimicrobial Drugs

Principles of Antimicrobial Activity – Selective Toxicity

The treatment of infection with antimicrobial drugs is based largely on the concept of selective toxicity; that is, treatments that damage or inhibit the micro-organism without damaging the host. This is sometimes referred to as the 'magic bullet' (a term popularised by the physician Paul Ehrlich), and is a feature shared with oncology where the aim is to do the same with malignant cells (Strebhardt and Ullrich 2008). There are some antimicrobials which have very poor selective toxicity which are actually used in the treatment of cancer; these are referred to as the antitumour antibiotics.

Because of the evolutionary relationship between humans and different types of micro-organism, some types of infection are inherently more difficult to treat than others. Those organisms which are more closely related to humans having fewer differences and so selective targets than those which are less distantly related. This is further complicated by illness, exposure to healthcare-associated organisms and the effect of treatments, all of which add to the complexity of treating infectious diseases. Additionally, the use of antimicrobial agents themselves has an effect on the microbiome of the person and the environment, and increases the risk of antimicrobial resistance.

You might note the use of the term *antimicrobial* rather than the more common *antibiotic*. That is because, strictly speaking, the term *antibiotic* only applies to substances produced by living organisms whereas the term *antimicrobial* covers both natural and purely synthetic products. Some antibiotics are somewhere in between, being semi-synthetic. These are usually natural products that are optimised in some way.

All life on earth can be categorised into one of two broad groups, prokaryotes and eukaryotes, depending upon whether they have a nucleus – prokaryotes being non-nucleated and eukaryotes having a nucleus. There are four main categories of micro-organism that are treated with antimicrobials.

Infection Prevention and Control in Healthcare Settings,
First Edition. Edward Purssell and Dinah Gould.
© 2023 John Wiley & Sons Ltd. Published 2023 by John Wiley & Sons Ltd.

- Bacteria
- Viruses
- Fungi
- Protozoa

Bacteria and another group of micro-organisms known as the archaebacteria are prokaryotes and only distantly related to humans, while fungi and protozoa are eukaryotes and much more closely related. As far as we are aware there are no medically significant archaebacteria, although this is an area of much research. Viruses are something else altogether, not really being directly related to humans at all.

The ability to damage, inhibit or kill the micro-organism without damaging the host requires that there be a structure or some kind of process in the micro-organism that is either missing or different from that in the host. If one looks at the evolutionary relationship of humans and these major groups of micro-organisms, one can see that the relationship between humans and bacteria is a very distant one. This means that there has been a lot of time for us to evolve to be different, hence there are a lot of selective targets and a relatively large number of drugs. Fungi and protozoa, on the other hand, are more closely related to humans, and so are biologically more similar and consequently there are fewer antifungal and antiprotozoal drugs.

Viruses are a special case, because by most definitions of 'life', they are not living organisms but instead are what are called 'obligate intracellular parasites'. This means that they cannot replicate on their own but need to use the replicative processes of the cells that they infect. This causes a particular problem for their treatment, because in order to stop a virus replicating, you will usually need to stop the cells in which they are residing from replicating or to damage it in some way. This may be satisfactory if infected cells can be specifically targeted leaving non-infected cells alone, but if not, then this might cause significant damage, depending upon the cell population concerned. This accounts for the relatively small number of antiviral drugs. Fortunately, in most cases the immune system is able to prevent serious viral infections.

Antibacterial Drugs

Bacteria are sometimes referred to as eubacteria ('eu' being Greek for 'true') to separate them from the archaebacteria which are very different. Because the relationship between humans and bacteria is a very distant one, there has been a lot of time for humans and bacteria to evolve to be different, hence there are a large number of antibacterial drugs which take advantage of the many differences between bacterial and human cells. These are shown in Table 5.1

There are many ways of identifying and classifying bacteria. The most basic is through staining and microscopy. This is useful because it helps with

Table 5.1 The main antibacterial targets.

General target action	Selectivity of target	Drug groups
Inhibition of bacterial cell wall synthesis	Human cells do not have a cell wall. The bacterial cell wall is made of a substance not produced by humans known as peptidoglycan	*Bind to penicillin-binding proteins (which build the cell wall):* β-lactams (penicillins, cephalosporins, monobactams, carbapenems) *Bind to peptidoglycan (the actual cell wall units):* Glycopeptides
Inhibition of protein synthesis	Bacterial ribosomes are a different size from human ribosomes. Humans have 80S ribosomes – small (40S) and large (60S) subunit; bacteria have 70S – small (30S) and large (50S)	*Bind to 30S subunit of the bacterial ribosome:* Aminoglycosides, tetracyclines *Bind to 50S subunit of the bacterial ribosome:* Macrolides, lincosamides, chloramphenicol, oxazolidinones, streptogramins
Disruption of membranes	Binds to Gram-negative lipopolysaccharide and bacterial membranes, but can also bind to human membranes, a possible cause of toxicity	Polymyxin B, colistin, daptomycin
Inhibition of nucleic acid synthesis	Preferentially binds to prokaryotic RNA polymerase over human enzymes	Rifamycins
	Inhibits type II topoisomerases, DNA gyrase and topoisomerase IV, these enzymes are thought to be different from those in humans	Fluoroquinolones
	Disrupts the DNA of microbial cells, inactive until modified, an action that only happens in anaerobic bacteria and protozoa	Metronidazole
Inhibition of folic acid synthesis (antimetabolites)	Bacteria synthesise folic acid, humans get folic acid from the diet	Sulfonamides, trimethoprim

identification but also sometimes suggests treatment. For example, those bacteria which do not retain Gram stain ('Gram negatives') have an outer membrane which prevents large molecules such as glycopeptides from reaching their target.

Not all antibacterial antimicrobials can be used to treat all bacteria. It is important for the clinician to understand which drug can be used to treat a specific infection caused by a particular bacterium in the specific context of the patient. For example, treating an infection in a skin wound is different from treating an infection with the same organism in an implantable device. Furthermore, because of the differences between the conditions in the body and those in the laboratory, it is not always possible to predict from laboratory reports how easy a given infection will be to treat.

Antiviral Drugs

Because viruses use host cells to replicate, it is difficult to develop drugs that target viruses alone, or virally infected cells, without damaging adjacent or similar healthy cells. Probably the most widely used antiviral drug is aciclovir. This acts as a guanosine analogue but, unlike guanosine, when incorporated into the new viral DNA, it prevents the next nucleoside being added. Its selective action comes from it being taken in an inactive form, and it is activated only by viral thymidine kinase enzymes and not their human equivalents, so it remains inactive in uninfected cells. It has activity against viruses that can activate it in this way, notably herpes simplex virus (HSV) types 1 and 2, and varicella zoster virus. Another virus for which effective treatment exists is influenza. The main drugs for this are the neuraminidase inhibitors oseltamivir and zanamivir, which inhibit the neuraminidase enzyme found on the viral surface and which allows the release of virus from infected cells and movement within the respiratory tract.

The virus which has the greatest number of drugs to treat it is HIV. This is partly due to the large amount of research into anti-HIV drugs and partly to some unique properties of HIV, particularly the presence of the viral enzymes reverse transcriptase, protease and integrase. These are either missing, or sufficiently different to human equivalents to make them selective targets. The main targets in HIV are shown in Table 5.2. Successful treatment of HIV normally requires at least three drugs from two classes, to reduce the risk of resistance developing. There is extensive guidance available from both national/international organisations, and the World Health Organization Consolidated Guidance on all aspects of the treatment of HIV (World Health Organization 2021a).

Antifungal Drugs

There are fewer selective targets in fungi than bacteria, reflecting the similarity of fungi to humans. Furthermore, serious fungal infections are rare, and often associated with underlying conditions that make treatment more difficult. Some fungi,

Table 5.2 The main anti-HIV targets.

Class of drug	Action	Examples
Nucleoside reverse transcriptase inhibitors	Inhibit viral reverse transcriptase which is not present in uninfected cells	Zidovudine, didanosine, zalcitabine, stavudine, abacavir, Truvada[*] (emtricitabine and tenofovir)
Non-nucleoside reverse transcriptase inhibitors		Efavirenz, nevirapine, delavirdine, etravirine, rilpivirine, doravirine
Protease inhibitors	Inhibit viral protease enzymes	Saquinavir, indinavir, ritonavir, nelfinavir, amprenavir, fosamprenavir
Integrase inhibitors	Inhibit viral integrase enzymes	Raltegravir, dolutegravir
Fusion inhibitors	Bind to the viral glycoprotein 41 (gp41) blocking 2nd step in the fusion pathway	Enfuvirtide

particularly those that grow as finger-like projections known as hyphae, such as *Aspergillus* spp., can also grow very quickly and be very invasive as a result of this method of growth. Antifungal prophylaxis is used to reduce the risk of fungal infections in some conditions, for example those resulting in immune suppression. Fluconazole is an example of a drug that is used in this way (Maertens et al. 2018).

The traditional mainstay of the antifungal drug group has been amphotericin, a very good antifungal but associated with significant side-effects. The main antifungal drug targets are shown in Table 5.3.

Table 5.3 The main antifungal targets.

General target action	Selectivity of target	Drug groups
Inhibition of ergosterol synthesis in cell membrane	Human cells contain cholesterol rather than ergosterol	*Inhibit conversion of lanosterol to ergosterol:* Azoles *Bind to ergosterol:* Polyenes
Block cell wall synthesis	Human cells do not have a cell wall	*Inhibit synthesis of β-1,3 glucans:* Echinocandins *Inhibit chitin synthesis:* Nikkomycin, polyoxins

Source: Scorzoni et al. (2017).

Antiprotozoal Drugs

The number of effective treatments for protozoal infections is much lower than those for bacterial infections. In part, this is due to the complex life cycles of many protozoans, and host–parasite–drug interactions, but it may also be at least partly due to the economics of producing these drugs which are most needed in relatively poor parts of the world (Khaw and Panosian 1995).

The Spectrum of Antimicrobials

This refers to the range of organisms that a particular therapeutic approach targets. Broad-spectrum drugs will treat a wide range of organisms, while narrow-spectrum drugs will treat fewer. Broad-spectrum treatment may be the result of using broad-spectrum antimicrobials, such as the carbapenems, or a combination of drugs. Although the use of broad-spectrum antimicrobials sounds like an attractive general strategy, it may be associated with the development of antimicrobial resistance as a result of their effects on other organisms in the microbiotica. One area where broad-spectrum antimicrobial therapy is warranted is infection in those who are severely immune suppressed.

Some drugs act in *synergy* with each other; that is, they have an additional additive effect from being given together. An example of this is ampicillin and gentamicin, in which the ampicillin damages the cell wall and the gentamicin then works inside the cell (Winstanley and Hastings 1990). Others come as combinations such as co-trimoxazole, a mixture of trimethoprim andsulfamethoxazole which work synergistically, or piperacillin/tazobactam, which is a mixture of the active drug piperacillin and the β-lactamase inhibitor tazobactam.

Targeted Versus Empiric Therapy

Empiric therapy is that based on experience rather than test results. In general, it is better to find out what is causing the infection before starting treatment, but this is not always possible, for example in the immune suppressed where treatment needs to begin immediately. Therefore, clinical experience is used to decide the likely organisms and treatments required. This often includes broad-spectrum antimicrobials, for example a broad-spectrum antibacterial with an antifungal.

Antimicrobial Resistance

Antimicrobial resistance refers to the capacity of micro-organisms to withstand the effects of antimicrobials or biocides that are intended to kill or inhibit them. There are two types of resistance.

- *Inherent resistance* – this is where the micro-organism is, and always has been, resistant to a particular antimicrobial. For example, Gram-negative bacteria are, and always have been, resistant to glycopeptide drugs such as vancomycin. This is due to the presence of an outer membrane that blocks access of the drug to the target in the cell wall. This type of resistance needs to be understood, but is not of great concern.
- *Acquired resistance* – this is where the micro-organism develops resistance, and so goes from being susceptible to being resistant. This type of resistance is of great concern, and is also an inevitable consequence of drug use.

Antimicrobial resistance has been identified by the World Health Organization as threatening 'the very core of modern medicine and the sustainability of an effective, global public health response to the enduring threat from infectious diseases' (World Health Organization 2015, p. 11). The development of resistance is an inevitable result of drug use. Antimicrobials are said to produce selective pressure; this means that using them kills susceptible organisms, leaving more resistant ones to grow. Thus, the resistant organisms are 'selected' and replace susceptible ones. In order for natural selection to operate in this way, there are three criteria that have to be met: there has to be variation in susceptibility to the drugs (some have to be more resistant); the resulting traits have to be heritable, or passed on to subsequent generations; and there has to be some advantage in the new state, sometimes referred to as *fitness*. Antimicrobial resistance usually meets these criteria, but not always. Sometimes resistant organisms grow less well when the antimicrobial is removed.

Variation in micro-organisms can be the result of mutation, remembering that many replicate very quickly. Even though mutation is rare, if you have very large number of organisms the actual number of mutations may be quite high. Another source of resistance genes is from producing organisms themselves. For example, a bacterium that produces an antibiotic against other bacteria must itself have resistance to that antibiotic, otherwise it will kill itself.

Microbial Genetics

There are three broad ways in which organisms reproduce their genome: asexual, sexual and limited sexual reproduction. Sexual reproduction is advantageous because it generates diversity, leading to the maintenance of beneficial mutations and the loss of deleterious mutations through natural selection. Asexual reproduction, or clonal reproduction, leads to cells that are essentially identical. Although bacteria are generally clonal in this way, as described in the next section, there are methods by which bacteria can gain genes. Many fungi reproduce through a mixture of both, normally asexual, leading to identical clones, but with occasional sexual reproduction.

The term *vertical gene transfer* refers to the transfer of genes from parent to child, while *horizontal gene transfer* is the acquisition of genes from a non-parent. There are a variety of ways in which bacteria can transfer genes horizontally (Heitman 2006).

Natural Transformation

Some bacteria are able to take up extracellular DNA from the environment. DNA is constantly being released into the environment from decomposing or disrupted cells, viral particles or through excretion from living cells. Some bacteria, known as *competent* bacteria, are able to take this up from the environment and either establish it as a plasmid or, more commonly, integrate it into the bacterial genome (Thomas and Nielsen 2005).

Conjugative Transfer

This occurs when two bacteria form a close physical relationship, leading to cell-to-cell junctions and development of a pore between the two cells which allows DNA to pass from one to the other. The most common genetic structures associated with this are plasmids, which are extrachromosomal DNA molecules. They normally contain genes that are stable, the plasmids themselves are self-replicating, and the genes that they express provide functions that are beneficial but not essential for cellular functioning (Frost et al. 2005).

Transduction

DNA transfer from one cell to another occurs as a result of infection with viruses that infect and replicate only in bacterial cells, known as *bacteriophages*. When infecting one cell, they inadvertently package cellular genes into their capsid, which they then pass on when infecting the next cell. If this recombines with the cellular chromosome, it can then be passed on to future generations (Frost et al. 2005).

Transposable elements

These are sequences of DNA sequences that are able to change their position within the genome, for example by moving from the chromosome to a plasmid. Once on a plasmid, they can then be spread horizontally to other bacteria. For example, the transposon Tn*1546*, which contains a cluster of genes known as *vanA* which confers vancomycin resistance in enterococci, is inherited clonally but also transferred horizontally (Gardete and Tomasz 2014), and has been found to be contained in plasmids in isolates of vancomycin-resistant *Staphylococcus aureus* (Sievert et al. 2008).

Methods of Resistance

Mechanism	Example
Destruction of the antibiotic molecule	β-lactamases that degrade β-lactam antibiotics such as penicillin
Chemical alterations of the antibiotic	Aminoglycoside-modifying enzymes that alter the drug
Decreased permeability	*Pseudomonas aeruginosa* has an outer membrane with low permeability for most drugs
Efflux	Mechanisms that 'pump' the drug out before it reaches toxic levels, sometimes referred to as efflux pumps
Target protection	*TetM* found in some bacteria dislodges tetracycline from its target in the ribosome
Target modification – mutations of the target site	Rifampin resistance may be due to point mutations in RNA polymerase gene
Target modification – enzymatic alteration of the target site	Macrolide resistance may be due to enzymatic modification resulting in methylation of the ribosome
Target modification – complete replacement or bypass of the target site	MRSA produces penicillin-binding proteins that do not bind β-lactams so well; vancomycin resistance is sometimes due to an alteration in the cell wall units so that they bind less well

Source: Munita and Arias (2016).

Measuring Resistance

The ability to treat bacterial infections with antimicrobials is assessed by susceptibility testing. This uses different combinations of antimicrobial and bacteria, and is based on the minimum inhibitory concentration (MIC), defined as 'the lowest concentration of an antibiotic required to inhibit the growth of an organism' (British Society for Antimicrobial Chemotherapy 2013; http://bsacsurv.org/science/mics). The MIC is compared to breakpoints, which are standardised concentrations of an antimicrobial which defines whether a particular species of bacteria is susceptible or resistant to that antimicrobial. These are provided in tables which give breakpoints for different antimicrobial and organism pairs. They are either given in mg/l. where direct concentrations are used, or a zone of inhibition (ZoI) in mm if the disc diffusion method is used.

Examples of these for *Staphylococcus aureus* are given in Table 5.4. This shows that for clindamycin, an MIC of equal to or less than 0.25 mg/l or a ZoI of equal to or larger than 26 mm suggests susceptibility while over 0.5 mg/l or less than 22 mm indicates resistance. For vancomycin there is no ZoI, and there are different MICs for *S. aureus* and coagulase-negative staphylococci such as *Staphylococcus epidermis*.

Table 5.4 Breakpoints for staphylococci and various drugs used to treat them.

Antibiotic	MIC breakpoint (mg/l)			Interpretation of zone diameters (mm)		
	R>	I	S<=	R = <	I	S >=
Clindamycin	0.5	0.5	0.25	22	23–25	26
Erythromycin	2	2	1	16	17–19	20
Vancomycin						
S. aureus	2		2			
Coagulase-negative staphylococci	4		4			

One important issue to note with regard to this is that laboratory conditions differ markedly to those at the site of infection. These tests are done on cultures of individual organisms which are exposed directly to the antimicrobial. A therapeutic concentration at the site of infection may be more difficult to achieve. For example, if there is necrotic tissue or pus it may be hard for the drug to reach the site of infection. For some drugs, notably aminoglycosides and glycopeptides, therapeutic drug monitoring is recommended (Abdul-Aziz et al. 2020). This is usually because the therapeutic range and the level at which toxicity can occur are quite close. It is important therefore to differentiate the *dose*, which is the amount of antimicrobial given to the patient, from the *exposure*, which includes the dose, mode of administration and the pharmacokinetics and pharmacokinetics at the site of infection (The European Committee on Antimicrobial Susceptibility Testing n.d.), as these may be very different. This is particularly so if the infection is in an area where there is pus, necrotic tissue or an implanted device, as the blood supply is likely to be poor.

World Health Organization Plan for the Prevention and Control of Antimicrobial Resistance

The WHO has developed a comprehensive plan for reducing the spread of antimicrobial resistance (World Health Organization n.d.). A key part of this plan is adopting a 'One Health' approach of integrating human, animal and environmental health, and encouraging the involvement of patients, the wider public, industry and policy makers. Key recommendations are as follows.

For Healthcare Professionals
- Prevent infections in the first place by ensuring hands, instruments and environment are clean.

- Only prescribe and dispense antibiotics when they are needed, according to current guidelines.
- Report antibiotic-resistant infections to the appropriate surveillance teams.
- Educate patients about how to take antibiotics correctly, antibiotic resistance and the dangers of misuse.
- Talk to patients about how they can prevent infections (for example, vaccination, hand washing, safer sex, and covering nose and mouth when sneezing).

For Industry

Invest in research and development of new antibiotics, vaccines, diagnostics and other tools. Antimicrobial research is expensive and, compared to many other drugs, provides a limited return for investors.

For Policy-makers

- Ensure that a robust national action plan to tackle antibiotic resistance is in place. This needs to address the specific needs of the country and the health service in each country.
- Improve surveillance of antibiotic-resistant infections.
- Strengthen policies, programmes and implementation of infection prevention and control measures.
- Regulate and promote the appropriate use and disposal of quality medicines.
- Make information available on the impact of antibiotic resistance.

There are similar recommendations for the public and animal health.

Damage to Host and Environmental Microbiome

In some parts of the body, particularly the large intestines, the established bacterial poplulations not only exclude other organisms but produce inhibitory substances, further preventing their growth. Antimicrobials can also select for antibiotic-resistant bacteria by increasing conjugation, transduction by bacteriophages and plasmid mobility, primarily through activation of bacterial cellular stress responses (Modi et al. 2014).

The use of antimicrobials alters the number and composition of the microbiotica. In particular, by removing or reducing susceptible bacterial species, they open niches for organisms that would not normally populate that part of the body. New infections that develop as a consequence of the effects of treatment with an antimicrobial are sometimes referred to as supra-infections.

One particularly important issue with regard to broad-spectrum antimicrobials is *Clostridium difficile* supra-infection. Although originally seen with clindamycin-associated colitis, a wide variety of other drugs can increase the risk, including cephalosporins, penicillins and fluoroquinolones. In order for *C. difficule* infection to occur, bacterial spores must be present in the environment or in the gut lumen, emphasising the importance of environmental cleanliness and hand hygiene to remove spores, and isolation of those with *C. difficile* to prevent contamination of the environment (Chilton et al. 2018).

Antimicrobial Stewardship

Antimicrobial stewardship is a key element of any antimicrobial resistance plan. It is defined as 'a coordinated program that promotes the appropriate use of antimicrobials (including antibiotics), improves patient outcomes, reduces microbial resistance, and decreases the spread of infections caused by multidrug-resistant organisms' (Association for Professionals in Infection Control and Epidemiology n.d.). It is not really restricting the use of antimicrobials, but ensuring that their use is rational. Infection control practitioners should be key members of antimicrobial stewardship teams, alongside doctors, nurses, pharmacists, microbiologists and infectious disease specialists.

Some antimicrobials are restricted, and it is important to check local policies regarding this. There are usually three levels of restriction.

1) Antimicrobals that can be freely prescribed.
2) Restricted antimicrobials that require approval from a microbiologist or infectious diseases expert. These are usually drugs that are new or expensive when other therapeutic options exist; or those where there is a particular need to protect the drug from the development of resistance.
3) Non-formulary antimicrobials which need to be approved by the Drug and Therapeutics Committee on a named patient basis. These are drugs not normally held in the local pharmacy.

Recommendations for antimicrobial stewardship refer to actions that can be taken before or at the time of prescription, or after prescription (World Health Organization 2021b).

Before Prescription
- Education of healthcare workers in the correct use of antimicrobials.
- Patient and public education.
- Institution-specific guidance for the treatment of common infections.
- Restricted use of certain antimicrobials.
- Checking reported antimicrobial allergies to ensure that these are really allergies.
- Close monitoring of local antimicrobial resistance patterns.

After Prescription
- Regular, prospective audits.
- Reassessment of antibiotic use.
- Ensuring that doses and routes of prescribed antibiotics are appropriate.
- Ensuring that the time of prescription is appropriate.

Future Trends in Antimicrobials

The future of antimicrobials lies in the development of new drugs, repurposing of those that already exist, and better understanding of the response to infection. This latter approach includes modulation of the immune response, such as the use of corticosteroids and immune suppressants where the immune system causes damage; and monoclonal antibodies and vaccines to boost immunity. The other key aspect of antimicrobial use is their control. Better diagnostics and targeting of therapy are essential to ensure that only those who will really benefit from them use antimicrobial drugs.

Suggested Activities

Exercise 5.1 Self-assessment

1 Complete the following sentences:
   A 'An antimicrobial drug is ....'
   B 'An antibiotic drug is ....'
   C 'The difference between them is ....'

2 Are the following statements true or false?
   A Viruses cannot replicate on their own.
   B All bacteria are dangerous to humans.
   C The spread of antimicrobial resistance is the result of the use of antimicrobials.
   D MRSA (methicillin-resistant *S. aureus*) cannot be treated at all.
   E Empiric therapy is often broad spectrum.
   F Broad-spectrum therapy is a good general treatment approach.
   G Antimicrobial resistance genes often occur naturally in the environment, or in the organisms that produce the antibiotic.

Exercise 5.2

Find some local or national guidance for the treatment of an infectious disease. Look at:

1 the criteria for treatment with antimicrobial drugs

2 the antimicrobials themselves and any special monitoring

3 the criteria for discontinuing these drugs.

Exercise 5.3

Read the local antimicrobial policy for a healthcare provider. Note any special procedures that are needed for prescribing different types of antimicrobial. Compare this to the information contained within a formulary such as the British National Formulary. It might also be possible that the healthcare organisation itself has its own formulary.

Exercise 5.4

For a number of different conditions, consider what is the most likely cause of each and how a definitive diagnosis is made. Where treatment is given on an empiric basis, that is without knowing for sure what the organism is, on what basis are the antimicrobials started and if necessary changed?

References

Abdul-Aziz, M.H., Alffenaar, J.-W.C., Bassetti, M. et al. (2020). Antimicrobial therapeutic drug monitoring in critically ill adult patients: a Position Paper. *Intensive Care Med.* 46: 1127–1153. https://doi.org/10.1007/s00134-020-06050-1.

Association for Professionals in Infection Control and Epidemiology (n.d.) Antimicrobial stewardship. https://apic.org/professional-practice/practice-resources/antimicrobial-stewardship

British Society for Antimicrobial Chemotherapy (2013). BSAC Methods for Antimicrobial Susceptibility Testing. https://bsac.org.uk/wp-content/uploads/2012/02/BSAC-disc-susceptibility-testing-method-Jan-2015.pdf

Chilton, C.H., Pickering, D.S., and Freeman, J. (2018). Microbiologic factors affecting *Clostridium difficile* recurrence. *Clin. Microbiol. Infect.* 24: 476–482. https://doi.org/10.1016/j.cmi.2017.11.017.

Frost, L.S., Leplae, R., Summers, A.O., and Toussaint, A. (2005). Mobile genetic elements: the agents of open source evolution. *Nat. Rev. Microbiol.* 3: 722–732. https://doi.org/10.1038/nrmicro1235.

Gardete, S. and Tomasz, A. (2014). Mechanisms of vancomycin resistance in *Staphylococcus aureus. J. Clin. Invest.* 124: 2836–2840. https://doi.org/10.1172/JCI68834.

Heitman, J. (2006). Sexual reproduction and the evolution of microbial pathogens. *Curr. Biol.* 16: R711–R725. https://doi.org/10.1016/j.cub.2006.07.064.

Khaw, M. and Panosian, C.B. (1995). Human antiprotozoal therapy: past, present, and future. *Clin. Microbiol. Rev.* 8: 427–439. https://doi.org/10.1128/CMR.8.3.427.

Maertens, J.A., Girmenia, C., Brüggemann, R.J. et al. (2018). European guidelines for primary antifungal prophylaxis in adult haematology patients: summary of the updated recommendations from the European conference on infections in Leukaemia. *J. Antimicrob. Chemother.* 73: 3221–3230. https://doi.org/10.1093/jac/dky286.

Modi, S.R., Collins, J.J., and Relman, D.A. (2014). Antibiotics and the gut microbiota. *J. Clin. Invest.* 124: 4212–4218. https://doi.org/10.1172/JCI72333.

Munita, J.M. and Arias, C.A. (2016). Mechanisms of antibiotic resistance. *Microbiol. Spectr.* 4: https://doi.org/10.1128/microbiolspec.VMBF-0016-2015.

Scorzoni, L., de Paula e Silva, A.C.A., Marcos, C.M. et al. (2017). Antifungal therapy: new advances in the understanding and treatment of mycosis. *Front. Microbiol.* 8: 36. https://doi.org/10.3389/fmicb.2017.00036.

Sievert, D.M., Rudrik, J.T., Patel, J.B. et al. (2008). Vancomycin-resistant *Staphylococcus aureus* in the United States, 2002–2006. *Clin. Infect. Dis.* 46: 668–674. https://doi.org/10.1086/527392.

Strebhardt, K. and Ullrich, A. (2008). Paul Ehrlich's magic bullet concept: 100 years of progress. *Nat. Rev. Cancer* 8: 473–480. https://doi.org/10.1038/nrc2394.

The European Committee on Antimicrobial Susceptibility Testing (n.d.) Clinical breakpoints – breakpoints and guidance. https://eucast.org/clinical_breakpoints.

Thomas, C.M. and Nielsen, K.M. (2005). Mechanisms of, and barriers to, horizontal gene transfer between bacteria. *Nat. Rev. Microbiol.* 3: 711–721. https://doi.org/10.1038/nrmicro1234.

Winstanley, T.G. and Hastings, J.G.M. (1990). Synergy between penicillin and gentamicin against enterococci. *J. Antimicrob. Chemother.* 25: 551–560. https://doi.org/10.1093/jac/25.4.551.

World Health Organization (2015). *Global Action Plan on Antimicrobial Resistance.* Geneva: World Health Organization.

World Health Organization (2021a). *Consolidated Guidelines on HIV Prevention, Testing, Treatment, Service Delivery and Monitoring: Recommendations for a Public Health Approach, 2021.* Geneva: World Health Organization.

World Health Organization (2021b). *Antimicrobial Stewardship Interventions: A Practical Guide.* Copenhagen: WHO Regional Office for Europe.

World Health Organization (n.d.). Antibiotic resistance. www.who.int/news-room/fact-sheets/detail/antibiotic-resistance.

6

Policies and Protocols for Infection Prevention and Control

Risk of Infection Associated with Healthcare

Healthcare-associated infections (HCAIs) are the most commonly reported untoward events affecting inpatients. Most are considered are preventable (Lancet 2015). Nevertheless, substantial risk has been identified for patients receiving healthcare. Risk factors include:

- shared facilities in premises where healthcare is delivered
- contact with different health workers carrying micro-organisms
- undergoing invasive procedures or having indwelling invasive devices in place
- consuming mass-produced food.

Attitudes in the UK regarding HCAIs have changed in recent years. At one time, HCAIs were regarded as an inevitable risk associated with receiving healthcare. Views began to change with a report issued by the National Audit Office (2000) highlighting the economic consequences of HCAIs for health services and impact on patients. Infection prevention and control has since become part of the clinical governance framework in acute and primary care and legislation has been put in place to reduce risks.

Infection Prevention and Control Strategies

Infection prevention and control should be incorporated into the care received by all patients and is essential in all settings where health and social care are delivered. Very sick patients are at greatest risk as they are managed with multiple indwelling devices. Long-stay patients have correspondingly increased exposure

Infection Prevention and Control in Healthcare Settings,
First Edition. Edward Purssell and Dinah Gould.
© 2023 John Wiley & Sons Ltd. Published 2023 by John Wiley & Sons Ltd.

to hospital pathogens, including those resistant to antimicrobial drugs which cause infections that are hard to treat. Outpatient clinics have traditionally been regarded as lower risk but more recently it has become apparent that cross-infection is possible in these settings (Bingham et al. 2016).

Today, many patients in the acute stages of illness receive care outside hospital while others managed in the community are at risk of infection because they have chronic conditions (e.g. diabetes, cancer). The 2020 COVID-19 pandemic drew attention to the vulnerability of frail older people in nursing homes and the importance of educating all health and social care workers to implement infection prevention and control strategies.

The chain of infection is broken by:

- *risk assessment* to enable care to be tailored to the needs of individual patients. For example, ensuring good glycaemic control and correcting electrolyte imbalance reduce the risk of surgical site infection
- *standard infection control precautions* to reduce risk of transferring infectious agents from recognised and unrecognised sources of infection. They include policies for decontamination (e.g. cleaning, disinfection, sterilisation) and safe sharps handling and disposal (Table 6.1). Premises where healthcare is delivered are required to apply the Code of Practice for preventing and controlling HCAIs under the Health Act (2006)
- *public health policies* to promote the health of the entire community (e.g. immunisation programmes, inspecting premises where food is produced and sold, notification of infectious diseases).

Risk Assessment

Risk assessment is the process employed to identify hazards and risk factors that have potential to cause harm. In the UK, risk assessment enables employers to fulfil their legal duty to protect staff from harm, injury and illness under Section 2 (1) of the Health and Safety at Work Act (1974). In healthcare settings, risk assessment is undertaken to safeguard patients and health workers. Applied to infection prevention and control, risk assessment involves:

Table 6.1 Potential sources of infection.

Blood and other body fluids
Secretions and excretions
Non-intact skin and mucous membranes
The environment and items in it that are likely to be contaminated

Table 6.2 Steps in risk assessment.

Step 1: Identify hazards.
Step 2: Determine which individuals could be harmed and how.
Step 3: Assess the risks and take action.
Step 4: Record the outcomes.
Step 5: Review the risk assessment.

- identifying tasks or activities that carry the risk of introducing or disseminating infection
- identifying individuals who are particularly susceptible to infection
- evaluating the risks identified and implementing precautions and controls.

The five steps involved in undertaking risk assessment are shown on Table 6.2. Box 6.1 applies risk assessment to infection prevention and control.

Standard Infection Control Precautions

Standard infection prevention and control precautions are required to protect patients and staff in all premises where healthcare is delivered (Table 6.3.)

Decontamination

All premises where healthcare is delivered are contaminated with potential pathogens transmissible to patients, including surfaces near and distant to patient care areas (Otter et al. 2011).

Box 6.1   Applying Risk Assessment to Infection Prevention and Control

Consider:

- The likelihood that an individual is carrying a particular micro-organism or that an item is contaminated based on knowledge of risk factors and local epidemiology (e.g. recent hospital or residential care increases the risk of carrying pathogens able to cause HCAI).
- The vulnerability of the individual patient to infection, taking into account health status and other risk factors (e.g. advanced age, immunosuppressive therapy).
- The potential for other patients or staff to be exposed to the organism and risk of transmission.

Source: Centers for Disease Control and Prevention (2021).

Table 6.3 Infection prevention and control policies.

Decontamination: cleaning, disinfection and sterilisation
Hand hygiene
Disposal of clinical waste
Segregation, handling and disposal of linen
Isolation of infectious and potentially infectious patients
Sharps handling and disposal

Decontamination is achieved at three levels:

- cleaning
- disinfection
- sterilisation.

Each level becomes progressively more effective but also more expensive, more difficult to perform and more likely to damage the item concerned.

Environmental Cleaning

Cleaning maintains the appearance, structure and efficient functioning of the clinical environment and its contents by reducing the number of micro-organisms present and preventing spread (Ayliffe et al. 1967). The method selected should not be more complex or expensive than necessary. In addition to expense, key considerations include the following.

- *How soon will recontamination occur?* Some areas/items (e.g. floors, drains, sluice hoppers) become recontaminated very rapidly. Cleaning rather than routine disinfection is usually the recommended approach for these, depending on local circumstances and events.
- *Will the area/item withstand the procedure?* Metal surfaces are corroded by hypochlorite disinfectants while delicate equipment (e.g. endoscopes) do not withstand autoclaving.
- *Will contact with the cleaning or decontaminating agent be possible for long enough?* Decontamination requires time to become effective. The length of time varies between different chemicals or type of heat applied.

Routine environmental disinfection is not usually practical because recontamination occurs very rapidly (Ayliffe et al. 1967). It may be necessary under specific circumstances (e.g. in an isolation room after a highly contagious patient has been discharged). Environmental cleaning in healthcare premises is a skilled activity undertaken by domestic staff who require training (Box 6.2).

Items should never be allowed to soak in cleaning fluids because micro-organisms can withstand the action of detergents and multiply to form reservoirs.

Box 6.2   Outline policy for good cleaning practice

- Use a fresh cleaning solution for each task, checking that it is of the required dilution.
- Apply the cleaning solution evenly to all surfaces, ensuring that all equipment (e.g. mopheads, wipes) is clean and dry before use. Avoid applying excess solution to prevent seepage into joins and cracks: damage and inadequate drying could result.
- Change the solution at regular intervals throughout cleaning to prevent micro-organisms accumulating, leading to recontamination.
- Allow enough time for the cleaning solution to penetrate surface soiling.
- Dispose of the solution via a sluice hopper. Avoid splashing to prevent environmental contamination.
- Never use washbasins in clinical areas to discard cleaning fluids.
- Dry surfaces thoroughly so that micro-organisms are unable to survive.
- Wash hands thoroughly after cleaning to prevent cross-contamination.

Cleaning cloths and mopheads can become heavily contaminated and inefficient practices lead to the redistribution of micro-organisms rather than their elimination. Colour-coded schemes have been recommended to reduce the risks of cross-contamination. Equipment is labelled with different colours according to the area where it is used (e.g. bathrooms, ward areas, operating theatre) and an item used in one area is never used elsewhere.

Risk assessment has been suggested as a way to optimise cleaning standards in healthcare premises (Box 6.3). The mechanical action of cleaning removes visible soiling and up to 80% of micro-organisms (Ayliffe et al. 1967). Detergent breaks down grease and the soil is diluted by water in the cleaning solution. A systematic

---

Box 6.3   Cleaning in Clinical Settings: A Risk Assessment and Systematic Approach

- *Step 1 Risk assessment*: inspect the area to identify soil, spillages and equipment that needs to be cleaned. Consider the risk profile of the patients and how contaminated the surfaces are likely to be.
- *Step 2 Plan cleaning*: assemble equipment and arrange the furniture to ensure access, particularly 'hard to reach areas'.
- *Step 3 Undertake cleaning*.
- *Step 4 Dry the area thoroughly to prevent cross-contamination*: moist surfaces transfer micro-organisms more effectively than dry ones.

Source: Assadian et al. (2021); Dancer and Kramer (2019); Marples and Towers (1979).

---

approach should be adopted, moving from least to most soiled locations to reduce risk of contamination.

High-touch surfaces (e.g. elevator buttons, computer keyboards, telephones) become heavily contaminated and need regular cleaning (Ledwoch et al. 2021). The frequency needs to be increased in specific circumstances to reduce risk. Norovirus may persist on high-touch surfaces during outbreaks (Lopman et al. 2012). Gram-negative and -positive bacteria can survive on mobile phones for up to six hours (Simmonds Cavanagh 2021).

Deep (terminal) cleaning is necessary when patients are discharged. Those admitted to a room previously used to isolate an infectious patient are more likely to become colonised or infected with the same pathogens (Otter et al. 2011). *Clostridioides difficile* presents a particular risk because the spores persist in the environment for months and are very difficult to destroy (Wilcox et al. 2017).

Decontaminating Clinical Equipment

Clinical equipment becomes heavily contaminated and many items in the clinical environment can operate as fomites (Kanamori et al. 2017). Examples are shown in Table 6.4. Many outbreaks of HCAI have been attributed to inadequate decontamination (Schabrun and Chipchase 2006). Wherever possible, items should be stored clean and dry. Soaking in disinfectant solutions is poor practice as the fluid is rapidly inactivated by organic matter and becomes heavily contaminated, setting up a reservoir of infection (Burdon and Whitby 1967). Portable equipment frequently moved between successive patients is a particular risk as it is often heavily contaminated (Livshiz-Riven et al. 2015) and not always cleaned between patients (Havill et al. 2011).

A system to determine the most appropriate method of decontaminating clinical equipment was developed by Spaulding in the 1950s (McDonnell and Burke 2011) and is still widely used today (Box 6.4). Items are classified as:

Table 6.4 Items in the clinical environment subject to heavy contamination: examples.

Baths
Bed linen
Bedpans and commodes
Catheter drainage bags
Flannels
Hoists
Mattresses
Urinals
Washbowls

> **Box 6.4   Selecting An Appropriate Approach to Decontaminating Clinical Equipment**
>
> - *Critical items* that penetrate skin/mucous membranes (e.g. needles, surgical instruments, urinary catheters) must be sterilised because infection risk is high.
> - *Medium-risk items* in contact with mucous membranes and those likely to become contaminated with readily transmissible pathogens should be disinfected or sterilised although they do not need to be sterile at the point of use with another patient (e.g. vaginal speculae, endoscopes, bedpans, infant feeding bottles, anaesthetic and respiratory equipment).
> - *Low-risk items* that contact skin without penetration require cleaning (e.g. mattresses, blood pressure cuffs, washbowls, linen).

- critical
- medium-risk
- non-critical.

Some modification to the above system may be necessary when dealing with specific patients or circumstances, e.g. equipment where contamination is possible with very high-risk pathogens such as prions (McDonnell and Burke 2011).

In many settings (e.g. family planning clinics, GP practices), nurses are responsible for cleaning and decontaminating clinical equipment and must be familiar with the principles of safe practice. Pre-cleaning is necessary because disinfection and sterilisation are ineffective in the presence of physical soiling. Care is necessary to avoid splashing and the creation of aerosols that could lead to cross-contamination. Plastic aprons and non-sterile disposable gloves should be worn to protect hands and unforms.

Disinfection

Disinfection is the destruction of vegetative micro-organisms but not spores. The aim is to reduce the number of vegetative micro-organisms to a level below the infective dose. 'Safe' levels vary according to circumstance, depending on the susceptibility of the patient and the virulence of the pathogen. Disinfection can be achieved with heat and chemicals. Heat disinfection is the method of choice whenever possible. It is rapid, cheaper than chemical disinfection and more easily controlled.

Heat Disinfection (Pasteurisation)

Most clinically significant micro-organisms are destroyed by exposure to moist heat between 50° and 70 °C for 20–30 minutes. Spores are more resistant to heat and under these conditions, many will not be destroyed. The disinfection temperature and time

---

Box 6.5   Procedure for Operating Heat Disinfectors

- Pre-clean items.
- Place items on the tray inside the disinfector, covering completely with water. Ensure that no air bubbles are trapped inside (e.g. in hollow-bore instruments).
- Check that the machine is not overloaded.
- Ensure that the water returns to the boil for at least five minutes after the items have been added, using a timer for accuracy.
- After processing, use clean forceps to raise the tray holding the items.
- Place the items on a clean surface and leave covered while they cool.
- Store the items in a dry, clean container.
- Change the water in the boiler daily.

---

commonly used during pasteurisation range from 60 °C for 10 minutes to 80 °C or above for one minute. Extra time is needed for cold instruments to reach the temperature necessary for disinfection and to become sufficiently cool to handle afterwards. In hospital, nurses are unlikely to be responsible for heat disinfection but in community settings they may be required to operate hot-water disinfectors (Box 6.5).

Cleaning and disinfection are often combined in dishwashers, washing machines and bedpan washers. Most contaminants are removed during the mechanical action of cleaning and any that persist are destroyed by heat.

Boiling

Boiling can be used to disinfect medium-risk items. Most bacteria and viruses are destroyed after a few minutes. Once the items are immersed, the water must return to the boil before timing begins. Boiling is not used much in high-income countries where other technologies are available but can be a practical method for use in the home.

Chemical Disinfection

An ideal disinfectant is effective, does not damage equipment or harm people and is inexpensive. Unfortunately, no chemical incorporating all these properties exists, rendering chemical disinfection an uncertain process. Many chemical disinfectants are toxic, corrosive, unstable in solution and readily deactivated by organic matter, plastics, rubber, detergents and hard water. When no alternative is available, compromise is required, taking into consideration factors that determine the effectiveness of chemical disinfectants. Speed and range of action are important. Good practice when using chemical disinfectants is shown in Box 6.6. Incorrect use can lead to outbreaks of infection (Weber et al. 2007).

Box 6.6   Good Practice when Using Chemical Disinfectants

- Use the correct concentration. A solution reconstituted below the recommended strength is not fully effective.
- Using higher concentrations is wasteful and not necessarily more efficacious (e.g. very high concentrations of alcohol evaporate before disinfection is achieved).
- Check the expiry date. Dilutions may deteriorate with age.
- Ensure satisfactory contact between the equipment and disinfecting solution. Disinfection cannot be achieved unless the solution has full, direct contact with all surfaces. It is essential to pre-clean items, ensure complete immersion and expel all trapped air bubbles.
- Ensure correct timing and remove the items from the disinfecting solution promptly to avoid reservoirs developing and risk of cross-contamination.

Control of Substances Hazardous to Health

The Control of Substances Hazardous to Health (COSHH) (2002) legislation requires employers to control substances that are hazardous to health. Hazardous substances are those that may damage health irrespective of whether harm is acute (immediate) or chronic (long-term). In healthcare, they include chemicals, body fluids and tissues. Many chemicals used in decontamination processes are hazardous. Managers need to consider whether an alternative substance can be used. If no alterative exists, under COSHH, the principles of good control practice must be applied (Box 6.7).

Different Types of Chemical Disinfectants

Hypochlorites
Hypochlorites are available in different dilutions, expressed as parts per million (ppm) of available chlorine (Table 6.5). They are rapidly effective against

Box 6.7   Control of Substances Hazardous to Health: Principles of Good Control Practice

- Minimise emissions, release and spread.
- Employ control measures proportionate to risk.
- Select effective options for control.
- Provide staff with personal protective equipment.
- Review the actions taken to effect control.
- Provide information and training to staff.
- Assess new measures and associated risks as they become available.

Table 6.5   Use of hypochlorites at different dilutions.

Uses	Dilution (%)	Available chlorine (ppm)
Blood/body fluids	1.0	10 000
General environmental use	0.1	1000
Infant feeding equipment	0.0125	125

bacteria, fungi and viruses but effectiveness is reduced in the presence of organic matter. At concentrations of 1000 ppm, they destroy spores and mycobacteria. Hypochlorites are very good general disinfectants but are corrosive at the concentrations necessary to decontaminate instruments and are readily inactivated by organic matter. It is, however, safe to use granular formulations containing sodium dichloroisocyanurate at 10 000 ppm to deal with spills of blood and body fluids as at this very high concentration, deactivation by organic matter is less likely. In the home, patients can use Domestos® or another brand of thick bleach (10 000 ppm) to deal with blood and body fluid spills but should be warned about safe handling.

Milton® (125–140 ppm) is safe for use in food preparation and to clean infant feeding bottles but items should not be allowed to soak. In the past, feeds have become contaminated in hospital milk kitchens (Ayliffe et al. 1970). Heat sterilisation or commercially prepared feeds are better options in hospital.

Phenolics
Phenolics are active against bacteria including mycobacteria and fungi but are not sporicidal. They are no longer much used in healthcare as their activity against viruses is limited and they are generally more effective for non-enveloped viruses. They are suitable as environmental disinfectants at concentrations of 1–2% and are stable in solution, not readily neutralised and cheap, but irritant to skin and corrosive.

Quaternary Ammonium Compounds
Quaternary ammonium compounds have natural detergent properties. They destroy most Gram-positive and -negative bacteria and enveloped viruses but not mycobacteria or spores. They are rapidly inactivated by organic matter and in weak dilution support the growth of bacteria. Quaternary ammonium compounds have been implicated in a number of outbreaks (Weber et al. 2007). They are sometimes used to disinfect low-risk items but overall their performance is inferior to that of hypochlorites and they are little used in healthcare.

Triclosan

Triclosan disrupts the synthesis of bacterial cell walls. It is active against Gram-positive bacteria but not very effective for Gram-negative bacteria and viruses. In healthcare it is used in hand hygiene products but its popularity is declining through concern about damage to the environment and toxicity (Halden et al. 2017).

Glutaraldehyde

Glutaraldehyde rapidly destroys vegetative bacteria, fungi and viruses. Mycobacteria are destroyed in 20–60 minutes and spores after 3–10 hours of exposure, depending on the formulation used, achieving sterilisation. Glutaraldehyde does not corrode metal and although it penetrates organic matter slowly, is not inactivated. Physical cleaning is necessary if instruments are contaminated with blood to avoid coagulation. Glutaraldehyde can be used to decontaminate equipment that would be damaged by heat (e.g. endoscopes) but must be handled with extreme care as it is highly toxic and can vaporise. It is highly irritant to skin and mucosae and can cause sensitisation reactions, including asthma and dermatitis. The use of glutaraldehyde requires good ventilation to allow fumes to dissipate and staff must wear protective clothing.

The serious health and safety issues associated with glutaraldehyde have prompted many organisations to seek alternatives.

Hydrogen Peroxide

Hydrogen peroxide disrupts cell membranes and DNA, destroying vegetative bacteria, fungi and viruses within one minute (Weber et al. 2016b). After prolonged contact, its effects are sporicidal. Hydrogen peroxide is inactivated by organic matter, corrosive to some metals and if used at high concentrations can irritate skin and mucous membranes. Hydrogen peroxide vapour is used to decontaminate isolation rooms formerly occupied by patients with MRSA, *C. difficile* and multidrug-resistant organisms but because of its toxicity, can only be used after they have been vacated (Box 6.8).

Box 6.8   'No-touch' Methods of Room Decontamination

Despite conventional cleaning, surfaces in clinical areas often remain heavily contaminated. 'No-touch' methods of room decontamination using hydrogen peroxide systems and ultraviolet light devices can reduce the numbers of pathogens on test surfaces under laboratory conditions and on environmental surfaces in clinical areas and have been recommended for terminal cleaning after patients have been discharged. There is less evidence that 'self-cleaning surfaces' (e.g. copper) can interrupt the chain of infection (Weber et al. 2016a).

Peracetic Acid

Peracetic acid is a combination of acetic acid and hydrogen peroxide. It destroys bacteria, fungi and viruses rapidly by denaturing proteins and destroys spores within 10 minutes (Deshpande et al. 2014). Peracetic acid is not readily inactivated by organic material. It is a very useful alternative to glutaraldehyde for high-level decontamination of delicate, heat-sensitive equipment (e.g. endoscopes) but is highly irritant to skin and mucous membranes.

Alcohols

Alcohols in 70% solution denature protein rapidly and destroy vegetative bacteria, including mycobacteria and fungi. Isopropanol and ethanol (ethyl alcohol) both destroy enveloped viruses within 30 seconds of application but ethanol is more effective against non-enveloped viruses (e.g. norovirus, rotavirus) (Kampf 2018). Alcohols are widely incorporated into sprays, impregnated into swabs and combined with emollients in the manufacture of highly effective handrubs and gels. The formulation does not appear to affect efficacy (Wilkinson et al. 2018). Alcohols are also used as surface disinfectants (e.g. dressing trolleys, stethoscopes). They evaporate quickly, leaving the surface dry, but penetrate organic matter poorly and are only suitable for use on physically clean surfaces.

Chlorhexidine Gluconate

Chlorhexidine was formulated to disinfect human tissue. It is non-toxic and non-corrosive but relatively expensive and more effective against Gram-positive than Gram-negative bacteria. It continues to destroy organisms for some time after application and is described as exhibiting residual effectiveness or substantivity (Russell and Day 1993). Chlorhexidine is not effective against mycobacteria, has limited activity against viruses and does not destroy spores. It is readily inactivated by organic matter and chemicals. It is unsuitable for environmental use because it is expensive and has such a narrow range of bactericidal activity but is widely combined with alcohol in handrubs and often used preoperatively as a skin antiseptic.

Octenidine

Octenidine is used to irrigate wounds and as a body wash. When used for preoperative skin preparation, it reduces the number of colony-forming units on patients' skin more effectively than soap and water (Tanner et al. 2012). At present, it is not widely used in healthcare.

Iodophors

Iodophors (e.g. povidone iodine) are used as skin antiseptics before orthopaedic procedures because they destroy spores. They have a broader spectrum than chlorhexidine but many people are allergic to iodine and patch testing is necessary before use. Povidone iodine is sometimes used in surgical scrubs and other hand hygiene preparations but is unpopular because it is harsh to skin.

Sterilisation

Sterilisation is the destruction of all micro-organisms and spores. It is necessary when the numbers surviving disinfection would be sufficient to establish infection, either because the organisms are highly virulent or because the patient is very susceptible. Indications for sterilisation are shown in Table 6.6. Sterilisation is rarely absolute and quality control is essential to ensure that adequate numbers of micro-organisms and spores are destroyed.

Methods of Sterilisation

A number of methods can be used to achieve sterilisation (Table 6.7). Heat is the most reliable and controllable and is the method of choice wherever practical. Chemicals (e.g. ethylene oxide, formaldehyde vapour) are used to sterilise items

Table 6.6   Indications for sterilisation.

Equipment that breaches the body's natural barriers to infection (e.g. surgical instruments, urinary catheters, injection needles, intravenous administration sets).
Dressing materials and topical applications that will be in contact with anatomical sites usually free of micro-organisms.
Situations in which contamination is possible with a large number of bacterial spores (e.g. *C. difficile, Bacillus anthracis*).
Equipment that has been in contact with extremely virulent pathogens (e.g. viral haemorrhagic fevers).

Table 6.7   Methods of sterilisation.

Heat
Dry heat: incineration, hot-air ovens, infrared convectors Moist heat under pressure: autoclaves
Radiation
Ultraviolet irradiation
X-rays
Gamma rays
Chemicals
Ethylene oxide gas
Formaldehyde gas
Glutaraldehyde
Peracetic acid
Filtration
Filters designed to remove all vegetative bacteria, spores and viruses from commercially prepared solutions

damaged at high temperature. Radiation is used to sterilise single-use items (e.g. syringes, needles, dressing packs). These methods are employed commercially by trained technicians, not usually in healthcare provider organisations.

Autoclaving

Autoclaving involves the use of steam under pressure and is the most reliable method of sterilising equipment. At atmospheric pressure, water boils at 100 °C. At higher than atmospheric pressure, water boils at a higher temperature if held in a closed container and the steam generated destroys vegetative micro-organisms and spores. Sterilisation is achieved at:

- 121 °C for 15 minutes
- 126 °C for 10 minutes
- 134 °C for 5 minutes.

Steam penetrates fabrics and porous objects rapidly, a property enhanced by the increased pressure. In an autoclave, air is removed by suction to create a vacuum before the steam enters, to ensure contact with all surfaces; failure of contact results in failure of sterilisation. In the commercial sector, equipment is autoclaved in large batches by technicians. In community clinics and general practice where small items of equipment are required in rapid succession, nurses may assume responsibility for operating small worktop autoclaves (Box 6.9).

Critical items (see Box 6.4) must be sterile at the point of use and either autoclaved inside a sealed packet or used immediately. Sterility is maintained

---

Box 6.9   Management and Use of Autoclaves

- Pre-clean all items with detergent and water: the presence of organic matter impedes contact of the surface with steam.
- Arrange items inside the autoclave, ensuring there is no contact between them; steam cannot reach surfaces that are touching. Open hinged instruments to allow maximum exposure of all surfaces. Do not overload the chamber.
- When the cycle is complete, remove items using sterile forceps and place in a sterile container.
- Wash cleaning brushes and store dry.
- Arrange for autoclaves to be serviced regularly by a trained technician according to the manufacturer's instructions. Autoclaves that are not functioning correctly may not sterilise.
- Test equipment at least weekly.
- Do not use small autoclaves to sterilise porous loads (e.g. dressing materials, fabrics) as steam penetration cannot be guaranteed in these devices.

indefinitely providing packs remain intact and dry. Medium-risk items that need to be sterilised but not sterile at the point of use (e.g. vaginal speculae) do not need pre-packaging.

Hot Air Ovens

Hot air ovens sterilise by maintaining pre-cleaned items at 170 °C for 60 minutes. Higher temperatures and longer exposure times are necessary than if an autoclave is used because air does not conduct heat as efficiently as steam. Items are cold when the cycle begins and need to cool before they are handled and this extends the length of the cycle. Consequently, hot air ovens are not practical when handling large batches of instruments or when a swift turn-round time is required and can only be used for items that are very heat resistant. They are unsuitable for plastics, rubber and many fabrics.

Recommendations for Handling Items Potentially Contaminated with Prions

Prions cause a group of diseases called the transmissible spongiform encephalopathies: Creutzfeldt–Jakob disease (CJD), scrapie and kuru. They are highly resistant to conventional methods of decontamination. Most chemical disinfectants, including glutaraldehyde, are ineffective. Prions are destroyed by immersion in sodium hypochlorite 2 M solution for two hours. Autoclaving is unreliable.

The main risk of transmission is through surgical procedures involving neurological tissues and the posterior eye. A number of other tissues are associated with medium levels of infectivity (e.g. anterior eye, cornea and lymphoid tissues such as the thymus, tonsils and spleen). Other tissues, including blood and blood products, are considered to have low levels of infectivity.

All surgical instruments used during procedures involving tissues with low levels of infectivity can be processed in the usual way. Those used during high- and medium-risk procedures on patients suspected of having CJD or at high risk (e.g. familial history) should be washed to remove soiling with care to avoid splashing and aerosol creation, then reprocessed prior to 'quarantining' in a plastic container with a sealed lid identified with the patient's details. The instruments can be used again on the same patient only. If the patient subsequently develops CJD, the instruments must be incinerated.

Single-Use Equipment

Items labelled as single-use must be discarded *after use*. The 2020 COVID pandemic raised questions about the possibility of repurposing equipment in short supply, e.g. single-use filtering facepiece respirators (Polkinghorne and Branley 2020), but advice issued by the Medicines and Healthcare products Regulatory Agency (2021) is unequivocal. Single-use items should never be reprocessed or reused as this could alter performance or jeopardise the safety of the patient or health worker. The legal implications are clear. Anybody who has reprocessed or reused a device intended for single use by the manufacturer assumes full responsibility for its safety and effectiveness.

Hand Hygiene

Hand hygiene is regarded as a leading infection prevention and control intervention. It is integral to clean and aseptic procedures, central to any infection prevention programme and audited in many countries as part of quality assurance. Most HCAIs are spread by direct contact via hands (Pittet et al. 2006). Hand hygiene breaks the chain of infection and reduces the numbers of bacteria available to cause cross-infection (Pittet et al. 2006). Most campaigns to promote adherence to hand hygiene increase the frequency at which hand hygiene is performed although their effectiveness is usually short-lived unless they are refreshed and there is only modest evidence that they prevent HCAI (Gould et al. 2018).

Micro-organisms on the skin fall into two categories.

- *Resident flora*: these bacteria persist in crevices in the skin and deep within the sebaceous and sweat glands and comprise the normal flora: micrococci, staphylococci and coryneforms. They are not easily dislodged and unlikely to contribute to cross-infection.
- *Transient skin flora*: these bacteria are readily acquired on the hands through contact with the environment and other people and are easily transferred to other people or fomites (Pittet et al. 2006), especially between moist surfaces (Marples and Towers 1979).

Most cross-infection via hands is caused by transient bacteria: staphylococci and Gram-negative opportunists (e.g. *Pseudomonas, Klebsiella* sp., *E.coli*). If they reach a susceptible site on a patient (e.g. open wound), they can cause infection. Even transient contact is enough to transfer large numbers of bacteria to a vulnerable patient (Casewell and Phillips 1977). Bacterial numbers are higher beneath rings, increasing risks of cross-infection if they are worn (Jacobson et al. 1985). Bacteria beneath long fingernails and artificial nails have been linked to outbreaks of Gram-negative infection (Moolenaar et al. 2000).

A range of products is available to undertake hand hygiene.

- *Soap and water*: soap has detergent properties and removes physical soiling. Hands should be dried thoroughly to reduce the risks of cross-infection.
- *Antiseptics* (e.g. chlorhexidine, iodophors) are used during preoperative hand preparation. Iodophors are sometimes used before orthopaedic procedures

because they are sporicidal. The residual effectiveness of chlorhexidine is particularly valuable during surgical procedures when the effects may have to last for several hours. These products are suitable for use on physically clean hands only.

- *Alcohol-based products* contain 70% ethanol or isopropanyl combined with emollients, sometimes with the addition of chlorhexidine. They are recommended for use in wards and other clinical areas (World Health Organization n.d.). Advantages are cosmetic acceptability, speed of use and good bactericidal activity but they have no detergent activity and are suitable for use on physically clean hands only. In clinical areas, handrub should be available at every bedspace.

Indications for hand hygiene include (Sax et al. 2007):

- before patient contact
- before clean or aseptic procedures
- after exposure to blood/body fluids
- after patient contact
- after touching the close patient environment (zone).

Hands should also be cleansed between activities involving the same patient that could lead to contamination (e.g. between perineal care and mouthcare) and if gloves are worn; gloves can tear or hands may become recontaminated when they are removed.

Hand hygiene products are only effective if contact is achieved with all surfaces of the hands. A special technique has been suggested to optimise the thoroughness of the hand hygiene event (Figure 6.1) (Ayliffe et al. 1978).

The effectiveness of hand hygiene should be optimised by not wearing rings, long nails or artificial nails.

Skin Care

Sore, dry hands are an occupational risk for health workers because frequent hand hygiene depletes the skin of lipids, disrupting its natural protective barrier. Actions that can be taken to protect hands are shown in Box 6.10. Damaged skin is colonised with large numbers of bacteria and should be covered with a waterproof dressing to reduce risks of cross-infection and protect the health worker from blood-borne infection.

Personal Protective Equipment

Personal protective equipment (PPE) is worn to:

- protect health workers from known risk of exposure to blood/body fluids and during contact with transmissible pathogens
- protect patients: gloves are worn as part of standard precautions and to reduce risk of infection during invasive procedures.

Steps 3–8 should take at least 15 seconds.

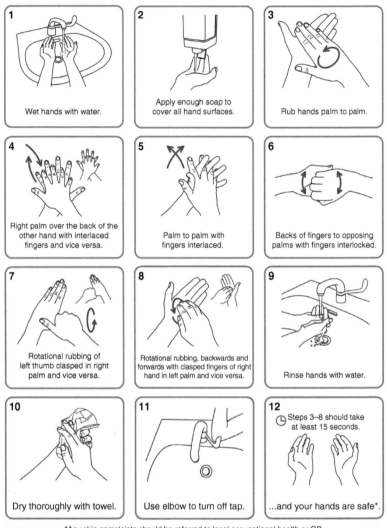

1 Wet hands with water.	**2** Apply enough soap to cover all hand surfaces.	**3** Rub hands palm to palm.
4 Right palm over the back of the other hand with interlaced fingers and vice versa.	**5** Palm to palm with fingers interlaced.	**6** Backs of fingers to opposing palms with fingers interlocked.
7 Rotational rubbing of left thumb clasped in right palm and vice versa.	**8** Rotational rubbing, backwards and forwards with clasped fingers of right hand in left palm and vice versa.	**9** Rinse hands with water.
10 Dry thoroughly with towel.	**11** Use elbow to turn off tap.	**12** Steps 3–8 should take at least 15 seconds. ...and your hands are safe*.

*Any skin complaints should be referred to local occupational health or GP.

Germs. Wash your hands of them.

Figure 6.1 Hand hygiene technique.

Box 6.10   Care of The Skin
• Use alcohol-based products containing emollients unless hands are visibly soiled. • Ensure that hands are wet before soap is applied, adjust the water temperature until it is comfortable, use soft, absorbent hand towels to dry hands thoroughly, pat hands dry, paying attention to areas between the fingers. • Check hands for signs of dryness, itching, redness, cracking and blistering at least once a day. • Apply hand moisturising creams containing emollients after hand hygiene and at the end of each working period. • Report any signs of skin damage to your manager or occupational health provider. *Source:* Royal College of Nursing (n.d.).

Gloves

Gloves were originally made from latex rubber but allergy among health workers and patients has promoted a switch to synthetic materials (e.g. nitrile, neoprene, polyvinyl chloride). They must meet British Standard EN 455 which requires them to be free of perforations (British Standards Institute 2000). Nevertheless, gloves should not be regarded as impermeable as they can tear or perforate during use and are not impermeable to viruses. Hands can be contaminated when gloves are used. Consequently, hand hygiene is still necessary when gloves are worn. Risk assessment should be undertaken before deciding whether gloves should be worn and whether sterile or non-sterile gloves are appropriate.

Non-sterile Disposable Gloves

Non-sterile disposable gloves (NSDGs) are worn for clean procedures (e.g. emptying a urinary catheter) and for added protection when contact is anticipated with blood, other body fluids or undertaking tasks that might lead to heavy contamination of the hands (e.g. emptying a stoma bag, caring for an incontinent patient). They are not necessary when bed-bathing patients, helping patients mobilise, to administer subcutaneous or intramuscular injections or manipulate vascular lines when there is no evidence of blood or leakage. NSDGs should be changed between patients and between procedures that could lead to contamination involving the same patient (e.g. between emptying a urinary catheter drainage bag and mouthcare).

There is confusion regarding the use of NSDGs and concerns that they are often used at the expense of hand hygiene through habit and social pressures (Jain et al. 2017). Excessive use increases the costs of healthcare, adds to the accumulation of clinical waste and land-fill and may be disliked by patients.

Sterile Gloves

Sterile gloves should be worn when there is risk of contaminating a susceptible site that would usually be free of micro-organisms (e.g. insertion point for central lines, urinary catheters). Double-gloving is advisable for high-risk procedures that could result in tearing or percutaneous injury to health workers (e.g. orthopaedic surgery, gynaecological surgery). Wearing an outer glove reduces damage to the inner one (Tanner and Parkinson 2006).

Masks

Masks were originally worn in operating theatres to protect patients from respiratory pathogens. Surgical facemasks made from paper are now worn to protect health workers from splashes of blood and body fluids and to protect patients from infections spread by droplet. They do not offer protection from aerosols because they are loose-fitting, allowing air to escape around the sides (Belkin 1997). The risk of spreading pathogens by direct contact may be increased because the paper becomes damp easily and there is risk of contamination when the mask is handled.

Filtering Face Piece Masks

Filtering face piece (FFP) masks offer protection from droplets and air-borne particles. Three levels of protection of are available: FFP1, FFP2 and FFP3 facemasks. These offer progressively higher levels of protection determined by the filtering device incorporated into the mask. The purpose of FFPs is to protect the wearer against harmful substances able to enter the airways when performing a specific task or working in a hazardous environment. To be effective, they must fit tightly to ensure that the seal between the mask and the face is adequate. Providing 'fit testing' is effective, FFP masks filter both the inflowing and outflowing air, protecting patients and health workers. Box 6.11 explains the safe use of face protection.

Aerosol-Generating Procedures

Some clinical procedures (Table 6.8) are considered to increase the risk of transmitting respiratory pathogens because they generate aerosols: minute respiratory particles small enough to remain suspended in the air for long periods of time and able to penetrate surgical facemasks.

There is considerable debate surrounding precisely which procedures generate aerosols (Klompas et al. 2021). Conversely, there is growing evidence that some procedures or use of equipment can generate aerosols that do not contain the patient's secretions and do not present risk of transmission (e.g. obtaining nose and throat swabs, administering humidified oxygen, administering medication via a nebuliser). During nebulisation, the aerosol originates from the fluid in the nebuliser chamber, not the patient, and does not carry virus particles from the patient. If a particle in the aerosol contacts a contaminated mucous membrane, it is no longer air-borne and is no longer part of an aerosol.

Box 6.11   Using Face Coverings Safely

- Hold the mask by its ties.
- Place the mask over your nose, mouth and chin.
- Position the strip against your nose.
- If fitting an FFP mask, check that it fits snugly by closing the filter surface and inhaling slowly; if the mask moulds around your face, it is properly positioned.
- Once you have fitted the face covering, avoid touching it until it is removed.
- Replace surgical masks every three hours; replace FFP masks every 3–8 hours.
- Dispose of the mask immediately after use.
- Perform hand hygiene.

Table 6.8   Aerosol-generating procedures.

Intubation
Extubation
Manual ventilation
Open suctioning
Cardiopulmonary resuscitation
Bronchoscopy
Surgery involving use of high-speed devices
Dental procedures
Non-invasive ventilation

The 2020 COVID-19 pandemic has reignited the importance of infection prevention and control measures in relation to aerosol-generating procedures (AGPs) (Box 6.12).

Box 6.12   Reducing the Risks Associated with Aerosol-Generating Procedures

- If possible, avoid undertaking AGPs with patients who have respiratory infections.
- Undertake the procedure in a well-ventilated room with the door closed.
- Wear non-sterile disposable gloves, fluid-resistant gowns and goggles.
- Use an FFP3 respiratory mask.
- Undertake hand hygiene before and after the procedure.

Aprons and Gowns

Uniforms become contaminated with potential pathogens, increasing the risk of cross-contamination (Mitchell et al. 2015). A range of specialised textiles has been developed to reduce risks. These include fabrics impregnated with substances that have antimicrobial properties and the ability to deflect splashes and sprays. Although effective in simulations, there is little evidence to demonstrate effectiveness under 'in-use' conditions. Nothing is known about how long the special effects persist (e.g. chemicals may be leached out with repeated washing) and they are expensive. At present, it is usual to wear a disposable plastic apron to protect the front of the uniform (the area most likely to become contaminated). Plastic is water repellent and offers protection from splashing, which cotton gowns do not (Wilson et al. 2007). Fluid-repellent gowns are available for use in operating theatres and other high-risk settings.

Eye Protection

Eye protection should be worn to prevent contamination when splashing with blood and other body fluids is likely.

Bare-Below-Elbow

Bare-below-elbow means not wearing artificial nails, nail polish, a wrist-watch or stoned rings and either wearing short-sleeved garments or being able to roll or push up sleeves (National Institute for Health and Care Excellence 2012). The reasoning behind bare-below-elbow is pragmatic: skin and natural nails can be washed free of contaminants much more easily than fabrics or other materials. Garments with disposable over-sleeves or loose, detachable three-quarter sleeves that can be drawn back are available for health workers with cultural objections to uncovered arms.

Contact Precautions

Contact precautions are recommended when patients have an infection that can be transmitted by contact with skin, mucous membranes, faeces, vomit, urine, wound drainage or multidrug-resistant organisms. Their use is controversial, some authorities arguing that providing standard precautions are properly executed, contact precautions should not be necessary (Curran 2015). Definitions of what constitute contact precautions vary in the literature and accounts of their effectiveness are conflicting. To be successful, implementation must be rigorous (Büchler et al. 2021).

Waste Disposal

Much of the clinical waste generated as a result of healthcare is classified as hazardous because it is likely to contain potential pathogens and toxic substances.

Waste from healthcare facilities must be segregated according to its need for special handling or disposal. In the United Kingdom this is done by colour of bag.

- Yellow bag: the contents require disposal by incineration only.
- Orange bag: the contents may be rendered safe if processed by means other than incineration.
- Yellow and black ('tiger') bag: the contents contain offensive/hygiene waste that is not infected.
- Black bag: household waste.

Most infectious waste can be placed in an orange bag; yellow bags are for waste that is both infectious and has additional characteristics requiring incineration. Orange bags must not contain chemicals, amalgam, medicines or anatomical wastes . Non-infected but offensive/hygiene waste, such as nappies, should be put in a yellow and black bag. It is important that waste is disposed of correctly to ensure that safety is maintained, and that cost and environmental impact are minimised.

Those handling waste need to consider the following factors.

- Training and information requirements.
- Personal hygiene.
- The correct segregation of waste.
- The provision and correct use of appropriate PPE.
- Immunisation.

Managers need to ensure that:

- appropriate procedures are used for handling waste
- packaging and labelling of waste are appropriate
- there is suitable transport on-site and off-site.

clear procedures are in place for dealing with accidents, incidents and spillages (Department of Health 2013).

Linen

Linen must be placed in the appropriate bag, depending on whether it is soiled, foul or infected. Linen used by a patient with a known infection should be placed in a red, water-soluble bag which is then put inside an outer polyester or nylon carriage bag, fastened and sealed when it is three-quarters full. Plastic aprons should be worn when changing beds to avoid contaminating uniforms and hands should be washed afterwards.

Laundries are required to adhere to guidelines for the safe handling of linen, disinfection, staff protection and dealing with effluent (Barrie 1994). Used linen is laundered at 65 °C for 10 minutes or 71 °C for three minutes, allowing adequate time to ensure that the washing solution mixes with the clothes and for heat to penetrate all items in the load. Linen used by a patient with a known infection is processed separately. The inner bag containing potentially infectious items should not be removed from the outer bag until the point of transfer to the washer-extractor. The high wash temperature and dilution in the washing machine remove and destroy the pathogens, rendering the linen safe to handle when the cycle is complete. Heat-labile items that cannot be subjected to temperatures higher than 40 °C require additional treatment, usually with sodium hypochlorite added during the penultimate rinse of the cycle. A final concentration of 150 ppm available chlorine must be achieved for a minimum of five minutes.

In nursing homes, residents' clothing should be laundered on the hottest cycle of the washing machine. Domestic washing machines likely to be available in nursing homes are not suitable for handling bedlinen. In domiciliary settings, contaminated clothing and linen should be washed with detergent on the hot wash cycle of a domestic washing machine to a temperature of 80 °C or on the highest temperature cycle otherwise possible. When dealing with contaminated fabrics, patients and their families should be aware that dilution is essential to wash away micro-organisms and to avoid overloading the washing machine. If washing by hand is unavoidable, household rubber gloves must be worn.

Many health workers launder their own uniforms in domestic washing machines, often at temperatures of 40 °C or lower Tumble-drying and ironing are necessary to remove vegetative bacteria (Patel et al. 2006).

Isolation Precautions

Isolation precautions fall into two categories.

- *Source isolation*: the patient is the source of infection and the aim is to protect other people.
- *Protective isolation* for patients who are highly susceptible to infection.

Source Isolation

For many micro-organisms, standard infection control precautions are sufficient to contain the risk of spread. These include pathogens spread by direct contact and in blood or other body fluids. Additional precautions called transmission-based precautions are necessary in the following circumstances.

- When a patient is known or suspected to be infected or colonised with pathogens readily transmitted person to person, e.g. rotavirus, norovirus, Group A streptococcus.

- When the pathogen is spread via the air-borne route, e.g. influenza, pulmonary tuberculosis, measles, chickenpox.
- When the pathogen is resistant to antimicrobials and the infection is hard to treat.
- When heavy environmental contamination is likely, e.g. Acinetobacter, *C. difficile* (the spores of *C. difficile* survive in the environment for long periods).
- For patients with pyrexia of unknown origin, especially those arriving from countries where serious infections are endemic, e.g. Ebola virus disease.

Source isolation is necessary in two situations: when a patient is known to be infected or colonised with a specific pathogen requiring transmission precautions and when infection or colonisation is suspected but has yet to be confirmed. Risk assessment should be undertaken when source isolation is contemplated because it can be distressing and may have a negative impact on patient outcomes (Stelfox 2003). A further complication is that in some countries, such as the UK, isolation facilities are not always readily available and use may have to be prioritised (Gould et al. 2018).

When undertaking risk assessment, it is important to remember that the aim is to isolate the source of the infection but this does not necessarily mean that the patient has to be confined to a single room, especially as there is no evidence that single room accommodation for patients with blood-borne infections and infections spread by contact reduces transmission. The use of single rooms for these patients is often justified on the grounds that it makes staff more aware that special precautions should be in place but this assumption is debatable.

Factors to be taken into account during risk assessment include the following.

- The patient's mental and physical condition. A patient carrying *C. difficile* who is continent could be managed safely on an open ward. For an incontinent patient with profuse diarrhoea, a single room would be desirable to contain environmental contamination.
- The presence of other highly susceptible patients in the same clinical setting.
- The number of patients who are infected or colonised with the same pathogen at the same time. Where clusters of infection occur, patients may be managed on the same ward or bay by a dedicated nursing team (cohorting).
- Local policy. The approach taken by different health providers is likely to vary according to the type of patients frequently admitted, their risk profiles and the prevalence of specific pathogens in the locality.

Protective Isolation

Patients who have undergone bone marrow and solid organ transplants are severely immunocompromised and highly susceptible to opportunistic infections. In the past, they were subjected to rigorous isolation precautions that could be distressing and expensive and were not evidence based (Hayes-Lattin et al. 2005). Today, many of the standard approaches to infection prevention and control routinely implemented in hospitals are considered sufficient to safeguard these patients.

Types of Isolation Facility

Single Rooms

Single-room accommodation with the door kept shut is recommended for patients whose infections are spread by the air-borne route. If the patient needs to leave the room, they should be educated to wear a mask and use a sputum pot when expectorating. If a single room is not available, patients should be managed under well-ventilated conditions.

Negative Pressure Rooms

Negative pressure rooms are used during source isolation to avoid transmission to people outside. Air moves from areas of high to low pressure. The air in negative pressure rooms is kept lower than the air pressure outside, preventing pathogens from flowing into adjacent areas when the door is opened. An exhaust system is used to suck contaminated air from the isolation room and release it outside the building, allowing contaminants to be diluted in the atmosphere.

Positive Pressure Rooms

Positive pressure rooms are used for patients in protective isolation. The air pressure in the isolation room is kept higher than that in the surrounding areas, preventing the incoming air from becoming contaminated.

Aseptic Technique

The term *asepsis* means free from infection. In healthcare, an aseptic technique is identified as one ensuring that only equipment and fluids that are not contaminated come into contact with susceptible body sites that in health are free of micro-organisms (National Institute for Health and Care Excellence 2012). Aseptic technique should be employed during any clinical procedure that bypasses the body's natural defences. It is possible to conduct straightforward, minor procedures aseptically without wearing sterile gloves or using a sterile field (e.g. emptying catheter drainage bags, changing intravenous administration sets). More complex procedures (e.g. inserting a urinary catheter or central venous line) require the use of sterile gloves and the creation of a sterile field (Box 6.13).

Clean Technique

Clean technique is a modification of aseptic technique employed when dealing with chronic wounds. The same principles are applied except that it is permissible

---

Box 6.13   Procedure for Aseptic Technique

- Perform hand hygiene.
- Check that the sterile pack is intact and free of moisture. Check that all other equipment (e.g. sachets of lotion) are intact and have not reached the expiry date.
- Protect clothing with a plastic apron.
- Use alcohol handrub to cleanse hands thoroughly.
- Open the outer pack so the sterile, inner pack slides onto a previously cleaned surface (e.g. dressing trolley, 'blue tray') without being touched.
- Create a sterile field by opening the inner pack without touching the inside or contents.
- Wear sterile gloves for all contact with the sterile field and its contents.
- Do not place non-sterile items on the sterile field.
- Perform hand hygiene.

---

for wounds to be treated with non-sterile fluids (e.g. tap water) and non-sterile gloves are worn. Clean technique is used for dressing most wounds healing by secondary intention (chronic wounds where there has been tissue loss) such as pressure ulcers and leg ulcers and for dry wounds and minor wounds (e.g. grazes). It should not be used to dress surgical wounds less than 48 hours old because a protective epithelial barrier has not yet formed over the wound surface.

Clean technique is not appropriate for patients who are immunocompromised and those with diabetes as they are at very high risk of infection.

Sharps Handling and Disposal
Sharps handling and disposal are discussed in Chapter 12.

Suggested Activities

Exercise 6.1 Self-assessment

1   Most healthcare-associated infections are considered preventable. True/False

2   Complete the sentence: 'Standard infection control precautions reduce risk of transferring infectious agents. . .'

3   Which of the following are potential sources of infection in healthcare settings?

A Blood
B Urine
C Skin and mucous membranes
D All the above

4 List the three methods of decontamination.

5 Which of the following require sterilisation or disinfection?
A Urinary catheters
B Endoscopes
C Mattresses
D Vaginal speculae

6 Disinfection is the destruction of vegetative micro-organisms and spores. True/False

7 What does the acronym COSHH stand for?

8 Items labelled as single-use can sometimes be recycled after special treatment. True/False

9 State the indications for hand hygiene.

10 When is source isolation necessary?

Exercise 6.2

How are decisions about isolating infectious and potentially infectious patients/ residents taken in your organisation? What types of patients are isolated most often? Do you agree with the decisions taken concerning isolation? What quality of care do these patients/residents receive? Could any improvements be made?

OR

What arrangements are in place for conducting hand hygiene audit in your clinical setting? Who collects the information? How is feedback received? Are these arrangements satisfactory? Could hand hygiene audit be improved?

Exercise 6.3

Obtain the systematic literature review reported by Livshiz-Riven et al. (2015) in the reference list. Read the review and address the following questions.

- How were the papers included in the review selected?
- What tool was used during critical appraisal?
- Are the review methods clearly described and reproducible?
- What are the messages for your organisation?

References

Assadian, O., Harbarth, S., Vos, M. et al. (2021). Practical recommendations for routine cleaning and disinfection procedures in healthcare institutions: a narrative review. *J. Hosp. Infect.* 113: 104–114. https://doi.org/10.1016/j.jhin.2021.03.010.

Ayliffe, G.A., Collins, B.J., Lowbury, E.J. et al. (1967). Ward floors and other surfaces as reservoirs of hospital infection. *J. Hyg.* 65: 515–536. https://doi.org/10.1017/s0022172400046052.

Ayliffe, G.A.J., Collins, B.J., and Pettit, F. (1970). Contamination of infant feeds in a Milton Milk kitchen. *Lancet.* 295: 559–560. https://doi.org/10.1016/S0140-6736(70)90783-X.

Ayliffe, G.A., Babb, J.R., and Quoraishi, A.H. (1978). A test for 'hygienic' hand disinfection. *J. Clin. Pathol.* 31: 923–928. https://doi.org/10.1136/jcp.31.10.923.

Barrie, D. (1994). How hospital linen and laundry services are provided. *J. Hosp. Infect.* 27: 219–235. https://doi.org/10.1016/0195-6701(94)90130-9.

Belkin, N.L. (1997). The evolution of the surgical mask: filtering efficiency versus effectiveness. *Infect. Cont. Hosp. Epidemiol.* 18: 49–57. https://doi.org/10.2307/30141964.

Bingham, J., Abell, G., Kienast, L. et al. (2016). Health care worker hand contamination at critical moments in outpatient care settings. *Am. J. Infect. Cont.* 44: 1198–1202. https://doi.org/10.1016/j.ajic.2016.04.208.

British Standards Institute (2000). Medical gloves for single use. Requirements and testing for freedom from holes. https://landingpage.bsigroup.com/LandingPage/Undated?UPI=00000000001402196

Büchler, A.C., Dangel, M., Frei, R. et al. (2021). Does high adherence to contact precautions lead to low in-hospital transmission of multi-drug-resistant micro-organisms in the endemic setting? *J. Hosp. Infect.* 116: 53–59. https://doi.org/10.1016/j.jhin.2021.07.002.

Burdon, D.W. and Whitby, J.L. (1967). Contamination of hospital disinfectants with pseudomonas species. *Br. Med. J.* 2: 153–155. https://doi.org/10.1136/bmj.2.5545.153.

Casewell, M. and Phillips, I. (1977). Hands as route of transmission for klebsiella species. *BMJ* 2: 1315–1317. https://doi.org/10.1136/bmj.2.6098.1315.

Centers for Disease Control and Prevention (2021). Environmental Cleaning Procedures. www.cdc.gov/hai/prevent/resource-limited/cleaning-procedures.html

Curran, E.T. (2015). Standard precautions: what is meant and what is not. *J. Hosp. Infect.* 90: 10–11. https://doi.org/10.1016/j.jhin.2014.12.020.

Dancer, S.J. and Kramer, A. (2019). Four steps to clean hospitals: LOOK, PLAN, CLEAN and DRY. *J. Hosp. Infect.* 103: e1–e8. https://doi.org/10.1016/j.jhin.2018.12.015.

Department of Health (2013). (HTM 07–01) Management and disposal of healthcare waste. www.england.nhs.uk/publication/ management-and-disposal-of-healthcare-waste-htm-07-01

Deshpande, A., Mana, T.S.C., Cadnum, J.L. et al. (2014). Evaluation of a sporicidal peracetic acid/hydrogen peroxide-based daily disinfectant cleaner. *Infect. Cont. Hosp. Epidemiol.* 35: 1414–1416. https://doi.org/10.1086/678416.

Gould, D.J., Drey, N.S., Chudleigh, J. et al. (2018). Isolating infectious patients: organizational, clinical, and ethical issues. *Am. J. Infect. Cont.* 46: e65–e69. https:// doi.org/10.1016/j.ajic.2018.05.024.

Halden, R.U., Lindeman, A.E., Aiello, A.E. et al. (2017). The Florence statement on triclosan and triclocarban. *Environ. Health Perspect.* 125: 064501. https://doi. org/10.1289/EHP1788.

Havill, N.L., Havill, H.L., Mangione, E. et al. (2011). Cleanliness of portable medical equipment disinfected by nursing staff. *Am. J. Infect. Cont.* 39: 602–604. https://doi. org/10.1016/j.ajic.2010.10.030.

Hayes-Lattin, B., Leis, J.F., and Maziarz, R.T. (2005). Isolation in the allogeneic transplant environment: how protective is it? *Bone Marrow. Transp.* 36: 373–381. https://doi.org/10.1038/sj.bmt.1705040.

Health Act (2006). www.legislation.gov.uk/ukpga/2006/28/contents

Health and Safety at Work Act (1974). www.legislation.gov.uk/ukpga/1974/37/contents

Jacobson, G., Thiele, J.E., McCune, J.H., and Farrell, L.D. (1985). Handwashing: ring-wearing and number of microorganisms. *Nurs. Res.* 34: 186–188.

Jain, S., Clezy, K., and McLaws, M.-L. (2017). Glove: Use for safety or overuse? *Am. J. Infect. Cont.* 45: 1407–1410. https://doi.org/10.1016/j.ajic.2017.08.029.

Kampf, G. (2018). Efficacy of ethanol against viruses in hand disinfection. *J. Hosp. Infect.* 98: 331–338. https://doi.org/10.1016/j.jhin.2017.08.025.

Kanamori, H., Rutala, W.A., and Weber, D.J. (2017). The role of patient care items as a fomite in healthcare-associated outbreaks and infection prevention. *Clin. Infect. Dis.* 65: 1412–1419. https://doi.org/10.1093/cid/cix462.

Klompas, M., Baker, M., and Rhee, C. (2021). What is an aerosol-generating procedure? *JAMA Surg.* 156: 113. https://doi.org/10.1001/jamasurg.2020.6643.

Lancet (2015). Health care-associated infections in the USA. *Lancet.* 385: 304. https:// doi.org/10.1016/S0140-6736(15)60101-5.

Ledwoch, K., Dancer, S.J., Otter, J.A. et al. (2021). How dirty is your QWERTY? The risk of healthcare pathogen transmission from computer keyboards. *J. Hosp. Infect.* 112: 31–36. https://doi.org/10.1016/j.jhin.2021.02.021.

Livshiz-Riven, I., Borer, A., Nativ, R. et al. (2015). Relationship between shared patient care items and healthcare-associated infections: a systematic review. *Int. J. Nurs. Stud.* 52: 380–392. https://doi.org/10.1016/j.ijnurstu.2014.06.001.

Lopman, B., Gastañaduy, P., Park, G.W. et al. (2012). Environmental transmission of norovirus gastroenteritis. *Curr. Opin. Virol.* 2: 96–102. https://doi.org/10.1016/j.coviro.2011.11.005.

Marples, R.R. and Towers, A.G. (1979). A laboratory model for the investigation of contact transfer of micro-organisms. *J. Hyg.* 82: 237–248. https://doi.org/10.1017/s0022172400025651.

McDonnell, G. and Burke, P. (2011). Disinfection: is it time to reconsider Spaulding? *J. Hosp. Infect.* 78: 163–170. https://doi.org/10.1016/j.jhin.2011.05.002.

Medicines and Healthcare products Regulatory Agency (2021). Single-use medical devices: implications and consequences of re-use. www.gov.uk/government/publications/single-use-medical-devices-implications-and-consequences-of-re-use

Mitchell, A., Spencer, M., and Edmiston, C. (2015). Role of healthcare apparel and other healthcare textiles in the transmission of pathogens: a review of the literature. *J. Hosp. Infect.* 90: 285–292. https://doi.org/10.1016/j.jhin.2015.02.017.

Moolenaar, R.L., Crutcher, J.M., Joaquin, V.H.S. et al. (2000). A prolonged outbreak of *pseudomonas aeruginosa* in a neonatal intensive care unit: did staff fingernails play a role in disease transmission? *Infect. Cont. Hosp. Epidemiol.* 21: 80–85. https://doi.org/10.1086/501739.

National Audit Office (2000). The Management and Control of Hospital Acquired Infection in Acute NHS Trusts in England. www.nao.org.uk/report/the-management-and-control-of-hospital-acquired-infection-in-acute-nhs-trusts-in-england

National Institute for Health and Care Excellence (2012). Healthcare-associated infections: prevention and control in primary and community care. www.nice.org.uk/guidance/cg139

Otter, J.A., Yezli, S., and French, G.L. (2011). The role played by contaminated surfaces in the transmission of nosocomial pathogens. *Infect. Cont. Hosp. Epidemiol.* 32: 687–699. https://doi.org/10.1086/660363.

Patel, S.N., Murray-Leonard, J., and Wilson, A.P.R. (2006). Laundering of hospital staff uniforms at home. *J. Hosp. Infect.* 62: 89–93. https://doi.org/10.1016/j.jhin.2005.06.002.

Pittet, D., Allegranzi, B., Sax, H. et al. (2006). Evidence-based model for hand transmission during patient care and the role of improved practices. *Lancet. Infect. Dis.* 6: 641–652. https://doi.org/10.1016/S1473-3099(06)70600-4.

Polkinghorne, A. and Branley, J. (2020). Evidence for decontamination of single-use filtering facepiece respirators. *J. Hosp. Infect.* 105: 663–669. https://doi.org/10.1016/j.jhin.2020.05.032.

Royal College of Nursing. n.d. Skin health. www.rcn.org.uk/clinical-topics/infection-prevention-and-control/skin-health

Russell, A.D. and Day, M.J. (1993). Antibacterial activity of chlorhexidine. *J. Hosp. Infect.* 25: 229–238. https://doi.org/10.1016/0195-6701(93)90109-D.

Sax, H., Allegranzi, B., Uçkay, I. et al. (2007). 'My five moments for hand hygiene': a user-centred design approach to understand, train, monitor and report hand hygiene. *J. Hosp. Infect.* 67: 9–21. https://doi.org/10.1016/j.jhin.2007.06.004.

Schabrun, S. and Chipchase, L. (2006). Healthcare equipment as a source of nosocomial infection: a systematic review. *J. Hosp. Infect.* 63: 239–245. https://doi.org/10.1016/j.jhin.2005.10.013.

Simmonds Cavanagh, R. (2021). Viability of hospital pathogens on mobile phone. *Am. J. Infect. Cont.* 50: 787–791. https://doi.org/10.1016/j.ajic.2021.11.003.

Stelfox, H.T. (2003). Safety of patients isolated for infection control. *JAMA* 290: 1899. https://doi.org/10.1001/jama.290.14.1899.

Tanner, J. and Parkinson, H. (2006). Double gloving to reduce surgical cross-infection. *Cochrane Database Syst. Rev.* 3: CD003087. https://doi.org/10.1002/14651858. CD003087.pub2.

Tanner, J., Gould, D., Jenkins, P. et al. (2012). A fresh look at preoperative body washing. *J. Infect. Prevent.* 13: 11–15. https://doi.org/10.1177/1757177411428095.

The Control of Substances Hazardous to Health Regulations. 2002. www.legislation. gov.uk/uksi/2002/2677/regulation/7/made

Weber, D.J., Rutala, W.A., and Sickbert-Bennett, E.E. (2007). Outbreaks associated with contaminated antiseptics and disinfectants. *Antimicrob. Agents Chemother.* 51: 4217–4224. https://doi.org/10.1128/AAC.00138-07.

Weber, D.J., Kanamori, H., and Rutala, W.A. (2016a). 'No touch' technologies for environmental decontamination: focus on ultraviolet devices and hydrogen peroxide systems. *Curr. Opin. Infect. Dis.* 29: 424–431. https://doi.org/10.1097/QCO.0000000000000284.

Weber, D.J., Rutala, W.A., Anderson, D.J. et al. (2016b). Effectiveness of ultraviolet devices and hydrogen peroxide systems for terminal room decontamination: focus on clinical trials. *Am. J. Infect. Cont.* 44: e77–e84. https://doi.org/10.1016/j.ajic.2015.11.015.

Wilcox, M.H., Ahir, H., Coia, J.E. et al. (2017). Impact of recurrent Clostridium difficile infection: hospitalization and patient quality of life. *J. Antimicrob. Chemother.* 72: 2647–2656. https://doi.org/10.1093/jac/dkx174.

Wilkinson, M.A.C., Ormandy, K., Bradley, C.R., and Hines, J. (2018). Comparison of the efficacy and drying times of liquid, gel and foam formats of alcohol-based hand rubs. *J. Hosp. Infect.* 98: 359–364. https://doi.org/10.1016/j.jhin.2017.09.024.

Wilson, J.A., Loveday, H.P., Hoffman, P.N., and Pratt, R.J. (2007). Uniform: an evidence review of the microbiological significance of uniforms and uniform policy in the prevention and control of healthcare-associated infections. Report to the Department of Health (England). *J. Hosp. Infect.* 66: 301–307. https://doi.org/10.1016/j.jhin.2007.03.026.

World Health Organization (n.d.). WHO guidelines on hand hygiene in health care. www.who.int/publications-detail-redirect/9789241597906

7

Healthcare-associated Infection

Healthcare-associated Infection

Healthcare-associated infection (HCAI) is defined as any infection contracted through treatment or contact with a health or social care setting or as a result of healthcare received in the community (National Institute for Health and Care Excellence 2016). It may originate outside an institution, be imported by patients, visitors or staff and then be transmitted to inpatients, residents or health workers. Clusters of staphylococcal infection tend to arise in hospitals whereas hospital outbreaks of norovirus ('winter vomiting') frequently originate in the community.

Healthcare-associated infection is the most common adverse event reported in healthcare (World Health Organization 2011). It is not a recent phenomenon but the pathogens responsible have changed since the second half of the eighteenth century when it was first identified as a problem (Selwyn 1991). HCAI is a major problem globally but the burden is highest in low-income countries where infection prevention practices suffer through lack of resources and there is a need to improve surveillance (Allegranzi et al. 2011).

The Consequences of Healthcare-associated Infection

Healthcare-associated infection causes avoidable morbidity, avoidable mortality and delays recovery. Over 4 million patients in Europe develop at least one HCAI annually and approximately 37000 die as a result (European Centre for Disease Prevention and Control 2013). Numbers are higher in low-income countries and the consequences are more serious.

Healthcare-associated infection increases the costs of healthcare. 'Hotel' costs increase through longer stay and readmission. Other factors contributing to increased expenditure include prescriptions for additional antimicrobial drugs,

Infection Prevention and Control in Healthcare Settings,
First Edition. Edward Purssell and Dinah Gould.

analgesia and consumables (e.g. dressing materials). Estimated costs vary. According to one source (Guest et al. 2020), HCAI costs the UK National Health Service over £1 billion annually, amounting to 1% of the total budget for healthcare. A recently conducted incidence study estimated that HCAI costs the UK £774 million annually (Manoukian et al. 2021). Individually, bloodstream infections are the most expensive but collectively, surgical site infections add most to the overall costs of HCAI because they are so common.

Other consequences of HCAI are decreased patient satisfaction, reduced public confidence in healthcare and increased risk of antimicrobial resistance (National Institute for Health and Care Excellence 2016).

Risk Factors

Risk of HCAI is increased in patients who are immunocompromised; suffer from chronic conditions, especially diabetes; have undergone an invasive procedure; are admitted to a critical care unit; and are older (Rodríguez-Acelas et al. 2017). Residents in nursing homes are at risk of acquiring and spreading HCAI (Box 7.1).

Preventing Healthcare-associated Infection

Attitudes towards HCAI have changed in recent years. Originally, HCAI was regarded as an inevitable risk of healthcare but today it is considered preventable (The Lancet 2015). Strategies include applying good fundamental infection prevention precautions such as hand hygiene; sensible use of gloves; isolating infectious patients; avoiding unnecessary use of antimicrobials to reduce the risks of antimicrobial resistance; and educating staff. Educating patients and the public is

---

Box 7.1 Healthcare-Associated Infections in Nursing Homes

Residents in nursing homes are at high risk of developing infection because of their age, likelihood of suffering from chronic conditions and loss of functional capacity, compounded by communal living and frequent contact with health workers, including those who attend to patients in other settings (e.g. at home or in community-based clinics). Colonisation frequently occurs, including by antimicrobially resistant organisms. Nursing homes frequently operate as reservoirs of HCAI and because they are very likely to move across sectors from nursing home to hospital and back, residents are likely to transfer pathogens across sectors.

Source: Adapted from Ludden et al. (2015).

also essential to avoid unnecessary antimicrobial prescribing for viral infections that will resolve without treatment.

The first step towards prevention is quantification of the problem (prevalence and incidence studies) and surveillance (monitoring).

Surveillance

Surveillance is the systematic, ongoing collection, collation and analysis of health-care data and feedback to staff to prompt appropriate action (World Health Organization 2011).The main purposes of surveillance are shown in Table 7.1.

Surveillance is the cornerstone of strategies to combat infectious disease. Population-based data inform public health policy while feedback encourages scrutiny and benchmarking of local against national data and identifies variations in infection rates that may in turn lead to scrutiny of local practice, remedial action and evaluation.

The value of surveillance was first demonstrated in the United States, where hospitals cannot be licensed without evidence that effective infection control policies are in place. A major study involving 338 hospitals, called the Study of the Efficacy of Nosocomial Infection Control (SENIC) project, demonstrated that surveillance with feedback to clinical staff could reduce HCAI by 32% (Haley et al. 1985).

Today, many sources of surveillance data are used. They include information from laboratory diagnoses, outbreak reports and serological tests. In many countries, surveillance is undertaken for key pathogens responsible for HCAI at national level. In the UK, surveillance programmes are in place for bloodstream infections caused by methicillin-resistant *Staphylococcus aureus* (MRSA),

Table 7.1 Purposes of surveillance.

- Establish baseline infection rates.
- Understand patterns and trends of infection within a population.
- Detect outbreaks or the emergence of a new pathogen.
- Estimate the magnitude of an infection.
- Identify the resources needed during and after a public health emergency.
- Evaluate public health programmes and infection prevention measures.
- Determine the nature and history of a disease.
- Monitor changes in infectious agents.
- Set research priorities.
- Support public health planning.
- Monitor changes in public health practice.

Source: Adapted from Thacker and Berkelman (1988).

methicillin-sensitive *Staphylococcus aureus* (MSSA), *Escherichia coli, Klebsiella* spp., *Pseudomonas* spp. and *Clostridioides difficile*. Surveillance gives infection prevention and control teams greater insight into the patterns of infection occurring in healthcare settings and draws attention to potential outbreaks. In addition to mandatory surveillance required at national level, many NHS trusts undertake additional surveillance activities.

Prevalence Studies

Prevalence is the number of people with an infection at a specific point in time (point prevalence) or over a specified period of time (period prevalence). Prevalence studies include both new and existing cases and are influenced by speed of recovery. The prevalence of HCAI appears greater if data collection takes place over a long period of time as patients usually stay in hospital longer, overestimating the number of cases reported. Estimates of prevalence for HCAI range from 5% to 10%. Numbers are highest in acute care where up to 3% of patients can be affected. Large-scale prevalence studies are challenging to organise. In the UK, the most recent statistics were compiled in 2011 (Public Health England 2012). Overall, 6.4% of inpatients in acute hospitals in England had at least one HCAI. Respiratory infections were the most common, accounting for 23% of all HCAIs reported, followed by urinary infections (17%), surgical site infections (16%), clinical sepsis (11%), gastrointestinal (9%) and bloodstream infections (7%).

Despite their limitations, prevalence studies are frequently used in service planning and to indicate the burden of disease and can have very positive outcomes. A series of midwifery-led point prevalence studies in women who had undergone caesarean sections in one NHS trust raised awareness of the high risk of surgical site infection, prompting changes that reduced infection rates from 26% to 8% (Baxter 2021).

Incidence Studies

Incidence is the number of new cases of a condition arising over a specified period of time in a population. Incidence studies provide more comprehensive information about the risk of developing infection than prevalence studies and are used to identify increases in transmission. The findings help determine which interventions should be undertaken to reduce spread. Incidence studies are more expensive and challenging to conduct than prevalence studies and for HCAI are usually undertaken for individual services or units, especially those where patients are considered at high risk.

The overall incidence of HCAI in the UK is estimated at 6%. A recent incidence study undertaken in two hospitals in Scotland over 12 months reported 250 cases of HCAI per 100 000 acute hospital beds (Box 7.2). The most frequently reported organisms in this incidence study were *E. coli, S. aureus* and norovirus. The

Box 7.2   Incidence of Healthcare-Associated Infection Reported in the Cost of Nosocomial Infection Study in Scotland

Site of infection	Cases per 100 000 occupied acute bed days
Urinary tract	51.2
Bloodstream	44.7
Lower respiratory tract	42.2
Gastrointestinal infection	39.2
Surgical site infection	35.3
Other HCAIs	13.6

Source: Adapted from Stewart et al. (2021b).

increased length of stay for patients who developed HCAI was 7.8 days (Stewart et al. 2021c). Risk factors were increased age, emergency admission, co-morbidity (cancer, cardiovascular disease, renal disease, diabetes) and admission to an intensive care unit (Stewart et al. 2021a).

Clinical Audit

Clinical audit is defined as a quality improvement process that seeks to improve patient care and outcomes through the systematic review of care compared to explicit, predetermined criteria and the implementation of change (Scrivener 2004). It is a well-established component of infection prevention programmes where it is frequently used to monitor and improve health workers' adherence to guidelines and protocols and the impact of new ones (Hay 2006). For some activities and issues, clinical audit takes place on an occasional basis when particular problems arise while others are routinely undertaken. Organisations vary in the number and scope of routine audits. In many countries, including the UK, hand hygiene and antimicrobial stewardship programmes are routinely audited across the health economy. Audits of the use of indwelling urinary catheters, management of intravenous lines, disposal of contaminated waste and occupational health policies (e.g. uptake of hepatitis B vaccination, screening after exposure to tuberculosis) are also undertaken routinely in many organisations.

Hand Hygiene Audit

Most HCAIs are spread by direct contact via hands (Pittet et al. 2006). Hand hygiene breaks the chain of infection, reduces the numbers of bacteria present on hands and is important for aesthetic reasons (Pittet et al. 2006). Most hand hygiene campaigns increase adherence although their effectiveness is usually short-lived and there is only modest evidence that they prevent HCAI (Gould et al. 2017).

Hand hygiene is usually audited by directly observing practice and the data are collected by manual documentation in line with WHO recommendations (World Health Organization 2009). This approach has been criticised because audit periods are usually brief (15–30 minutes), providing only a snapshot of practice at a single point in time, variation between auditors results in lack of standardised data and health workers increase hand hygiene frequency, temporarily inflating performance in response to becoming aware of being observed (Hawthorne effect). Advantages are that auditors witness errors in 'real time' and can plan educational interventions. Many organisations also monitor consumption of hand hygiene products but unless accompanied by observation, this is an unreliable measure because of spillage, wastage and use for unintended purposes.

Electronic automated hand hygiene monitoring systems obtain data more efficiently than manual audit, generate standardised data allowing meaningful comparisons across clinical areas and overcome the Hawthorne effect. Disadvantages are the expense of purchase, installation and maintenance, concerns from staff anxious about who will have access to the data and how the information will be used and inaccuracies related to system design and function – in some systems, proximity of the health worker to the bedside may register a hand hygiene opportunity which is ignored if the intention is to observe a sleeping patient without disturbing them. Electronic systems do not obviate the need for occasional manual audit to remind health workers about the importance of hand hygiene, identify where errors occur and institute education (Gould et al. 2017).

Pathogens Causing Healthcare-associated Infection

The main groups of pathogens responsible for HCAI are shown in Table 7.2.

Table 7.2   Pathogens frequently responsible for healthcare-associated infection.

- *Staphylococcus aureus*
- *Staphylococcus epidermidis*

Clostridioides difficile

Gram-negative bacilli, e.g. *E. coli, Klebsiella* spp., *P. mirabilis, Acinetobacter baumannii, Serratia*

Norovirus

Staphylococcus aureus

Staphylococcus aureus is a Gram-positive bacterium that produces the enzyme coagulase which is able to clot plasma. *S. aureus* is carried in the nose, throat, axillae, toe webs and perineum of 30–50% of healthy people without causing clinical infection. Asymptomatic carriage is clinically significant because the bacteria can be transferred to susceptible sites (e.g. from the nose to a wound) or from an asymptomatic carrier to a vulnerable patient, resulting in cross-infection. Skin lesions such as chronic wounds or cannula insertion points can become heavily colonised and are particularly likely to operate as reservoirs. Transmission is by direct and indirect contact, mainly via hands and fomites.

Staphylococcus aureus is the most common cause of pyogenic (pus-forming) infection. It causes boils, abscesses, septic fingers, styes, impetigo (inflammatory skin condition with pustules) and sticky eyes in neonates. In hospital, *S. aureus* is a major pathogen responsible for wound infections, bronchopneumonia and bloodstream infections (Tong et al. 2015). Some strains produce toxins that cause extensive cellular damage, e.g. toxic shock syndrome (TSS) associated with the use of vaginal tampons and food intoxication.

The statutory bodies in the UK have conducted mandatory surveillance of MSSA bloodstream infections with monthly reporting since 2011.

Methicillin-resistant Staphylococcal Infection

Methicillin-resistant *Staphylococcus aureus* emerged in the 1960s. It carries a gene conferring resistance to β-lactam antibiotics including flucloxacillin and also to cephalosporins and carbapenem. It causes the same types of infections as methicillin-sensitive *S. aureus*, is spread in the same way and is not usually more virulent but causes problems because infections are difficult to treat with routinely used antibiotics and can be extremely difficult to eradicate. Most people become asymptomatic carriers, especially if they are healthy, but operate as reservoirs and are a risk to seriously ill patients. MRSA was a serious problem in healthcare premises throughout the 1980s and 1990s worldwide. The statutory bodies in the UK have conducted mandatory surveillance of MRSA bloodstream infections with monthly reporting since 2005.

Since 2008 there has been a dramatic decline in the number of reported cases of MRSA but it is still responsible for infections that are serious and readily transmissible. The guidelines for infection and prevention and control in the UK were updated in 2021 (Coia et al. 2021). Risk-based screening for MRSA is undertaken for new hospital admissions. Those testing positive are required to undergo decolonisation (Box 7.3). Swabs should be obtained from at least two sites (e.g. nose, perineum, wound, entry site of an indwelling device).

Patients who have undergone decolonisation treatment can be screened again 2–3 days later to determine whether it was effective but surgery should not be

---

Box 7.3   Example Topical Decolonisation Programme for Patients Testing Positive for Methicillin-Resistant *S. aureus*

- Daily shower or bed-bath with a topical agent, e.g. Octenisan®, chlorhexidine gluconate body wash 4% or chlorhexidine gluconate body wipes 2% for five days.
- Hair wash with the topical agent on two occasions during the decolonisation programme (recommended days 2 and 4). Usual styling products can then be applied.
- Application of mupirocin ointment 2% to external nares twice a day over five days.
- Daily change of flannels, towels, personal items of clothing and bedclothes advisable.
- Where patients have dermatitis, eczema or any other skin condition, this should also be treated.

---

delayed if a positive test is obtained. In the event of an outbreak not controlled despite the introduction of infection prevention and control measures, staff may be screened, liaising with the occupational health department if possible. The guidelines recommend developing local policies for staff decolonisation programmes and whether or not staff should be allowed to work. Environmental sampling should only be undertaken if an outbreak occurs, not routinely. Terminal cleaning with hydrogen peroxide vapour or ultraviolet light technology is recommended when a patient with MRSA is discharged.

Decolonisation is effective long term in 50–60% cases but may have to be repeated if patients are readmitted. Adherence to the regimen can be poor for patients undertaking decolonisation at home before elective admission because topical application can have a drying effect on skin and hair. Patients carrying MRSA have reported feelings of stigma (blame for their condition, exclusion and rejection) and poor mental health which can be compounded by isolation (Rump et al. 2017). The updated MRSA guidelines emphasise the importance of providing information and support for patients who screen positive for MRSA. Plasmid-mediated resistance to mupirocin has been reported and is associated with decolonisation failure (Patel et al. 2009).

Treatment of Methicillin-resistant *Staphylococcus aureus*

Traditionally, the drug of choice for MRSA has been the glycopeptide vancomycin; newer therapies include clindamycin, minocycline, linezolid or doxycycline which avoid the toxicities associated with vancomycin. Combined therapy may be tried if single therapy has not been effective. Rifampicin and sodium fusidate may be effective together. Other drugs include linezolid, quinupristin combined with dalfopristin, and tigecycline. Topical mupirocin is usually used to eradicate skin and nasal carriage in both patients and staff but other drugs, such as cream containing chlorhexidine and neomycin, are needed for mupirocin-resistant MRSA.

Vancomycin-resistant MRSA was first detected in the United States in 2002. Its prevalence is increasing, especially in Africa and Asia. Stringent infection prevention measures including antimicrobial stewardship are essential to contain global spread (Wu et al. 2021).

Community-acquired Methicillin-resistant *Staphylococcus aureus*

Community-acquired methicillin-resistant *S. aureus* (CA-MRSA) infections are defined as MRSA infections occurring in otherwise healthy populations lacking risk factors. Initially, most reports were of infections in children but infections have since been reported in sports teams, prisons and among healthy people in the community lacking risk factors. CA-MRSA mainly causes skin and soft tissue infections but serious, life-threatening, invasive infections such as bacteraemia and necrotising pneumonia have also been described (Maree et al. 2007). Many CA-MRSA strains carry genes for Panton-Valentine leukocidin (PVL) which is an exotoxin lethal to leucocytes able to cause tissue necrosis. This virulence factor appears to be responsible for the ability to cause invasive infections.

Occasional outbreaks of CA-MRSA have been reported in hospitals imported from the community (McManus et al. 2021). Most infections have been limited to localised areas of skin and soft tissues but occasionally more serious infections occur, sometimes resulting in mortality. The bacteria are able to survive on different surfaces and fomites are likely to be important in transmission (Desai et al. 2011).

Coagulase-negative Staphylococci

Some species of staphylococci do not produce coagulase and are described as coagulase-negative staphylococci (CNSs). *Staphylococcus epidermidis* is the CNS most frequently responsible for HCAI. It is a commensal carried in the nose and on the skin of healthy people. Many of these infections are related to the formation of biofilms (Box 7.4).

Coagulase-negative staphylococci in biofilms can cause serious infections involving peritoneal dialysis catheters, prosthetic heart valves and orthopaedic implants (Box 7.5). If they gain access to the bloodstream via intravascular devices, septicaemia results. Infections are difficult to eradicate because CNSs are naturally resistant to many antibiotics and the biofilm protects them from the host defence mechanisms (Becker et al. 2014).

Box 7.4   Biofilms

Planktonic micro-organisms living freely in the environment can attach to surfaces where they cover themselves in a slimy glycoprotein matrix called a biofilm. Biofilms can develop over the tissues (e.g. dental plaque) and over indwelling and inserted medical devices (e.g. urinary catheters, pacemakers). The biofilm provides physical protection from host defences and antimicrobial drugs, enabling the micro-organisms to reproduce and form a large colony. These conditions are optimal for plasmid exchange and the presence of the biofilm encourages the development of antimicrobial resistance. Biofilms can become highly complex, eventually harbouring different types of micro-organisms. As the biofilm matures, micro-organisms may seed to other parts of the body.

Source: Adapted from Donlan (2001).

Box 7.5   Biofilms and Implanted Medical Devices

Biofilm formation leading to serious infection is becoming an increasing hazard for patients who require implanted medical devices. Many of these patients are already at high risk because they are immunocompromised. Rates of infection following prosthetic joint replacement are very low but as the population ages and more people require this type of surgery and live with their implanted device for longer, the total number of those who develop infections will increase correspondingly.

Source: Adapted from Uçkay et al. (2009).

Clostridioides difficile

Clostridioides difficile is an anaerobic, Gram-positive spore-forming bacillus. Patients become colonised by ingesting bacteria and through direct and indirect contact via hands and fomites. The inoculating dose is small and environmental reservoirs are common. The bacterium releases toxins causing diarrhoea that ranges from mild to severe and can be life threatening. The toxins disrupt the ecology of the normal bowel flora, usually after the patient has received broad-spectrum antibiotics, particularly ampicillin, clindamycin or the cephalosporins. Other risk factors include increasing age, co-morbidity and taking proton pump inhibitors.

Clostridioides difficile is the most common cause of infectious diarrhoea in hospitals and nursing homes and can result in high levels of morbidity and mortality, contributing to the costs of healthcare. Symptoms usually commence when the patient is taking antibiotics but the incubation period is very variable. As a result, the condition may not be diagnosed until after they have left hospital and the source of the infection is often unknown. Symptoms frequently return after treatment because spores persist in the gut. Diagnosis is confirmed by the presence of the toxin in the faeces.

The incidence of *C. difficile* is increasing. Globally, it represents a major infection prevention challenge and a drain on healthcare resources, and decreases quality of life (Wilcox et al. 2017). Environmental contamination plays an important role in transmission. High-touch surfaces (e.g. bed tables, call buttons) can operate as reservoirs and spread occurs by direct and indirect contact via hands and fomites. Deep cleaning (e.g. hydrogen peroxide systems) is necessary to control outbreaks because spores persist for long periods in the environment. There is increased risk of infection if the patient is admitted to a bedspace formerly occupied by a patient with *C. difficile*. Antibiotic policies to control the use of broad-spectrum antibiotics and early discontinuation of antibiotics are important factors in control.

The number of outbreaks caused by *C. difficile* has increased in recent years and cases have become more complex (Leffler and Lamont 2015). About 0.5% percent of the population carry the bacteria (Manzoor et al. 2017) and carriage rate is higher among those recently discharged from hospital.

Streptococcal Infections

Streptococci are Gram-positive, chain-forming cocci that do not sporulate. The different serotypes are classified into Lancefield groups which aid laboratory diagnosis. There are two groups.

- Alpha-haemolytic streptococci
- Beta-haemolytic streptococci

Streptococcus pyogenes (Group A Streptococcus)

Group A streptococcus, also called group A streptococci (GAS) or *Streptococcus pyogenes*, causes a wide range of infections, some mild (e.g. sore throats, skin infections) and some invasive life-threatening diseases including puerperal fever and necrotising fasciitis (Box 7.6).

Group A streptococci spread through the tissues by releasing toxins, resulting in generalised infection. Scarlet fever is pharyngitis with a rash induced by the toxin. The toxins may also induce hypersensitivity reactions, for example glomerulonephritis and rheumatic fever developing up to four weeks after infection. Transmission is via respiratory droplets, discharge from skin lesions and via fomites. Environmental reservoirs are common and in some outbreaks bedside

---

Box 7.6   Necrotising Fasciitis

Necrotising fasciitis is a rare but serious infection involving the subcutane-ous tissues and fascia of the skin. It is caused by a range of pathogens including Group A streptococcus, clostridia, Gram-negative bacteria and fungi. It is a rare condition but the incidence is increasing and in the UK, approximately 500 new cases are reported annually. The organisms travel through the subcutaneous tissues causing erythema and swelling, damaging blood vessels and causing disproportionate pain. As the infection progresses, oedema develops in response to tissue damage accompanied by haemor-rhagic swelling. Necrotising fasciitis can occur at any anatomical location but is most likely to affect the perineum, lower extremities, postoperative wounds, abdomen, oral cavity and neck. Patients require aggressive debride-ment of the affected area and intravenous antimicrobials, depending on the causative organism. Mortality is over 20% because of the severity of the condition and because the early signs and symptoms are non-specific, delaying diagnosis.

Source: Adapted from Diab et al. (2020).

---

curtains have been identified as the source of infection (Mahida et al. 2014). Asymptomatic carriage in the throat is common, especially in children. The bacteria have also been isolated from the nose, vagina and perianal area. Invasive Group A streptococcus (iGAS) can cause serious infection sporadically and in clusters in the community, hospitals and nursing homes (Curran 2012). Mortality is high, especially in older people with chronic conditions.

Control measures during outbreaks include screening staff to exclude carriers and isolating infected patients until antibiotic therapy has become effective. Deep environmental cleaning to remove reservoirs is recommended to control out-breaks (Steer et al. 2012). GAS, iGAS and scarlet fever are notifiable diseases.

Streptococcus agalactiae (Group B Streptococcus)

This organism can cause serious infection in neonates. Most people acquire immunity by the time they reach adulthood but the bacteria live harmlessly in the gut and female urogenital tract and can be transmitted to the baby before or dur-ing delivery. Transmission can occur from an index (first identified) case to other neonates, resulting in a cluster of infections (MacFarquhar et al. 2010).

Streptococcus pneumoniae

Streptococcus pneumoniae (pneumococcus) is a respiratory tract commensal able to cause a wide range of mild infections and severe life-threatening invasive disease. Infections can be acquired in hospital but the majority are community acquired (see Chapter 10).

Viridans Group Streptococci

The viridans group of streptococci are commensals in the mouth, gut and urogenital tract. They can cause infective endocarditis via the bloodstream in patients with previously damaged heart valves. Infection has also been reported following dental treatment.

Enterococci

Enterococci are Gram-positive bacteria forming part of the commensal flora in the large intestine. They can survive in the environment for long periods and may persist after cleaning. The two most important species are *Enterococcus faecalis* and *E. faecium*. Most enterococcal infections are caused by *E. faecalis*. Enterococci are weakly pathogenic but can cause serious infections (e.g. septicaemia, endocarditis, wound infections, urinary tract infections and occasionally pneumonia) in vulnerable patients, especially those with indwelling devices. Patients in intensive care and specialist units (e.g. renal, haematology, liver units) are most often infected (Cookson et al. 2006). Transmission is by contact with contaminated surfaces.

Key infection prevention measures include contact precautions, cohorting during outbreaks and surveillance of patients at risk. Enterococci are intrinsically resistant to some antibiotics and the mainstay of treatment has been vancomycin. Vancomycin resistance emerged in the 1980s and vancomycin-resistant enterococci (VRE) are now a global problem, affecting the most vulnerable patients, increasing length of hospital stay and frequently causing outbreaks. Mortality is 17–50% (Monteserin and Larson 2016).

Gram-Negative Infections

Gram negative bacteria are opportunistic bacteria able to survive in minute traces of moisture with very little nourishment. They include coliforms, *Acinetobacter* and *Pseudomonas*.

- *Klebsiella* spp.
- *E. coli*
- *Proteus mirabilis*
- *Acinetobacter baumanni*
- *Serratia*
- *Burkholderia cepacia*

These bacteria multiply rapidly in warm, damp environments and are a leading cause of HCAI. Environmental reservoirs can harbour large numbers of bacteria, sometimes leading to outbreaks (Aranega-Bou et al. 2019). They are frequently isolated on the hands of staff, patients' skin and items in close patient contact. They may ascend to the bladder, colonise the gut and appear in the faeces, and can be transferred from the oropharynx to the lower respiratory passages, causing pneumonia (Desai et al. 2016). Cross-infection occurs readily and over the years many outbreaks have been reported, especially in intensive care and neonatal units (Luo et al. 2021). Coliforms are naturally resistant to many antimicrobials.

Strict adherence to the fundamental principles of infection prevention and control is necessary, including hand hygiene and avoiding environmental contamination to prevent reservoirs developing. Problems are compounded by the ability of coliforms to develop resistance to antimicrobials. Reservoirs include other patients who are infected or colonised. Transmission occurs readily via hands and fomites.

Guidelines for the prevention and control of multidrug-resistant Gram-negative bacteria emphasise the importance of sound fundamental infection prevention measures, isolating patients in single rooms where possible, cohort nursing in outbreak situations and deep cleaning when patients are discharged using a hydrogen peroxide system if available. Screening is recommended in high-risk areas (e.g. intensive care) (Wilson et al. 2016).

Coliforms can cause significant problems outside hospital. *E. coli* is the most common cause of urinary infections in the community and is also the most common organism causing bacteraemia in many countries, resulting in high risk of morbidity and mortality. Infection is usually localised, often originating in the urinary tract. Risk factors include poorly managed urinary infections and urinary catheterisation (Abernethy et al. 2017). National mandatory surveillance for *E. coli* bloodstream infections was introduced in the UK in 2011 demonstrates that 80% of cases originate outside hospital.

Carbapenemase-producing Enterobacteriaceae
Enterobacteriales, particularly *Klebsiella* spp. and *E. coli,* can develop plasmid-mediated resistance to carbapenem. Carbapenemase-producing enterobacteriales (CPEs) are now endemic in some hospitals and there is evidence that waste water is an important reservoir (Mathers et al. 2018). CPEs constitute a major global health problem and the number of outbreaks in hospitals and nursing homes is increasing (Legeay et al. 2019), operating as a drain on healthcare resources (Otter et al. 2017). Ten percent of those colonised become infected. Treatment options are limited and the mortality rate is high (26–44%). Risk factors include repeated hospital admission, previous antibiotic treatment,

admission to intensive care and having an indwelling medical device. CPE is controlled through sound fundamental infection prevention and control precautions, identifying and eliminating potential reservoirs, screening patients at high risk (rectal swabs), promptly isolating cases and treating colonised and symptomatic patients with linezolid.

Other Gram-negative Bacilli
Pseudomonas aeruginosa
Pseudomonas aeruginosa is a notorious opportunistic Gram-negative bacillus able to colonise and cause infections in wounds, the urinary tract, the insertion points of invasive devices and bloodstream infections (Walker and Moore 2015). It is able to form biofilms, leading to heavy contamination and environmental reservoirs (Walker and Moore 2015). Outbreaks are often linked to water systems, including hospital sinks, drains, taps and showers (Box 7.7), and are frequently reported from neonatal units (Jefferies et al. 2012). *Pseudomonas* bloodstream infections are subject to mandatory surveillance in England.

Acinetobacter baumannii
Acinetobacter baumannii is a Gram-negative aerobic opportunistic bacillus able to cause infection in the immunocompromised. Multivariate-resistant strains have been reported (Coelho et al. 2006). *A. baumanniii* is able to tolerate dry conditions and survive for prolonged periods on surfaces. It has been associated with numerous outbreaks, especially in burns units, and frequently causes ventilator-associated respiratory infections and bloodstream infections. *A. baumannii* is of increasing concern because of its growing resistance to antimicrobials and disinfectants (Milani et al. 2021).

Box 7.7   Reducing Risks of *Pseudomonas* Infection from Sinks in Healthcare Premises

Splashes from sinks contaminated with *Pseudomonas* spp. or other Gram-negative bacteria can travel over a metre and contaminate the environment of nearby patients. The U-bend and sink traps are the main reservoirs because they are heavily soiled and perpetually damp. Consequently, these locations become heavily contaminated and the bacteria form protective biofilms. The number of sink-related outbreaks has increased in recent years. Some health providers have created 'waterless' wards by removing sinks and plumbing from clinical areas (Hopman et al. 2017) or replacing conventional sinks with ones fitted with heating elements to destroy bacteria or chemical decontamination treatments.

Burkholderia cepacia

Burkholderia cepacia complex is a group of Gram-negative opportunistic bacteria widely distributed in soil and water. The bacteria have very simple growth requirements and are inherently resistant to many antimicrobials. Most outbreaks have been reported from patients who are immunocompromised. Those with cystic fibrosis are at particular risk and infection can result in serious pulmonary disease that is hard to treat and often fatal. *B. cepacia* is often difficult to isolate in the laboratory and can spread rapidly by cross-infection. Outbreaks are often traced to contaminated fluids, including disinfectants. Contamination appears to occur during manufacture, identifying the need for stricter quality control and regulation during production (Häfliger et al. 2020).

Fungi as Causative Agents of Healthcare-associated Infection

The incidence of serious HCAI caused by fungi (mycoses) is increasing. These infections are most likely to occur in severely immunocompromised patients in critical care units.

Invasive Candidiasis

Invasive candidiasis is the most serious fungal disease reported in high-income countries. At least 15 species are able to cause deep-seated infection and of these, *Candida albicans* is the most common. Invasive infection occurs because the organism either contaminates a susceptible site directly or reaches it via the bloodstream. Resistance to antifungal agents and mortality are high (Kullberg and Arendrup 2015).

Candida auris

Candida auris is a yeast first isolated in 2009 and since reported worldwide. It has caused a number of major outbreaks of invasive mycoses, often causing wound or bloodstream infections. Control is challenging because diagnosis is difficult. *Candida auris* is multidrug resistant and can form biofilms, enabling it to survive well on inanimate surfaces (Lamoth and Kontoyiannis 2018). Increasing incidence is probably related to the number of severely immunocompromised patients in intensive care units (de Cássia Orlandi Sardi et al. 2018). The hospital environment becomes heavily contaminated with spores and environmental decontamination is considered to be important in control. Immunocompromised patients are most at risk and most cases have been reported from intensive care units.

Norovirus

Norovirus is an RNA virus causing acute gastroenteritis. It is a global problem. Nausea, vomiting and diarrhoea develop after an incubation period of only

10–15 hours with no prodrome. The virus is spread readily via contact with faeces and aerosols released during vomiting and by direct and indirect contact via fomites. Health workers and cleaners can transmit the virus (Overbey et al. 2021).

Control is difficult because norovirus is highly transmissible, survives well on inanimate surfaces, including high-touch surfaces (e.g. elevator lift buttons, door handles), the infective dose is very low and people who are asymptomatic can shed large numbers of the virus. Outbreaks are extremely common in hospital and nursing homes. Control is challenging because items in the clinical environment become heavily contaminated (Nenonen et al. 2014). Outbreaks are also frequently reported in the community, particularly in 'closed' environments (e.g. nursing homes, schools, prisons, cruise ships), and although norovirus is often described as causing 'winter vomiting', it can occur at any time of year (Ahmed et al. 2014). Most infections resolve spontaneously within 48–72 hours in healthy people but dehydration can be severe in older people with chronic conditions and some deaths have been reported.

In hospitals and nursing homes, the burden of disease is high. In the UK, reported outbreaks have been linked to 13 000 patients with 3400 staff becoming ill, 8900 days of ward closure and the loss of over 15 500 bed-days annually (Harris et al. 2014).

Guidelines for the management of norovirus in healthcare settings in England were updated in 2012 (Box 7.8). Practice varies between settings and more research is required to establish effectiveness (Currie et al. 2016).

Norovirus infection is also a risk following the ingestion of bivalve shellfish (e.g. mussels). These creatures feed by filtering particles from the surrounding water, which in coastal waters can be contaminated (Hassard et al. 2017).

The Infection Prevention and Control Service

Infection prevention and control is the responsibility of everybody working in healthcare. All staff need to understand the fundamental principles and apply them in their workplace. Ensuring that staff receive the appropriate education is the responsibility of the infection prevention and control team.

The Infection Prevention and Control Team

The need for an infection prevention and control team (IPCT) with dedicated staff was first recognised in the UK in the 1950s. Early initiatives were considered successful and the service became established in many other countries (Jenner and Wilson 2000). Most infection prevention specialists are nurses. In many hospitals, the number of infection prevention nurses employed is calculated as one nurse

---

Box 7.8   Guidelines for The Management of Norovirus in Healthcare Settings

- Avoid admissions and transfers from affected bays and wards.
- Keep doors to isolation rooms and bays closed with signage to restrict entry.
- Prepare for reopening by planning the earliest date for a terminal clean.
- Arrange terminal cleaning before reopening rooms and bays.
- Ensure that all staff and visitors have been advised about the outbreak and how norovirus is transmitted.
- Maintain records of all symptomatic patients and staff.
- Monitor all affected patients for signs of dehydration and correct as necessary.
- Use non-sterile disposable gloves and aprons to prevent contamination with faeces and vomit.
- Masks can be worn to reduce risk from droplets and aerosols.
- Ensure adherence to hand hygiene, including patients.
- Remove exposed foods (e.g. fruit bowls) and discourage eating and drinking by staff in clinical areas.
- Monitor environmental cleaning and disinfection. Frequently touched surfaces should be treated with detergent and disinfectant containing 1000 ppm available chlorine.
- Use disposables wherever possible and decontaminate all other equipment immediately after use.
- Deal with spillages of faeces and vomit wearing PPE and decontaminate the area with an agent containing 1000 ppm available chlorine.

Source: Adapted from Norovirus Working Party (2012).

---

per 250 beds. This figure is based on epidemiological work undertaken by Haley et al. (1985). Some countries also employ hospital epidemiologists to lead the service. These are medically trained personnel who have received training in infection prevention. In other countries, including the UK, IPCTs are nurse led. Table 7.3 outlines the responsibilities of IPCTs.

Infection Control Link Nurses

Infection control link nurse schemes were introduced in the 1990s (Teare and Peacock 1996). They are made up of ward-based staff who work closely with IPCTs and operate as links between the IPCT and their own clinical area. They facilitate liaison, operate as local resources for infection prevention issues, provide ward-based education and undertake audit (e.g. hand hygiene). Clinical staff

Table 7.3   Responsibilities of infection prevention and control teams.

- Develop and implement IPCT programmes.
- Formulate and disseminate guidelines.
- Co-ordinate continuous education and training.
- Establish surveillance for HCAIs.
- Detect and manage outbreaks.
- Monitor and audit IPC practices and standards.
- Promote access to the infrastructure, materials and equipment necessary for effective IPC.
- Report infection-related data to senior managers, statutory bodies overseeing IPC and the public.

report satisfaction with link nurse schemes (Williams et al. 2013) and there is some evidence that they can be effective (Sopirala et al. 2014).

The Infection Prevention and Control Committee

The IPC committee oversees IPC policy throughout the organisation and leads the planning, monitoring and evaluation of all aspects of IPC. In addition to senior IPC team members, representatives from key services serve on the committee to bring together individuals with expertise in different areas of healthcare (e.g. senior medical and nursing staff, occupational health, hospital engineers, laboratory staff).

Infection Prevention and Control Regulations, Policies, Guidelines and Standards

In high-income countries, IPC is centrally organised by statutory bodies with legislation in place to ensure safe practice. In the UK, the Health and Social Care Act (2008) includes the Code of Hygiene which governs standards of IPC in organisations delivering healthcare. In England, the Department of Health and NICE publish policy documents on issues related to HCAI. These take the form of reports, safety bulletins, codes of practice and health notices sent as recommendations. Guidance is sought from experts including medical microbiologists, specialist nurses and pharmacists before publication and in response to specific enquiries from manufacturers. Recommendations are implemented by IPC teams to meet local requirements.

In the US, responsibility for IPC is taken by the Centers for Disease Control (CDC). The WHO provides international guidelines and in many countries additional recommendations are provided by professional bodies. In the UK, these include the Healthcare Infection Society, the Infection Prevention Society and the Royal College of Nursing. In the US, there are the Association for Professionals in Infection Control and Epidemiology (APIC) and the Society for Healthcare Epidemiology of America (SHEA).

Suggested Activities

Exercise 7.1 Self-assessment

1 Healthcare-associated infections can be acquired in which of the following: nursing homes; acute hospitals; community clinics; private hospitals; the domiciliary setting?

2 HCAI is the most common adverse event reported in healthcare.
   True/False

3 Explain the difference between prevalence and incidence.

4 Clinical audit is defined as which of the following?
   A A quality improvement process
   B Used in health services to improve patient care
   C A rigorous, highly controlled exercise
   D Only of any value if it is used to drive change

5 Biofilms develop exclusively over living tissues.
   True/False

6 Which of the following are Gram-negative bacteria?
   A *Pseudomonas* spp.
   B *Staphylococcus epidermidis*
   C *Klebsiella spp.*
   D *Candida auris*

7 Which of the following are Gram-positive bacteria?
   A Beta-haemolytic streptococci
   B Carbapenemase-producing Enterobacteriaceae
   C *Acinetobacter baumannii*
   D Group A streptococci

8 *Clostridioides difficile* is:
   A Gram positive
   B Able to form spores

C Able to form toxins
D Transmitted via hands and fomites

9 *Staphylococcus aureus* is:
   A Gram positive
   B Able to form spores
   C Able to form toxins
   D Transmitted via hands and fomites

10 Enterococci are:
   A Able to form spores
   B Able to develop antimicrobial resistance
   C Able to cause wound infections
   D Transmitted via hands and fomites

Exercise 7.2

What are the main causes of healthcare-associated infection causing problems in your clinical setting? Select one of the above and consider the following.

- What are the problems that have arisen?
- How have these problems been tackled so far?
- Identify lessons for future clinical practice, policy and education in your organisation

Exercise 7.3

Look at an epidemiological dataset, for example data on *Clostridium difficile* infections. These are provided by some national and international bodies, for example the UK Health Security Agency (https://www.gov.uk/government/collections/clostridium-difficile-guidance-data-and-analysis) and the European Centre for Disease Prevention and Control (https://atlas.ecdc.europa.eu/public/index.aspx). Look at a dataset for your country, or a country of interest. Think about what it is telling you, and consider why rates may differ between countries. In particular look for how infections are defined and identified, if reporting is mandatory or voluntary, and whether numbers show incidence (the number of new infections), or the prevalence (the number of cases at a given point in time).

References

Abernethy, J., Guy, R., Sheridan, E.A. et al. (2017). Epidemiology of Escherichia coli bacteraemia in England: results of an enhanced sentinel surveillance programme. *J. Hosp. Infect.* 95: 365–375. https://doi.org/10.1016/j.jhin.2016.12.008.

Ahmed, S.M., Hall, A.J., Robinson, A.E. et al. (2014). Global prevalence of norovirus in cases of gastroenteritis: a systematic review and meta-analysis. *Lancet. Infect. Dis.* 14: 725–730. https://doi.org/10.1016/S1473-3099(14)70767-4.

Allegranzi, B., Nejad, S.B., Combescure, C. et al. (2011). Burden of endemic health-care-associated infection in developing countries: systematic review and meta-analysis. *Lancet.* 377: 228–241. https://doi.org/10.1016/S0140-6736(10)61458-4.

Aranega-Bou, P., George, R.P., Verlander, N.Q. et al. (2019). Carbapenem-resistant Enterobacteriaceae dispersal from sinks is linked to drain position and drainage rates in a laboratory model system. *J. Hosp. Infect.* 102: 63–69. https://doi.org/10.1016/j.jhin.2018.12.007.

Baxter, E. (2021). A midwifery-led prevalence programme for caesarean section surgical site infections. *J. Hosp. Infect.* 109: 78–81. https://doi.org/10.1016/j.jhin.2020.12.008.

Becker, K., Heilmann, C., and Peters, G. (2014). Coagulase-negative staphylococci. *Clin. Microbiol. Rev.* 27: 870–926. https://doi.org/10.1128/CMR.00109-13.

de Cássia Orlandi Sardi, J., Silva, D.R., Soares Mendes-Giannini, M.J., and Rosalen, P.L. (2018). Candida auris: epidemiology, risk factors, virulence, resistance, and therapeutic options. *Microbial. Pathogen.* 125: 116–121. https://doi.org/10.1016/j.micpath.2018.09.014.

Coelho, J.M., Turton, J.F., Kaufmann, M.E. et al. (2006). Occurrence of carbapenem-resistant *Acinetobacter baumannii* clones at multiple hospitals in London and Southeast England. *J. Clin. Microbiol.* 44: 3623–3627. https://doi.org/10.1128/JCM.00699-06.

Coia, J.E., Wilson, J.A., Bak, A. et al. (2021). Joint Healthcare Infection Society (HIS) and Infection Prevention Society (IPS) guidelines for the prevention and control of meticillin-resistant Staphylococcus aureus (MRSA) in healthcare facilities. *J. Hosp. Infect.* 118: S1–S39. https://doi.org/10.1016/j.jhin.2021.09.022.

Cookson, B.D., Macrae, M.B., Barrett, S.P. et al. (2006). Guidelines for the control of glycopeptide-resistant enterococci in hospitals. *J. Hosp. Infect.* 62: 6–21. https://doi.org/10.1016/j.jhin.2005.02.016.

Curran, E.T. (2012). Outbreak column 5: *streptococcus pyogenes* (group a streptococci) (GAS). *J. Infect. Prevent.* 13: 206–210. https://doi.org/10.1177/1757177412460896.

Currie, K., Curran, E., Strachan, E. et al. (2016). Temporary suspension of visiting during norovirus outbreaks in NHS boards and the independent care home sector in Scotland: a cross-sectional survey of practice. *J. Hosp. Infect.* 92: 253–258. https://doi.org/10.1016/j.jhin.2015.10.018.

Desai, R., Pannaraj, P.S., Agopian, J. et al. (2011). Survival and transmission of community-associated methicillin-resistant Staphylococcus aureus from fomites. *Am. J. Infect. Cont.* 39: 219–225. https://doi.org/10.1016/j.ajic.2010.07.005.

Desai, S., Policarpio, M.E., Wong, K. et al. (2016). The epidemiology of invasive pneumococcal disease in older adults from 2007 to 2014 in Ontario, Canada:

a population-based study. *CMAJ Open.* 4: E545–E550. https://doi.org/10.9778/cmajo.20160035.

Diab, J., Bannan, A., and Pollitt, T. (2020). Necrotising fasciitis. *BMJ* 369: m1428. https://doi.org/10.1136/bmj.m1428.

Donlan, R.M. (2001). Biofilm formation: a clinically relevant microbiological process. *Clin. Infect. Dis.* 33: 1387–1392. https://doi.org/10.1086/322972.

European Centre for Disease Prevention and Control (2013). Point prevalence survey report: Acute care hospitals. www.ecdc.europa.eu/en/healthcare-associated-infections-acute-care-hospitals/surveillance-disease-data/report

Gould, D.J., Creedon, S., Jeanes, A. et al. (2017). Impact of observing hand hygiene in practice and research: a methodological reconsideration. *J. Hosp. Infect.* 95: 169–174. https://doi.org/10.1016/j.jhin.2016.08.008.

Guest, J.F., Keating, T., Gould, D., and Wigglesworth, N. (2020). Modelling the annual NHS costs and outcomes attributable to healthcare-associated infections in England. *BMJ Open.* 10: e033367. https://doi.org/10.1136/bmjopen-2019-033367.

Häfliger, E., Atkinson, A., and Marschall, J. (2020). Systematic review of healthcare-associated Burkholderia cepacia complex outbreaks: presentation, causes and outbreak control. *Infect. Prevent. Pract.* 2: 100082. https://doi.org/10.1016/j.infpip.2020.100082.

Haley, R.W., Culver, D.H., White, J.W. et al. (1985). The efficacy of infection surveillance and control programs in preventing nosocomial infections in US hospitals. *Am. J. Epidemiol.* 121: 182–205. https://doi.org/10.1093/oxfordjournals.aje.a113990.

Harris, J.P., Adams, N.L., Lopman, B.A. et al. (2014). The development of web-based surveillance provides new insights into the burden of norovirus outbreaks in hospitals in England. *Epidemiol. Infect.* 142: 1590–1598. https://doi.org/10.1017/S0950268813002896.

Hassard, F., Sharp, J.H., Taft, H. et al. (2017). Critical review on the public health impact of norovirus contamination in shellfish and the environment: a UK perspective. *Food. Environ. Virol.* 9: 123–141. https://doi.org/10.1007/s12560-017-9279-3.

Hay, A. (2006). Audit in infection control. *J. Hosp. Infect.* 62: 270–277. https://doi.org/10.1016/j.jhin.2005.09.008.

Health and Social Care Act 2008. www.legislation.gov.uk/ukpga/2008/14/contents

Hopman, J., Tostmann, A., Wertheim, H. et al. (2017). Reduced rate of intensive care unit acquired gram-negative bacilli after removal of sinks and introduction of 'water-free' patient care. *Antimicrob. Res. Infect. Cont.* 6: 59. https://doi.org/10.1186/s13756-017-0213-0.

Jefferies, J.M.C., Cooper, T., Yam, T., and Clarke, S.C. (2012). Pseudomonas aeruginosa outbreaks in the neonatal intensive care unit – a systematic review of risk factors and environmental sources. *J. Med. Microbiol.* 61: 1052–1061. https://doi.org/10.1099/jmm.0.044818-0.

Jenner, E. and Wilson, J. (2000). Educating the infection control team – past, present and future. A British prespective. *J. Hosp. Infect.* 46: 96–105. https://doi.org/10.1053/jhin.2000.0822.

Kullberg, B.J. and Arendrup, M.C. (2015). Invasive candidiasis. *N. Engl. J. Med.* 373: 1445–1456. https://doi.org/10.1056/NEJMra1315399.

Lamoth, F. and Kontoyiannis, D.P. (2018). The Candida auris alert: facts and perspectives. *J. Infect. Dis.* 217: 516–520. https://doi.org/10.1093/infdis/jix597.

Leffler, D.A. and Lamont, J.T. (2015). *Clostridium difficile* infection. *N. Engl. J. Med.* 372: 1539–1548. https://doi.org/10.1056/NEJMra1403772.

Legeay, C., Hue, R., Berton, C. et al. (2019). Control strategy for carbapenemase-producing Enterobacteriaceae in nursing homes: perspectives inspired from three outbreaks. *J. Hosp. Infect.* 101: 183–187. https://doi.org/10.1016/j.jhin.2018.10.020.

Ludden, C., Cormican, M., Vellinga, A. et al. (2015). Colonisation with ESBL-producing and carbapenemase-producing Enterobacteriaceae, vancomycin-resistant enterococci, and meticillin-resistant Staphylococcus aureus in a long-term care facility over one year. *BMC Infect. Dis.* 15: 168. https://doi.org/10.1186/s12879-015-0880-5.

Luo, K., Tang, J., Qu, Y. et al. (2021). Nosocomial infection by Klebsiella pneumoniae among neonates: a molecular epidemiological study. *J. Hosp. Infect.* 108: 174–180. https://doi.org/10.1016/j.jhin.2020.11.028.

MacFarquhar, J.K., Jones, T.F., Woron, A.M. et al. (2010). Outbreak of late-onset group B streptococcus in a neonatal intensive care unit. *Am. J. Infect. Cont.* 38: 283–288. https://doi.org/10.1016/j.ajic.2009.08.011.

Mahida, N., Beal, A., Trigg, D. et al. (2014). Outbreak of invasive group a streptococcus infection: contaminated patient curtains and cross-infection on an ear, nose and throat ward. *J. Hosp. Infect.* 87: 141–144. https://doi.org/10.1016/j.jhin.2014.04.007.

Manoukian, S., Stewart, S., Graves, N. et al. (2021). Bed-days and costs associated with the inpatient burden of healthcare-associated infection in the UK. *J. Hosp. Infect.* 114: 43–50. https://doi.org/10.1016/j.jhin.2020.12.027.

Manzoor, S.E., McNulty, C.A.M., Nakiboneka-Senabulya, D. et al. (2017). Investigation of community carriage rates of Clostridium difficile and Hungatella hathewayi in healthy volunteers from four regions of England. *J. Hosp. Infect.* 97: 153–155. https://doi.org/10.1016/j.jhin.2017.05.014.

Maree, C.L., Daum, R.S., Boyle-Vavra, S. et al. (2007). Community-associated methicillin-resistant *Staphylococcus aureus* isolates and healthcare-associated Infections1. *Emerg. Infect. Dis.* 13: 236–242. https://doi.org/10.3201/eid1302.060781.

Mathers, A.J., Vegesana, K., German Mesner, I. et al. (2018). Intensive care unit wastewater interventions to prevent transmission of multispecies Klebsiella pneumoniae Carbapenemase-producing organisms. *Clin. Infect. Dis.* 67: 171–178. https://doi.org/10.1093/cid/ciy052.

McManus, B.A., Aloba, B.K., Earls, M.R. et al. (2021). Multiple distinct outbreaks of Panton-valentine leucocidin-positive community-associated meticillin-resistant Staphylococcus aureus in Ireland investigated by whole-genome sequencing. *J. Hosp. Infect.* 108: 72–80. https://doi.org/10.1016/j.jhin.2020.11.021.

Milani, E.S., Hasani, A., Varschochi, M. et al. (2021). Biocide resistance in Acinetobacter baumannii: appraising the mechanisms. *J. Hosp. Infect.* 117: 135–146. https://doi.org/10.1016/j.jhin.2021.09.010.

Monteserin, N. and Larson, E. (2016). Temporal trends and risk factors for healthcare-associated vancomycin-resistant enterococci in adults. *J. Hosp. Infect.* 94: 236–241. https://doi.org/10.1016/j.jhin.2016.07.023.

National Institute for Health an d Care Excellence (2016). Healthcare-associated infections. www.nice.org.uk/guidance/qs113/resources/healthcareassociated-infections-pdf-75545296430533

Nenonen, N.P., Hannoun, C., Svensson, L. et al. (2014). Norovirus GII.4 detection in environmental samples from patient rooms during nosocomial outbreaks. *J. Clin. Microbiol.* 52: 2352–2358. https://doi.org/10.1128/JCM.00266-14.

Norovirus Working Party (2012). Guidelines for the management of norovirus outbreaks in acute and community health and social care settings. www.gov.uk/government/publications/norovirus-managing-outbreaks-in-acute-and-community-health-and-social-care-settings

Otter, J.A., Burgess, P., Davies, F. et al. (2017). Counting the cost of an outbreak of carbapenemase-producing Enterobacteriaceae: an economic evaluation from a hospital perspective. *Clin. Microbiol. Infect.* 23: 188–196. https://doi.org/10.1016/j.cmi.2016.10.005.

Overbey, K.N., Hamra, G.B., Nachman, K.E. et al. (2021). Quantitative microbial risk assessment of human norovirus infection in environmental service workers due to healthcare-associated fomites. *J. Hosp. Infect.* 117: 52–64. https://doi.org/10.1016/j.jhin.2021.08.006.

Patel, J.B., Gorwitz, R.J., and Jernigan, J.A. (2009). Mupirocin resistance. *Clin. Infect. Dis.* 49: 935–941. https://doi.org/10.1086/605495.

Pittet, D., Allegranzi, B., Sax, H. et al. (2006). Evidence-based model for hand transmission during patient care and the role of improved practices. *Lancet. Infect. Dis.* 6: 641–652. https://doi.org/10.1016/S1473-3099(06)70600-4.

Public Health England (2012). Healthcare associated infections (HAI): point prevalence survey, England. www.gov.uk/government/publications/healthcare-associated-infections-hcai-point-prevalence-survey-england

Rodríguez-Acelas, A.L., de Abreu Almeida, M., Engelman, B., and Cañon-Montañez, W. (2017). Risk factors for health care-associated infection in hospitalized adults: systematic review and meta-analysis. *Am. J. Infect. Cont.* 45: e149–e156. https://doi.org/10.1016/j.ajic.2017.08.016.

Rump, B., De Boer, M., Reis, R. et al. (2017). Signs of stigma and poor mental health among carriers of MRSA. *J. Hosp. Infect.* 95: 268–274. https://doi.org/10.1016/j.jhin.2016.09.010.

Scrivener, R. (ed.) (2004). National Institute for Clinical Excellence, Royal College of Nursing, University of Leicester, Commission for Health Improvement. In: *Principles for Best Practice in Clinical Audit.* Abingdon: Radcliffe Medical.

Selwyn, S. (1991). Hospital infection: the first 2500 years. *J. Hosp. Infect.* 18: 5–64. https://doi.org/10.1016/0195-6701(91)90004-R.

Sopirala, M.M., Yahle-Dunbar, L., Smyer, J. et al. (2014). Infection control link nurse program: an interdisciplinary approach in targeting health care-acquired infection. *Am. J. Infect. Cont.* 42: 353–359. https://doi.org/10.1016/j.ajic.2013.10.007.

Steer, J.A., Lamagni, T., Healy, B. et al. (2012). Guidelines for prevention and control of group A streptococcal infection in acute healthcare and maternity settings in the UK. *J. Infect.* 64: 1–18. https://doi.org/10.1016/j.jinf.2011.11.001.

Stewart, S., Robertson, C., Kennedy, S. et al. (2021a). Personalized infection prevention and control: identifying patients at risk of healthcare-associated infection. *J. Hosp. Infect.* 114: 32–42. https://doi.org/10.1016/j.jhin.2021.03.032.

Stewart, S., Robertson, C., Pan, J. et al. (2021b). Epidemiology of healthcare-associated infection reported from a hospital-wide incidence study: considerations for infection prevention and control planning. *J. Hosp. Infect.* 114: 10–22. https://doi.org/10.1016/j.jhin.2021.03.031.

Stewart, S., Robertson, C., Pan, J. et al. (2021c). Impact of healthcare-associated infection on length of stay. *J. Hosp. Infect.* 114: 23–31. https://doi.org/10.1016/j.jhin.2021.02.026.

Teare, E.L. and Peacock, A. (1996). The development of an infection control link-nurse programme in a district general hospital. *J. Hosp. Infect.* 34: 267–278. https://doi.org/10.1016/S0195-6701(96)90107-3.

Thacker, S.B. and Berkelman, R.L. (1988). Public health surveillance in the United States. *Epidemiologic. Rev.* 10: 164–190. https://doi.org/10.1093/oxfordjournals.epirev.a036021.

The Lancet (2015). Health care-associated infections in the USA. *Lancet.* 385: 304. https://doi.org/10.1016/S0140-6736(15)60101-5.

Tong, S.Y.C., Davis, J.S., Eichenberger, E. et al. (2015). Staphylococcus aureus infections: epidemiology, pathophysiology, clinical manifestations, and management. *Clin. Microbiol. Rev.* 28: 603–661. https://doi.org/10.1128/CMR.00134-14.

Uçkay, I., Pittet, D., Vaudaux, P. et al. (2009). Foreign body infections due to *Staphylococcus epidermidis. Ann. Med.* 41: 109–119. https://doi.org/10.1080/07853890802337045.

Walker, J. and Moore, G. (2015). Pseudomonas aeruginosa in hospital water systems: biofilms, guidelines, and practicalities. *J. Hosp. Infect.* 89: 324–327. https://doi.org/10.1016/j.jhin.2014.11.019.

Wilcox, M.H., Ahir, H., Coia, J.E. et al. (2017). Impact of recurrent Clostridium difficile infection: hospitalization and patient quality of life. *J. Antimicrob. Chemother.* 72: 2647–2656. https://doi.org/10.1093/jac/dkx174.

Williams, L., Burton, C., and Rycroft-Malone, J. (2013). What works: a realist evaluation case study of intermediaries in infection control practice. *J. Adv. Nurs.* 69: 915–926. https://doi.org/10.1111/j.1365-2648.2012.06084.x.

Wilson, A.P.R., Livermore, D.M., Otter, J.A. et al. (2016). Prevention and control of multi-drug-resistant gram-negative bacteria: recommendations from a joint working party. *J. Hosp. Infect.* 92: S1–S44. https://doi.org/10.1016/j.jhin.2015.08.007.

World Health Organization (2009). *Guide to the Implementation of the WHO Multimodal Hand Hygiene Improvement Strategy*. Geneva, Switzerland: World Health Organization.

World Health Organization (2011). *Report on the Burden of Endemic Health Care-Associated Infection Worldwide*. Geneva, Switzerland: World Health Organization.

Wu, Q., Sabokroo, N., Wang, Y. et al. (2021). Systematic review and meta-analysis of the epidemiology of vancomycin-resistance Staphylococcus aureus isolates. *Antimicrob. Res. Infect. Cont.* 10: 101. https://doi.org/10.1186/s13756-021-00967-y.

8

Urinary Tract Infection

Urinary Tract Infections

Urinary tract infections are the most common infections in hospital and community settings. Women are more susceptible than men because of the shorter length of the female urethra and its closer proximity to the perineum, which is the most common source of the pathogens responsible. By the time they have reached the age of 24 years, one in three women will have experienced at least one episode of urinary tract infection requiring treatment and many will have had recurrent infections (Foxman 2002). Risk factors in the general population are age over 65 years, pregnancy, recent sexual activity and obesity. Patients who are immunocompromised or diabetic and those with renal abnormalities or chronic wounds are also at increased risk.

Urinary tract infection is the most common reason for prescribing antimicrobials and this in turn is a driver for antimicrobial resistance. These infections can have very serious consequences. The bacteria may gain access to the bloodstream and multiply in sufficient numbers to cause bloodstream infection. The incidence of bloodstream infection caused by *Escherichia coli* is increasing in community settings, probably related to *E. coli* urinary tract infections, and carries a high risk of morbidity and mortality (Abernethy et al. 2017).

Pathogenesis of Urinary Tract Infection

In health, the bladder is kept free of micro-organisms. The epithelial cells lining its internal surface resist bacterial adhesion and any bacteria that succeed in gaining access via the narrow urethra are diluted as the bladder fills and are flushed out during micturition. The presence of a urinary catheter overcomes these defences and because urinary catheters are so frequently used, catheter-associated

Infection Prevention and Control in Healthcare Settings,
First Edition. Edward Purssell and Dinah Gould.

urinary tract infection (CAUTI) is among the most common healthcare-associated infections. In some areas, such as care of the elderly, rehabilitation and psychiatry, UTI is the most common infection (European Centre for Disease Prevention and Control 2013). Total direct hospital costs of CAUTI in English hospitals have been estimated at £54.4 million per year (Smith et al. 2019). Bloodstream infection (bacteraemia) occurs in 5% of catheterised patients, possibly in response to trauma when the catheter is introduced in some cases.

Pathogens Causing Urinary Tract Infections

The pathogens most commonly responsible for urinary tract infections are shown on Table 8.1. Most are caused by Gram-negative bacilli. Patients who have been catheterised for a long time are also at high risk of *Candida* urinary tract infection.

Pathogens able to cause CAUTI can be acquired endogenously or exogenously. Endogenous infection occurs if contamination is from the patient's own urethral meatus, rectum, vagina or another site (e.g. infected or colonised wound). Exogenous infection is usually via the hands of staff when the catheter is inserted or when the apparatus is manipulated. Catheterised patients operate as reservoirs of infection and cross-infection is a risk to other patients (Nicolle 2014). Clusters of infection have been reported (Su et al. 2003) and there is evidence that transmission occurs via the hands of health workers (Schaberg et al. 1976).

Most *E. coli* urinary tract infections are caused by a few serotypes that carry a surface antigen (antigen K), which confers protection against phagocytes. Some strains of *Proteus* are equipped with pili enabling them to adhere to the bladder epithelium and ascend the ureters to the kidneys, causing pyelonephritis (infection of the renal pelvis of the kidney).

Table 8.1 Bacteria responsible for urinary tract infections.

Gram-negative bacteria
Escherichia coli
Pseudomonas spp.
Klebsiella spp.
Proteus spp.
Serratia marcescens

Gram-positive bacteria
Staphylococcus epidermidis
Staphylococcus aureus
Enterococcus faecalis

Diagnosing Urinary Tract Infection

Diagnosis is made according to the clinical signs and symptoms of infection and the findings of laboratory investigations. Patients who are not catheterised usually complain of frequency, dysuria, urgency and suprapubic pain. They may also notice that the urine has developed an odour. This is particularly common with infections caused by *Pseudomonas*. Patients may also notice that the urine appears cloudy. This is owing to the presence of neutrophils (pyuria). If infection is severe, patients feel generally unwell, are often pyrexial and the urine is blood-stained (haematuria). Urinary tract infection should be suspected if an older, previously lucid patient becomes restless or disoriented or if a previously continent patient loses continence. Patients who are catheterised do not experience frequency or dysuria and the diagnosis is reached on the basis of laboratory investigations.

Dipstick tests can be used to give a presumptive diagnosis of urinary tract infection. They detect the presence of neutrophils, blood and nitrites released by the action of bacterial enzymes on nitrate in the urine. Urinary tract infection is confirmed when 100 000 bacteria are present in 1 ml (10^5 per ml) of freshly voided urine. The presence of neutrophils is an indicator that the body has responded to the presence of bacteria and mounted an inflammatory response, helping to confirm the presence of infection. For catheterised patients, UTI is diagnosed if there are at least 10^5 bacteria per ml in a specimen taken from the sampling port on the drainage system. False-positive diagnosis is very common. For patients who are not catheterised, this can be caused by inadequate cleansing of the urethral meatus before the urine was voided. For catheterised patients, contamination may occur if the specimen is obtained from the outlet of the drainage bag instead of the specimen port or if aseptic technique is breached when the specimen is obtained. Contamination from the specimen container is also possible during transit. Contaminated specimens are more likely to contain a large number of different micro-organisms. On the laboratory report, this is often described as 'mixed bacterial growth'. Neutrophils are unlikely to be present in large numbers in contaminated specimens.

Treating Urinary Tract Infection

Symptomatic infection of the lower urinary tract requires antimicrobial treatment. Narrow-spectrum antimicrobials are the treatment of choice to reduce risks of antimicrobial resistance. Nitrofurantoin or trimethoprim are usually given. Asymptomatic infections in women who are not pregnant are sometimes mild and self-limiting. In these cases, antimicrobial treatment can be delayed to allow symptoms to resolve (National Institute for Health and Care Excellence 2018). Trimethoprim is not recommended for pregnant women in the first trimester because there is a risk of foetal harm.

Bacteriuria

Bacteriuria is the presence of bacteria in urine. Asymptomatic bacteriuria occurs in the absence of any of the signs and symptoms of infection. It is very common among older people, especially those in nursing homes, regardless of whether they are catheterised. Asymptomatic bacteriuria occurs within 24–48 hours of catheterisation but is not associated with increased morbidity or mortality and can disappear spontaneously if the catheter is removed (Benton et al. 2006). Patients should be monitored carefully nevertheless, as nearly a quarter of those with asymptomatic bacteriuria develop urinary tract infection within 10 days. Routine specimen taking and culture, antimicrobial treatment and prophylaxis are not recommended, however (Smith et al. 2008), as treatment does not prevent recurrence (Trautner and Darouiche 2004) and taking antimicrobials increases the risk of *Clostridioides difficile* colonisation and infection.

Sources of Bacteria in Catheterised Patients

Until the 1960s, urine draining from catheters was collected in open-necked glass bottles. When the 'closed' system of drainage into plastic catheter bags was introduced, lower infection rates were reported (Thornton 1970). However, micro-organisms can still gain access:

- when the catheter is inserted
- by migrating from the drainage bag to the bladder. In 15–20% of catheterised patients with bacteriuria, the organisms are the same as those isolated from the drainage bag (Garibaldi et al. 1974). Migration occurs upwards along the inside of drainage tubing (interluminal route) or via the periurethral space between the outer wall of the catheter and the bladder (intraluminal route)
- when the 'closed' system is broken. This is inevitable when emptying the drainage bag, taking specimens, undertaking catheter washouts to alleviate mechanical blockage, if the drainage bag and tubing become disconnected by accident and when the drainage bag and catheter are changed. Drainage systems are often fitted with flutter valves, drip chambers or airlocks but laboratory modelling studies indicate that these devices do not eliminate bacterial migration completely (Nickel et al. 1985).

Once the urine has become contaminated, some bacteria remain floating freely in suspension but others settle to form a biofilm over the catheter and drainage apparatus, protecting them from the host defences. Although the bacteria trigger an inflammatory response, the action of neutrophils migrating to the site is decreased and the presence of a foreign body causes irritation and trauma, leading to pathogenic invasion (Trautner and Darouiche 2004).

Risk Factors for Catheter-associated Urinary Tract Infection

Urinary catheterisation is considered short term if the catheter is removed within three days and long term if catheterisation continues for over three months (Royal College of Nursing 2021). Risk of CAUTI increases with the length of time the catheter remains in place (Aaronson et al. 2011). Long-term catheterisation is associated with very high risk of infection and related complications. It should be avoided unless there is no alternative (Melzer and Welch 2017; National Institute for Health and Care Excellence 2018).

Complications of Urinary Catheterisation

Urinary catheterisation leads to high risk of CAUTI and other complications (Table 8.2).

Preventing Complications Associated with Urinary Catheterisation

The most effective way of preventing complications is to avoid urinary catheterisation if at all possible. Unfortunately, urinary catheterisation is frequently undertaken without rationale, especially for older female patients admitted via the accident

Table 8.2 Complications of urinary catheterisation.

Trauma and inflammation leading to urethritis and urethral stricture
Renal calculi
Pyelonephritis
Encrustation
Catheter blockage
Leakage
Pain
Bloodstream infection

Source: Garibaldi et al. (1974); Toughill (2005); Wilde et al. (2017).

Table 8.3 Indications for urinary catheterisation.

Relieve urinary retention.

Monitor fluid balance during critical illness to prevent occlusion by blood clots after specific procedures (e.g. transurethral prostatectomy).

Instil medication (e.g. chemotherapy).

Maintain skin integrity and facilitate continence when all other approaches have failed.

Provide comfort during end-of-life-care.

---

department: it has been estimated that up to 65% of catheters are inserted and left in place unnecessarily (Murphy et al. 2015). In England, 18% of inpatients have a urinary catheter and in nursing homes 10% of residents have an indwelling urethral catheter (McNulty 2009). Common reasons for use in this setting include intractable incontinence and to manage healing of a sacral wound. Data from the NHS Safety Thermometer (NHS Digital n.d.) indicate that 8% of patients in the community live with an indwelling urethral catheter. The use of indwelling urethral catheters varies considerably between centres, indicating scope for improved practice (Shackley et al. 2017). Appropriate reasons for inserting a urinary catheter are shown in Table 8.3.

Avoiding Overuse of Long-term Urinary Catheters

When the long-term use of a catheter is contemplated, risk assessment is essential to ensure that no feasible alternative exists, determine the most suitable type of catheter and drainage system and consider factors that could place the individual patient at particular risk of infection (e.g. compromised immune status) and identify whether infection could present an especially serious outcome for an individual patient (e.g. patients having one kidney).

A number of alternatives to indwelling urinary catheters exist. These include condom drainage systems, intermittent urinary catheterisation and incontinence aids and garments. Suprapubic catheters are thought to reduce the risk of infection because the catheter is inserted through the abdominal wall, preventing bacterial migration via the urethra, but they do not prevent other problems related to the use of long-term catheters (Prinjha et al. 2016).

Strategies to reduce the duration of catheterisation include the following.

- *Trial without catheter (TWOC)*: the catheter is removed and the patient's ability to empty the bladder is monitored. Local studies have demonstrated that TWOC can reduce the duration of catheterisation (Dawson et al. 2017).
- *'Stop orders' and reminder systems*: the catheter is removed when specific clinical criteria are met or after a predetermined period of time (e.g. first postoperative day). Rates of CAUTI can be reduced and recatheterisation is seldom necessary (Meddings et al. 2014).

Catheter Management

In hospital, successful management and the unnecessary use of urinary catheters depend on good communication between members of the multidisciplinary team and careful record keeping (Murphy et al. 2015). The use of catheter passports can improve management (Box 8.1).

In community settings, managing the care of patients with long-term indwelling urinary catheters consumes a considerable amount of nursing time (Forde and Barry 2018). Choice of the most suitable catheter and drainage apparatus and their management are important.

Catheter Material

Catheters are manufactured from a range of different materials. Traditionally, latex was used for catheters intended for short-term use but latex is irritant and may cause allergy (Belfield 1988). More expensive catheters, including those suitable for longer-term use, are manufactured from inert materials (e.g. Teflon®, silicone, silicone–Teflon® combinations, elastomers and hydrogels) because their smooth finish is less likely to cause encrustation or irritation (Cox 1990). Hydrogel-coated catheters are particularly well tolerated because they absorb fluid, becoming softer and less irritant. Catheters with novel coatings such as silver alloy or antimicrobials are available but their impact on CAUTI remains to be verified in well-controlled trials and there is a need for further product development and research to design and test innovative catheter materials (Feneley et al. 2012).

Catheter Length

Catheter length should be determined according to length of the urethra. The standard catheter length is 40 cm for males and 25 cm for females. Male-length

---

Box 8.1   Catheter Passports

Catheter passports are a key source of clinical information. They should be kept up to date and include all relevant clinical information (e.g. why catheterisation was undertaken, type of catheter in use, size and length, date of insertion/last changed and details of catheter-related equipment) and document plans for future care (e.g. trial without catheter). Their use helps to prevent unnecessarily prolonged catheterisation and promotes consistency of care, especially when patients move between wards or across sectors.

Source: Adapted from Codd (2014).

catheters are not suitable for women because they are more likely to kink and drag, leading to accidental disconnection, and are more difficult to conceal beneath clothing.

Catheter Gauge

Catheter gauge is measured with a unit called a charrière (Ch). One Ch measures 0.33 mm. Catheters of 12–30 Ch are available for adults. Smaller sizes are used for children. The optimal gauge is 12–14 Ch for adult males and 10–12 Ch for adult females. Larger gauges are not usually necessary as a 12 Ch catheter can drain 100 litres of fluid over 24 hours, a capacity far exceeding physiological requirement. However, larger gauges may be required to meet the needs of specific types of patients. After prostate surgery, an irrigation catheter or a larger gauge catheter (18–30 Ch) is necessary to drain blood clots. Experience may demonstrate that some patients produce urine containing large quantities of debris. Whistle-tip catheters, which have enlarged drainage holes, are suitable for these patients. Fitting a larger gauge catheter than that required will irritate the urethral mucosa, promoting bypassing and leakage, and may cause discomfort.

Balloon Size

Balloons on self-retaining catheters are available in two standard sizes: 10 and 30 ml. The larger size might be necessary for a woman with weak pelvic muscles catheterised long term or in men to prevent bleeding from the prostate bed following surgery, but the smaller size is recommended for routine use. Large balloons are more likely to irritate the bladder mucosae and cause trauma (Roe and Brocklehurst 1987), induce leakage and damage to the bladder neck. Balloons should be filled with sterile water, not saline, which may crystallise, blocking the inflation channel and making deflation and removal more difficult. The balloon must always be inflated according to the manufacturer's instructions as over- or underinflated balloons become misshapen and increase risk of trauma to the bladder mucosae.

Choice of Drainage Bag

The design of drainage bags is important. They should be fitted with a sampling port to allow specimens to be aspirated without breaking the closed system and have sufficient tubing to allow the bag to hang free. Many catheters have airlocks or other devices to reduce the risk of backflow. Some patients catheterised long term at home use a system fitted with a valve. This allows the bladder to fill and be emptied intermittently, avoiding the need for a drainage system. Other patients prefer a leg bag worn discreetly under clothing. The volume that can be held in a leg bag is relatively small and at night a larger volume bag is necessary. This should be fitted as an extension onto the leg bag drainage system, not used to replace it.

There is no evidence that instilling antiseptic into drainage bags prevents infection.

Catheter Insertion

Catheter insertion should be undertaken aseptically using sterile gloves and equipment. Sterile local anaesthetic or lubricating gel can be instilled before the procedure to reduce discomfort and risk of trauma.

Meatal Cleansing

The urethral meatus should be washed with soap and water during usual bathing or showering. Applying antiseptics has been associated with increased rates of bacteriuria, probably because handling forces perineal bacteria into the urethra when the catheter is manipulated during the process (Burke et al. 1981).

Catheter Replacement

Manufacturers suggest that catheters intended for short- or medium-term use should be replaced within 28 days and those intended for long-term use should be replaced every three months. More frequent replacement is not encouraged because it can result in transient bacteraemia and very frequent replacement has been associated with high rates of CAUTI. Antimicrobial prophylaxis is not recommended for replacement because of the risk of antimicrobial resistance.

Positioning of the Drainage System

The drainage bag should remain at a lower level than the patient to allow the urine to drain under gravity and be supported to prevent dragging that could damage the urethra or bladder. The outlet should always hang clear of the floor.

Emptying

Patients managed with sealed drainage systems are less likely to develop CAUTI, emphasising the importance of keeping the system closed (Platt et al. 1983). It is necessary to achieve a balance between overfrequent opening, which increases the risk of contaminating the urine, and allowing the drainage bag to become overfull and unsightly. Hand hygiene and the use of non-sterile disposable gloves are important because hands are often contaminated when the tap is handled (Glenister 1987). The urine should be drained into a disposable receptable if possible or into a receptacle that can be put into a bedpan washer afterwards to prevent risk of cross-infection.

Changing Drainage Bags

Manufacturers provide advice about optimal frequency of drainage bag changes. Use for 5–7 days is often suggested. Prompt disposal is necessary to avoid risks of cross-infection. They should be changed more frequently if they become discoloured, contain sediment, if offensive odour develops or if they become damaged.

Reducing Risks of Encrustation and Blockage

Encrustation and blockage are reported in 50% of all patients catheterised long term (Getliffe 1994, 2003). Encrustation is most likely to occur for patients who have frequent infections caused by bacteria that form biofilms readily (e.g. *Proteus mirabilis*, *Klebsiella* spp., *E.coli*, *Enterococcus* spp.). They release an enzyme called urease which is able to degrade urinary urea into ammonium ions which cause the urine to become alkaline, precipitating calcium and magnesium salts out of solution. The salts give rise to crystalline deposits over the inner surface of the catheter and drainage apparatus. Blockage arises when the precipitated salts occlude the eyes of the catheter and often causes leakage around the outside of the catheter.

Monitoring urinary pH in patients known to be at risk helps to identify incipient problems (Getliffe 2003). Catheter patency solutions can be used to alleviate catheter blockage if encrustation is a recurrent problem (Box 8.2). A leaking

---

Box 8.2   Catheter Patency Solutions

Catheter patency solutions contain a weakly acidic chemical (citric acid) which reacts with and dissolves crystalline deposits in the catheter and drainage system. They can be used to extend the lifespan of the catheter when the frequency of catheter changes caused by blockage from encrustation has become unacceptable. If experience demonstrates that a patient's catheter regularly becomes occluded, a patency solution could be used to extend its life instead of resorting to a catheter change. Patency solutions are issued on prescription and should only be used after careful patient assessment and when there is evidence that blockage is caused by encrustation and not some other factor. They should not be used to try and prevent CAUTI.

Source: Adapted from Yates (2018).

catheter should never be replaced with one that has a larger Ch because it will increase pain and may cause bladder spasm, exacerbating leakage.

Leakage and blockage are best avoided as they frequently result in visits to the accident department (Tay et al. 2016).

Preventing Dehydration

Older people are at high risk of dehydration through the physiological changes that accompany ageing. Many patients presenting in the accident department are dehydrated and mortality is higher for this group. Preventing dehydration reduces the risks of encrustation, CAUTI and bloodstream infection because increased fluid intake generates larger volumes of urine and dilutes the nutrients within it that are necessary to support bacterial growth (Stickler and Feneley 2010). A quality improvement initiative to improve hydration in nursing homes in south-east England has reduced the incidence of urinary tract infection by a third (Omar et al. 2019).

Bundles to Reduce Risks of Catheter-associated Urinary Tract Infection

Catheter-associated UTI prevention bundles can be effective in situations where no alternative to long-term catheter use exists (Saint et al. 2016). An example is shown in Box 8.3.

Box 8.3   Bundle to Prevent Catheter-Associated Urinary Tract Infection

- Cleanse the perineum to reduce the number of micro-organisms present. There is no evidence that antiseptics offer any advantage over soap and water.
- Instil sterile lubricant into the urethra to ease passage of the catheter and reduce risk of trauma.
- Adopt strict aseptic technique when inserting the catheter, changing and emptying the drainage bag and to obtain specimens.
- Avoid breaking the 'closed' system of drainage.
- Perform hand hygiene before and after manipulating the system.
- Position the drainage bag below the level of the bladder to avoid reflux.
- Secure the catheter to the patient's body to avoid kinking and urethral tension.
- Use a catheter bag stand to prevent the bag contacting the floor.
- Undertake meatal care with soap and water twice a day as part of routine hygiene (e.g. bathing, showering).
- Use an individual measuring device to empty the drainage bag for individual patients.
- Wear non-sterile disposable gloves to empty the drainage bag.

- Change drainage bags when they become discoloured, contain sediment, if offensive odour develops or if they become damaged.
- If a leg bag is used, add a larger overnight drainage bag when the patient is ready for bed.
- Encourage the patient to drink and ensure adequate hydration.

Patient Education

Patients experiencing recurrent urinary infections can be advised to ensure adequate oral intake of fluids to avoid dehydration. Currently, there is no evidence that cranberry juice can prevent urinary infection (National Institute for Health and Care Excellence 2018). Those with an established infection should be advised to complete the course of antibiotics if they have been prescribed. Paracetamol or ibuprofen can be taken for pain. Patients with pyelonephritis managed at home may be prescribed codeine for pain and should be advised to contact the health services if symptoms persist or if they are unable to tolerate oral fluids because of severe vomiting. They may have to be admitted as day cases for the intravenous administration of antimicrobials.

Long-term catheterisation can have far-reaching consequences for patients. It has a major impact on body image as well as causing psychological and emotional concerns. Individuals may be reluctant to leave the home to work or attend social activities and sexual activity can be difficult (Prinjha et al. 2016). Patients frequently report lack of information about health-related and practical issues such as where to obtain replacement catheters. They need to be educated individually to ensure that they are competent and confident and should receive full details of all the equipment they need and how to obtain supplies (Royal College of Nursing 2021). Products should be discreet to promote dignity and privacy and not place unnecessary restrictions on lifestyle.

Other important information includes who to contact if problems arise and how to dispose of equipment safely. Disposal in household rubbish is usually possible but it may be necessary to arrange special collection.

Suggested Activities

Exercise 8.1 Self-assessment

1   Finish the sentence: 'Risk factors for urinary tract infection include . . .'

2   Which of the following are able to cause urinary tract infection?
   A *Staphylococcus epidermidis*
   B *Neisseria gonorrhoeae*

C *Escherichia coli*
D *Candida albicans*

3 Which of the following are likely to be documented on a laboratory report for a patient with a confirmed urinary tract infection?
A Mixed bacterial growth
B Large numbers of neutrophils
C Presence of nitrites
D 10^5 bacteria identified per ml of urine

4 Explain briefly how bacteria can gain access to the bladder of a patient who has an indwelling urinary catheter.

5 Asymptomatic bacteriuria always requires antimicrobial treatment.
True/False

6 Urinary catheterisation is justified for which of the following?
A Promotion of comfort during end-of-life-care
B Encouraging a large sacral wound to heal
C Monitoring haemodynamic balance in a critically ill patient
D None of the above

7 What does the abbreviation TWOC stand for?

8 Which of the following can be caused by long-term urinary catheterisation?
A Encrustation of the catheter and drainage system with calcium salts
B Encrustation of the catheter and drainage system with sodium deposits
C Blockage of the eyes of the catheter
D Infection of the renal pelvis of the kidney

9 Catheter patency solutions should not be used routinely for all patients catheterised long term.
True/False

10 Maintaining adequate hydration is necessary to avoid urinary tract infection. Explain why.

Exercise 8.2

Investigate the use of urinary catheters in your clinical setting. Based on information contained in this chapter, do you think that good practice is consistently achieved? Identify any improvements that could be introduced to break the chain of infection, avoid other complications and how the impact of the changes could be monitored.

Exercise 8.3

Access the paper by Saint et al. (2016) on the reference list at the end of this chapter. What levels of evidence are used to underpin the recommendations for the care of catheterised patients recommended by the authors? To what extent do the findings demonstrate external validity (ability to be generalised to other patient populations)?

References

Aaronson, D.S., Wu, A.K., Blaschko, S.D. et al. (2011). National incidence and impact of noninfectious urethral catheter related complications on the surgical care improvement project. *J. Urol.* 185: 1756–1760. https://doi.org/10.1016/j.juro.2010.12.041.

Abernethy, J., Guy, R., Sheridan, E.A. et al. (2017). Epidemiology of Escherichia coli bacteraemia in England: results of an enhanced sentinel surveillance programme. *J. Hosp. Infect.* 95: 365–375. https://doi.org/10.1016/j.jhin.2016.12.008.

Belfield, P.W. (1988). Urinary catheters. *BMJ (Clin. Res. Ed.)* 296: 836–837.

Benton, T.J., Young, R.B., and Leeper, S.C. (2006). Asymptomatic bacteriuria in the nursing home. *Ann. Long-Term Care: Clinic. Care. Aging.* 14: 17–22. www.hmpgloballearningnetwork.com/site/altc/article/5963.

Burke, J.P., Garibaldi, R.A., Britt, M.R. et al. (1981). Prevention of catheter-associated urinary tract infections. *Am. J. Med.* 70: 655–658. https://doi.org/10.1016/0002-9343(81)90591-X.

Codd, J. (2014). Implementation of a patient-held urinary catheter passport to improve catheter management, by prompting for early removal and enhancing patient compliance. *J. Infect. Prevent.* 15: 88–92. https://doi.org/10.1177/1757177413512386.

Cox, A.J. (1990). Comparison of catheter surface morphologies. *Br. J. Urol.* 65: 55–60. https://doi.org/10.1111/j.1464-410X.1990.tb14662.x.

Dawson, C.H., Gallo, M., and Prevc, K. (2017). TWOC around the clock: a multimodal approach to improving catheter care. *J. Infect. Prevent.* 18: 57–64. https://doi.org/10.1177/1757177416668584.

NHS Digital (n.d.) NHS Safety Thermometer. https://digital.nhs.uk/services/closed-services/nhs-safety-thermometer

European Centre for Disease Prevention and Control (2013). Point Prevalence Survey of Healthcare-Associated Infections and Antimicrobial Use in European Acute Care Hospitals: 2011–2012. www.ecdc.europa.eu/en/publications-data/point-prevalence-survey-healthcare-associated-infections-and-antimicrobial-use-0

Feneley, R.C.L., Kunin, C.M., and Stickler, D.J. (2012). An indwelling urinary catheter for THE 21st century. *BJU Internat.* 109: 1746–1749. https://doi.org/10.1111/j.1464-410X.2011.10753.x.

Forde, L. and Barry, F. (2018). Point prevalence survey of indwelling urinary catheter use and appropriateness in patients living at home and receiving a community nursing service in Ireland. *J. Infect. Prevent.* 19: 123–129. https://doi.org/10.1177/1757177417736595.

Foxman, B. (2002). Epidemiology of urinary tract infections: incidence, morbidity, and economic costs. *Am. J. Med.* 113: 5–13. https://doi.org/10.1016/S0002-9343(02)01054-9.

Garibaldi, R.A., Burke, J.P., Dickman, M.L., and Smith, C.B. (1974). Factors predisposing to bacteriuria during indwelling urethral catheterization. *N. Engl. J. Med.* 291: 215–219. https://doi.org/10.1056/NEJM1974080 12910501.

Getliffe, K.A. (1994). The characteristics and management of patients with recurrent blockage of long-term urinary catheters. *J. Adv. Nurs.* 20: 140–149. https://doi.org/10.1046/j.1365-2648.1994.20010140.x.

Getliffe, K. (2003). Managing recurrent urinary catheter blockage: problems, promises, and practicalities. *J. Wound Ostomy Continence Nurs.* 30: 146–151. https://doi.org/10.1067/mjw.2003.120.

Glenister, H. (1987). The journal of infection control nursing. The passage of infection. *Nurs. Times* 83: 68–73.

McNulty, C.A. (2009). Reducing urinary catheter related infections in care homes: a review of the literature. *J. Infect. Prevent.* 10: 70–75. https://doi.org/10.1177/175717 7408098180.

Meddings, J., Rogers, M.A.M., Krein, S.L. et al. (2014). Reducing unnecessary urinary catheter use and other strategies to prevent catheter-associated urinary tract infection: an integrative review. *BMJ Qual. Saf.* 23: 277–289. https://doi.org/10.1136/bmjqs-2012-001774.

Melzer, M. and Welch, C. (2017). Does the presence of a urinary catheter predict severe sepsis in a bacteraemic cohort? *J. Hosp. Infect.* 95: 376–382. https://doi.org/10.1016/j.jhin.2017.01.003.

Murphy, C., Prieto, J., and Fader, M. (2015). 'It's easier to stick a tube in': a qualitative study to understand clinicians' individual decisions to place urinary catheters in acute medical care. *BMJ Qual. Saf.* 24: 444–450. https://doi.org/10.1136/bmjqs-2015-004114.

National Institute for Health and Care Excellence (2018). Urinary tract infection (lower): antimicrobial prescribing. www.nice.org.uk/guidance/ng109.

Nickel, J.C., Grant, S.K., and Costerton, J.W. (1985). Catheter-associated bacterium. *Urol.* 26: 369–375. https://doi.org/10.1016/0090-4295(85)90185-2.

Nicolle, L.E. (2014). Catheter associated urinary tract infections. *Antimicrob. Resist. Infect. Cont.* 3: 23. https://doi.org/10.1186/2047-2994-3-23.

Omar, F., Khan, A., Wilson, P. et al. (2019). Preventing Escherichia coli bacteraemia through optimized hospital hydration: an inpatient survey on drinks consumption on care of elderly wards. *J. Hosp. Infect.* 103: 170–171. https://doi.org/10.1016/j.jhin.2019.03.011.

Platt, R., Murdock, B., Frank Polk, B., and Rosner, B. (1983). Reduction of mortality associated with nosocomial urinary tract infection. *Lancet.* 321: 893–897. https://doi.org/10.1016/S0140-6736(83)91327-2.

Prinjha, S., Chapple, A., Feneley, R., and Mangnall, J. (2016). Exploring the information needs of people living with a long-term indwelling urinary catheter: a qualitative study. *J. Adv. Nurs.* 72: 1335–1346. https://doi.org/10.1111/jan.12923.

Roe, B.H. and Brocklehurst, J.C. (1987). Study of patients with indwelling catheters. *J. Adv. Nurs.* 12: 713–718. https://doi.org/10.1111/j.1365-2648.1987.tb01374.x.

Royal College of Nursing (2021). Catheter Care Guidance for Health Care Professionals. www.rcn.org.uk/professional-development/publications/catheter-care-guidance-for-health-care-professionals-uk-pub-009-915

Saint, S., Greene, M.T., Krein, S.L. et al. (2016). A program to prevent catheter-associated urinary tract infection in acute care. *N. Engl. J. Med.* 374: 2111–2119. https://doi.org/10.1056/NEJMoa1504906.

Schaberg, D.R., Weinstein, R.A., and Stamm, W.E. (1976). Epidemics of nosocomial urinary tract infection caused by multiply resistant gram-negative bacilli: epidemiology and control. *J. Infect. Dis.* 133: 363–366. https://doi.org/10.1093/infdis/133.3.363.

Shackley, D.C., Whytock, C., Parry, G. et al. (2017). Variation in the prevalence of urinary catheters: a profile of National Health Service patients in England. *BMJ Open* 7: e013842. https://doi.org/10.1136/bmjopen-2016-013842.

Smith, P.W., Bennett, G., Bradley, S. et al. (2008). Shea/Apic guideline: infection prevention and control in the long-term care facility. *Infect. Cont. Hosp. Epidemiol.* 29: 785–814. https://doi.org/10.1086/592416.

Smith, D.R.M., Pouwels, K.B., Hopkins, S. et al. (2019). Epidemiology and health-economic burden of urinary-catheter-associated infection in English NHS hospitals: a probabilistic modelling study. *J. Hosp. Infect.* 103: 44–54. https://doi.org/10.1016/j.jhin.2019.04.010.

Stickler, D.J. and Feneley, R.C.L. (2010). The encrustation and blockage of long-term indwelling bladder catheters: a way forward in prevention and control. *Spinal. Cord.* 48: 784–790. https://doi.org/10.1038/sc.2010.32.

Su, L.-H., Ou, J.T., Leu, H.-S. et al. (2003). Extended epidemic of nosocomial urinary tract infections caused by *Serratia marcescens*. *J. Clin. Microbiol.* 41: 4726–4732. https://doi.org/10.1128/JCM.41.10.4726-4732.2003.

Tay, L.J., Lyons, H., Karrouze, I. et al. (2016). Impact of the lack of community urinary catheter care services on the emergency department. *BJU Int.* 118: 327–334. https://doi.org/10.1111/bju.13430.

Thornton, G.F. (1970). Bacteriuria during indwelling catheter drainage: II. Effect of a closed sterile drainage system. *JAMA* 214: 339. https://doi.org/10.1001/jama.1970.03180020059010.

Toughill, E. (2005). Indwelling urinary catheters: common mechanical and pathogenic problems. *Am. J. Nurs.* 105: 35–37. https://doi.org/10.1097/00000446-200505000-00025.

Trautner, B.W. and Darouiche, R.O. (2004). Role of biofilm in catheter-associated urinary tract infection. *Am. J. Infect. Cont.* 32: 177–183. https://doi.org/10.1016/j.ajic.2003.08.005.

Wilde, M.H., McMahon, J.M., Crean, H.F., and Brasch, J. (2017). Exploring relationships of catheter-associated urinary tract infection and blockage in people with long-term indwelling urinary catheters. *J. Clin. Nurs.* 26: 2558–2571. https://doi.org/10.1111/jocn.13626.

Yates, A. (2018). Using patency solutions to manage urinary catheter blockage. *Nurs. Tim.* 114: 18–21.

9

Wound Infections

The skin is the body's major barrier against invading pathogens. Infection is a risk when it is no longer intact. Breaches occur as a result of:

- surgical intervention
- accidental trauma
- an underlying metabolic condition causing a chronic wound (e.g. pressure ulcers, leg ulcers, diabetic foot ulcers).

Wound Repair

Wound repair takes place in four stages which overlap, especially if healing is impaired or infection develops.

- *Haemostasis*: the immediate reaction to trauma. Blood loss is reduced by initiation of the clotting cascade.
- *The inflammatory response*: this is a defensive phase in which micro-organisms are destroyed and the wound bed prepares to regenerate tissue (4–6 days).
- *The proliferative phase*: connective tissue and new blood capillaries grow to fill the wound space (5–24 days).
- *Maturation*: the new tissue gains strength and flexibility although it never regains its former tensile strength (25 days–2 years).

Healing

Healing can occur by:

- primary intention
- secondary intention

Infection Prevention and Control in Healthcare Settings,
First Edition. Edward Purssell and Dinah Gould.
© 2023 John Wiley & Sons Ltd. Published 2023 by John Wiley & Sons Ltd.

Healing by Primary Intention

Healing by primary intention occurs when tissue loss is minimal. Most surgical wounds heal by primary intention. If the wound is large, the edges are held together by sutures, wound adhesive or wound closure devices (e.g. Steri-Strips™) to encourage healing.

Healing by Secondary Intention

Healing by secondary intention takes place when tissue loss has occurred and new cells grow upwards from the wound bed to replace it. Chronic wounds, burns and surgical wounds where there has been extensive tissue loss heal by secondary intention. Tissue repair proceeds more slowly than for wounds healing by primary intention, depending on the amount of tissue that needs to be regenerated. A moist environment is essential for healing (National Institute for Health and Care Excellence 2016).

New epithelial cells migrate readily over moist living tissue but in chronic lesions the wound surface may become dry or covered in debris and the epithelial cells migrate towards moist areas below the surface, disrupting the healing process, which can be protracted. Healing by secondary intention for surgical wounds is often unplanned but is occasionally the method of choice following colorectal, vascular or plastic surgery where tissue loss has been extensive or wounds are heavily infected. Unplanned healing by secondary intention is inevitable if dehiscence has occurred. Healing takes a long time, and patients require a great deal of nursing support (Chetter et al. 2017).

Surgical Site Infection

Surgical site infections (SSIs) are defined as infections that arise within 30 days of undergoing surgery or within one year if the patient has received an implantable device (e.g. prosthetic joint replacement). They develop when the number and activity of bacteria in the wound overwhelm the patient's immune system, resulting in tissue breakdown and delayed healing. Globally, 300 000 million people undergo surgical procedures every year, placing them at risk. According to the European Centre for Disease Control, SSIs account for 19.6% of all healthcare-associated infections reported in Europe but this is likely to be an underestimate as the signs and symptoms of infection may not become apparent until after the patient has been discharged and is excluded from surveillance data.

Three categories of SSI are recognised.

- *Superficial incisional* SSIs when infection is limited to the area of skin around the incision.

- *Deep incisional* SSIs occurring beneath the incision in the muscle and surrounding tissues.
- *Organ or space* SSIs involving an organ or a space between organs.

Signs and Symptoms of Surgical Site Infection

- Swelling
- Erythema
- Pus or bleeding
- Unpleasant odour
- Pain which may become throbbing if infection is severe
- Pyrexia
- Enlarged lymph nodes

Severe SSI may result in delayed healing and abscess formation. Dehiscence occurs if the bacteria break down collagen, undermining the strength of the regenerating tissues.

Identifying Surgical Site Infection

If SSI is suspected, a swab or sample of pus aspirated from the wound should be sent to the laboratory for microscopy and culture. Oral antibiotics are sufficient to treat minor SSIs. Intravenous administration is necessary for severe infections. Abscesses (localised collections of necrotic tissue, bacteria and neutrophils contained within a fibrin network) should be incised and drained as they may exert enough pressure to force bacteria into the surrounding tissues, blood or lymphatic vessels, resulting in septicaemia. Antimicrobials cannot penetrate a mass of purulent tissue and are ineffective. Staphylococci are the pyogenic bacteria most likely to cause abscesses. If dehiscence has occurred, the tissues must be left to heal by secondary intention.

Categories of Surgical Wounds

Four categories are recognised, each with a different risk of infection (Table 9.1).

Impact of Surgical Site Infections

Impact on the patient depends on whether the SSI is superficial or involves the deeper tissues. Superficial SSIs usually resolve after a course of oral antibiotics. They cause short-term discomfort but can still be a source of anxiety, distress and inconvenience. SSIs involving the deeper tissues and organ spaces are a leading cause of morbidity and mortality. Patients who have developed severe SSI experience marked pain, isolation and insecurity (Andersson et al. 2010). Impact on the

Table 9.1   Categories of wounds.

- *Clean wounds*: no inflammation or lapse in aseptic technique during surgery and no entry into the respiratory and gastrointestinal tracts (e.g. orthopaediac and cardiac operations, neurosurgery). Infection rate: 1–5%.
- *Clean-contaminated wounds*: wounds generated by surgical procedures that involve entering the respiratory or gastrointestinal tract without significant spillage (e.g. gastrointestinal surgery, abdominal hysterectomy, prostatic resection). Infection rate: 4–8%.
- *Contaminated wounds*: evidence of acute inflammation without pus or where gross spillage has occurred from a hollow internal organ or an otherwise clean operation where there has been a major breach of aseptic technique, recent traumatic wounds, open fractures and large bowel surgery. Infection rate: 10–15%.
- *Dirty wounds*: surgery where there is pre-existing infection (e.g. drainage of an abscess). Infection rate: 20–40%.

physical, emotional, social and economic aspects of life can be profound and many patients are ill-equipped to cope at home (Tanner et al. 2013).

The mean additional hospital stay for a patient with a serious SSI is 10 days and costs to the health service are considerable (Jenks et al. 2014). They include prolonged hospital stay, readmission, additional surgery, postdischarge care (e.g. community nursing services), the use of consumables (e.g. extra analgesia, dressing materials) and longer waiting lists (Badia et al. 2017).

Bacteria Causing Wound Infection

Surgical site infection is usually caused by a single organism but in the case of chronic wounds or secondary infection in acute surgical wounds, a number of different organisms is usually isolated (Brown 2018).

The bacteria most often responsible for SSI are shown in Table 9.2.

Risk Factors for Surgical Site Infection

Risk of developing SSI is influenced by patient-related (endogenous) factors and exogenous factors (external to the patient). Often, both sets of factors interact to

Table 9.2   Bacteria causing wound infections.

- *Staphylococcus aureus*
- *Staphylococcus epidermidis*
- Gram-negative bacilli, e.g. *Escherichia coli, Pseudomonas aeruginosa, Klebsiella* spp.
- *Streptococcus* spp.
- *Clostridium perfringens* (gas gangrene)

Table 9.3   Interventions to enhance surgical outcomes.

- Ensure optimal fluid and electrolyte balance
- Correct negative nitrogen balance
- Correct low haemoglobin level
- Control underlying metabolic disorders (e.g. diabetes mellitus)
- Maintain normal body temperature throughout the perioperative period
- Encourage the patient to learn and practise deep breathing and leg exercises
- Provide information to promote postoperative recovery and rehabilitation

influence individual risk (Korol et al. 2013). For patients undergoing elective surgery, it is possible to reduce many of the risks of SSI through preoperative assessment and intervention (Table 9.3).

Most SSIs originate in the operating theatre when the tissues are exposed but secondary infection occurring in the ward or after the patient has been discharged is also possible. Numerous studies have investigated risk factors for SSIs and prevention and concluded that some are more readily modified than others (Moucha et al. 2011). One of the earliest and most influential research studies highlighting risk factors for SSI is presented in Box 9.1.

The first major research study to examine SSI was reported from Canada (Cruse 1973). Incidence was determined prospectively in an 850-bed hospital over a period of five years. A 10-year follow-up was later published (Cruse and Foord 1980). All wounds were examined daily until the 28th postoperative day. Altogether, 23 649 wounds were inspected.

Preoperative Risk Factors for Surgical Site Infection
Age
Age increases risk of SSI (Korol et al. 2013) but as older people are more likely to suffer from pre-existing health conditions, it is impossible to disentangle age as an independent risk factor (Ridgeway et al. 2005).

Box 9.1   Risk factors for surgical site infection: results of an early epidemiological study (Cruse 1973).

The overall SSI rate was 4.8% but there was considerable variation depending on wound category.

Clean wounds	1.8%
Clean-contaminated wounds	8.9%
Contaminated wounds	21.5%
Dirty wounds	28.5%

Pre-existing Health Conditions

Underlying ill health, especially conditions likely to depress the immune response, is an important risk factor. The relationship between diabetes and SSI is well established and has been attributed to reduced phagocytic activity (Zhang et al. 2015) and impaired glycaemic control (Anderson et al. 2014). Patients with existing infection (e.g. urinary infection, pneumonia) are at increased risk of SSI, probably because bacteria seeded from the primary site of infection are carried in the bloodstream to the wound. The association appears to be especially marked in patients undergoing prosthetic joint replacement (David and Vrahas 2000). Wherever possible, infection should be treated before surgery is undertaken.

Immunosuppressive Treatment

Treatment that depresses the immune response (e.g. steroids, cancer chemotherapy) increases risk of SSI. If patients are receiving immunosuppressive therapy, it should cease preoperatively if possible (WHO 2018).

Obesity

Cruse (1973) identified an association between SSI and obesity: for clean wounds overweight people had an infection rate of 13% compared with 1.8% for those whose body weight was ideal. This association has since been established for colorectal procedures (Paulson et al. 2017), caesarean section (Ward et al. 2008) and orthopaedic operations (Moucha et al. 2011). There are a number of contributory factors. Excess adipose tissue complicates wound closure and healing is further impaired because adipose tissue has a poor blood supply (Waisbren et al. 2010). Gram-negative bacteria flourish in moist skinfolds and can be transferred into the wound, causing secondary infection. Elective patients should be encouraged to lose weight before surgery if necessary.

Undernourishment

The inflammatory response, immunological response and tissue repair depend on adequate supplies of protein. A negative nitrogen balance impedes healing and increases the opportunity for infection to supervene. Not surprisingly, Cruse and Foord (1980) established a clear relationship between undernourishment and SSI. Taking low levels of serum albumen as an indicator of undernourishment, Hennessey et al. (2010) established that hypoalbuminemia is a major risk factor for SSI following gastrointestinal surgery and is associated with deeper SSI and extended hospital stay. In their global recommendations for the prevention of SSI, the WHO (2018) suggest correcting undernutrition preoperatively where possible, through nutritional supplements and, if necessary, enteral feeding.

Length of Preoperative Stay

When patients are admitted to hospital, their existing skin flora is replaced by hospital-acquired strains that are more likely to be resistant to antimicrobials. SSI is not only more likely but often difficult to treat. Cruse and Foord (1980) reported an infection rate of 1.1% for patients admitted one day before surgery compared with 2% for those in hospital for a week before surgery. The trend towards day-case surgery and shorter postoperative stay has now reduced this risk.

Carriage of Staphylococcus aureus

Patients carrying *S. aureus* are at increased risk of developing SSI. Preoperative application of mupirocin reduces risk (Bode et al. 2010). Preoperative screening for methicillin-resistant *S. aureus* and decolonising carriers has reduced the number of staphylococcal infections.

Cigarette Smoking

Cigarette smoking increases the risk of SSI. Smoking impairs tissue regeneration, possibly by constricting the peripheral blood vessels and reducing blood supply and tissue oxygenation. Risk is highest if smoking occurs on the day of surgery (Nolan et al. 2017).

Nature of the Surgical Procedure and Site

Surgical site infection is closely associated with the nature of the operation (Coello et al. 2005). Skin is heavily colonised with micro-organisms (Reichel et al. 2011). Numbers are lowest on the arms and legs (10^2–10^3/cm^2) but much higher on the forehead (10^6/cm^2), between the webs of the toes (10^9/cm^2) and in areas that tend to be moist (e.g. axillae, groin, perineum), increasing risks of colonisation and infection at these sites. Consequently, secondary wound infections are very common. Open surgery carries a higher risk of SSI than minimally invasive ('keyhole') procedures (Caroff et al. 2019). For some operations (e.g. caesarean section), risk has been reported to increase when emergency surgery is necessary but not reported for others (e.g. gastrointestinal procedures) (Aghdassi et al. 2021).

The incidence of SSI following bowel surgery is very high (Paulson et al. 2017). Mechanical bowel preparation with colonic washouts and the use of purgatives is recommended to reduce the risk of endogenous infection with Gram-negative bacteria (WHO 2018).

Surgical Technique

The technique and skill of the individual undertaking the procedure are important. National SSI surveillance in the UK has demonstrated considerable variation for the same procedure between organisations and is most marked for gastrointestinal surgery.

Conditions in the Operating Theatre

Conditions in the operating theatre influence risk of SSI. Skin scales carrying large numbers of bacteria are shed during friction against clothing. They become air-borne, settle onto the gloved hands of staff, drapes or instruments and can be transferred into the wound (Whyte et al. 1982). Skin scales originating from staff present a greater risk than those originating from the patient (Hoffman et al. 2002). Contaminated particles can also be released from surfaces in the operating room or escape when power tools are used (e.g. orthopaedic surgery). Skin shedding is a particular risk for staphylococcal infection.

Duration of the Procedure

Duration of the operation influences the amount of time the tissues are exposed to potential sources of contamination. Consequently, longer operations tend to be associated with higher rates of SSI (Leong et al. 2006). Duration often reflects the complexity of the procedure and the required surgical expertise and increases the risk of lapses in asepsis and other complications. Tissues are likely to be manipulated more during lengthy, complicated operations, increasing opportunities for surgical error and contamination. Minimally invasive techniques have helped to reduce these risks.

Wound Drainage

Body fluids collecting in the tissues (e.g. blood, serous exudates, bile) provide an ideal environment for bacterial growth and multiplication. Wound drainage was introduced to reduce this risk; however, it has since been argued that the presence of the drain itself may lead to SSI because it allows bacteria from the skin to migrate into the wound along the external or internal surface of the tubing. In the study by Cruse and Foord (1980), a drain inserted through the incision increased the incidence of SSI. This finding has since been corroborated in more recent studies and is an area of ongoing research (Barbadoro et al. 2016).

In the meantime, there are suggestions that risk can be reduced by inserting the drain through a separate incision so that shortening and other manipulation can be undertaken independently of wound dressing changes. Employing closed suction drainage into a sealed, sterile reservoir is also recommended (Reiffel et al. 2013).

Presence of Sutures and Other Foreign Bodies

The presence of a foreign body increases risk of SSI. The normal immunological defence mechanisms can usually cope with small numbers of bacteria but are likely to be overwhelmed in the presence of foreign material. Sutures, especially multibraided types, trap bacteria (Beldi et al. 2009). The increasing use of wound adhesives is overcoming this problem. Risks are increased for patients who have received cardiac implants or prosthetic devices (Coello et al. 2005).

Preventing Surgical Site Infections

Surgical site infections are considered preventable because rates differ among surgeons performing the same procedure, indicating that there is scope for improving individual performance (Troughton et al. 2019). Numerous guidelines for prevention have been developed. In the UK, comprehensive recommendations are offered by the National Institute for Health and Care Excellence (2020).

Instruments and Equipment

All instruments and equipment used for invasive procedures must be sterile. Packs must be stored in a cool dry place and checked to ensure that they are intact before use.

Preoperative Hair Removal

Although hair is heavily contaminated with potential pathogens, shaving increases the risk of SSI, especially if undertaken several hours before surgery. Razors cause small abrasions which become heavily colonised, increasing the number of microorganisms present to contribute to cross-infection. Consequently, it has been recommended that hair should only be removed if it will obscure the site of the incision, using clippers to avoid abrasions (National Institute for Health and Care Excellence 2020; World Health Organization 2018). Depilatory creams are not recommended because there is no evidence that they are more effective at reducing risks of SSI than clippers (Tanner et al. 2011).

Hair should be removed outside the operating theatre to avoid environmental contamination using a single-use electric or battery-operated clipper that can be disinfected between patients. Clippers fitted with a vacuum-assisted hair collection device save time and remove trimmings (Edmiston et al. 2016).

Preoperative Showering

Micro-organisms on the skin can enter the incision and increase risk of SSI but there is no evidence that antiseptic preoperative showering reduces SSI (Webster and Osborne 2015), although in some centres patients are still requested to shower with antiseptic, usually chlorhexidine (Tanner and Khan 2008). Both NICE and WHO recommend preoperative showering or bathing with plain soap (National Institute for Health and Care Excellence 2020; WHO 2018).

Surgical Hand Antisepsis

The aim of surgical hand antisepsis is to remove transient micro-organisms and residents deep in the stratum corneum (Tavolacci et al. 2006). Thorough antisepsis is important because the effects may have to last for hours. The number of bacteria able to contribute to SSI increases because they are leached out of the deeper layers of the stratum corneum and subungual spaces (beneath the finger nails) when hands sweat inside surgical gloves, especially if the operation is protracted. Gloves frequently become perforated, allowing micro-organisms to escape into the open tissues (Beldi et al. 2009).

There is no evidence that one type of antiseptic reduces SSI more effectively than another. Chlorhexidine gluconate can reduce the number of colony-forming units (CFUs) on the hands more effectively than povidone iodine but CFUs are a proxy measure of infection, not evidence that infection has occurred. Alcohol handrubs with additional antiseptic ingredients can reduce CFUs better than chlorhexidine. There is tentative evidence that a three-minute scrub can reduce CFUs on the hand compared to a two-minute scrub. There is no evidence that using nail picks or brushes reduces CFUs on the hands (Tanner and Parkinson 2006; Tanner et al. 2016).

Operating Room Ventilation

Ventilation systems in operating theatres are designed to reduce the number of air-borne particles available to contaminate the wound. The pressure of the air in a conventionally ventilated operating room is kept higher than in the surrounding ancillary rooms and corridors. The air entering is forced through filters and flows into the surrounding lower-pressure areas outside. It is completely replaced about every 20 minutes. Laminar systems employ ultrafiltration to offer greater protection. They are used when prostheses are inserted during orthopaedic surgery as SSI has especially serious consequences for these patients (Charnley 1970).

Initially, lower rates of SSI were reported when laminar airflow was introduced (Lidwell et al. 1982) but later studies have been unable to identify a relationship between microbiological quality of operating room air and SSI (Stacey and Humphreys 2002) and a recent Cochrane review could establish no difference in SSI rates for a range of different procedures conducted under laminar flow compared to conventional ventilation (Bischoff et al. 2017). Consequently, the need for expensive ventilation systems is now questioned (Parvizi et al. 2017).

Irrespective of the type of ventilation used, the system must undergo regular, planned maintenance by the estates department (Box 9.2).

Minimising activity by restricting the number of staff present in the operating theatre and avoiding unnecessary door opening and people entering and leaving have traditionally been encouraged to enable the operating team to concentrate and to prevent disruption of the air flow. There is tentative evidence from laboratory simulations that staff activity can influence the number of air-borne particles, especially around the operating and instrument tables (Annaqeeb et al. 2021).

Antimicrobial Prophylaxis

The purpose of surgical antimicrobial prophylaxis is to prevent any organisms that gain access to the incision multiplying in sufficient numbers to cause SSI. NICE

Box 9.2   Maintaining ventilation in the operating theatre

Good practice includes the following factors.

- Theatre etiquette: keeping doors into the operating theatre closed while operations are in progress and restricting the number of people present. Spectators should use a viewing gallery.
- Regularly maintaining the operating environment with checks to ensure that air filters are in good working order.
- Cleaning all surfaces daily to prevent dust settling.
- Cleaning between cases.
- Keeping equipment stored in the theatre to a minimum to prevent dust accumulating and interruptions by others needing to retrieve it.

(2019) recommends antibiotic prophylaxis for clean-contaminated and contaminated cases and for prosthetic joint surgery. Administration is usually performed when anaesthesia is induced. The WHO recommends administration within 120 minutes of making the incision, taking into account the half-life of the specific antimicrobial (WHO 2018). Choice of antimicrobial depends on the type of bacteria most likely to cause infection in a given type of wound (Bratzler et al. 2013).

Skin Disinfection

Antiseptics are applied to the skin immediately before the surgical incision is made to reduce the numbers of bacteria able to contaminate it. Risk is decreased if the skin is cleansed preoperatively with a combined chlorhexidine and alcohol preparation compared to povidone iodine (Darouiche et al. 2010; Tuuli et al. 2016). The WHO recommends skin disinfection with chlorhexidine (WHO 2018). A recent trial has indicated that a new skin antiseptic, olanexidine, may also be effective (Obara et al. 2020).

Temperature

Maintaining the patient's normal body temperature during the surgical procedure decreases risk of SSI (Seamon et al. 2012). Fall in body temperature, especially during major surgery, promotes SSI, particularly in older people and those with pre-existing disease. Current recommendations suggest maintaining temperature at 36 °C throughout the perioperative period (National Institute for Health and Care Excellence 2020).

Theatre Attire
Scrubs
Micro-organisms are continually shed from skin through friction with clothing. Operating room staff wear sterile scrubs to reduce the risk of transferring skin

scales into the incision but some still manage to escape at the neckline, wrists and ankles and through pores in the material. Closely woven fabric helps to prevent shedding and as micro-organisms are transferred more readily between moist surfaces than dry ones, fluid-resistant scrubs are advisable (Whyte et al. 1990).

A range of textiles are being developed for use in healthcare, some with antimicrobial properties and the ability to deflect splashes. They are effective in simulations but there is little evidence to demonstrate effectiveness under 'in use' conditions (Mitchell et al. 2015).

Masks

Surgical facemasks were originally worn to prevent respiratory pathogens entering the wound. It is not clear if they are of any real value but they are still used because they help protect staff from splashing and risks of blood-borne infection (Lipp and Edwards 2014).

Gloves

Sterile gloves are worn to prevent the transfer of micro-organisms from hands into the incision. If gloves become perforated, the risk of SSI increases and the risk of blood-borne infection to clinicians is greater (Beldi et al. 2009). Double gloving is recommended to protect both when risks are very high (Tanner and Parkinson 2006). All blood spillages should be dealt with as soon as they occur.

Head Coverings

Head coverings prevent hair and any associated bacteria falling into the incision but there is no evidence that they are necessary for staff outside the scrub team who have no immediate patient contact during the preocedure.

Overshoes

Occasional visitors to the operating theatre are sometimes requested to wear overshoes but there is no evidence that they are of any value (Humphreys et al. 1991). Handling shoes to position and remove them is likely to result in hands becoming contaminated.

Postoperative Care

In the operating theatre, the wound is occluded by a sterile dressing. This should remain in place for at least 48 hours to avoid exposing the open tissues to the risk of exogenous infection. After the first 48 hours, the dressing can be removed to allow inspection of the wound. It can be replaced by an occlusive waterproof dressing allowing the patient to bath or shower, cleansing the incision with normal saline if necessary. Antiseptics are unnecessary as the contact time with the wound is unlikely to be sufficient to destroy micro-organisms. Absorptive dressings are required if the wound leaks serous fluid.

The frequency of dressing changes depends on the amount of leakage. Cross-infection is possible when wounds are dressed. Risk is reduced by hand hygiene before and after changing dressings. Hand hygiene is important regardless of whether non-sterile disposable gloves are used.

Information for Postoperative Surgical Patients
Today, many patients undergo surgical procedures as day cases and for those who are admitted, hospital stay is usually short. Consequently, patient education is essential to ensure smooth recovery after discharge (Box 9.3). Patients need to know:

• how to look after the incision and surrounding tissues
• how to reapply dressings
• where to obtain new supplies of dressing materials if necessary
• where to seek advice.

Guidelines and Bundles to Reduce Risks of Surgical Site Infections

Clinical guidelines have been developed by NICE, WHO and professional organisations (National Institute for Health and Care Excellence 2020; World Health Organization 2018). A summary is provided in Box 9.4. The effectiveness of bundled interventions to reduce risks of SSI for specific patient groups has been evaluated in

---

Box 9.3   Postoperative care after leaving hospital

Patients need to know that a newly created wound will probably look moist. Excessive weeping and the appearance of pus or blood indicate SSI requiring medical or nursing advice. Some pain is normal because the skin and underlying tissues have been traumatised but sudden increase in pain or throbbing could indicate infection. It should be possible to control anticipated levels of pain with a simple analgesic (e.g. paracetamol). Feeling generally unwell and pyrexia indicate SSI and patients should seek medical or nursing advice. Patients discharged while still taking antibiotics need to be informed about the importance of finishing the course even if they feel well and of avoiding alcohol if taking metronidazole (which can react with alcohol, causing unpleasant side-effects).

Dressing materials should be stored in a secure, dry place and hands should be washed before and after changing dressings. Small dressings can be wrapped and disposed of with normal household waste but special arrangements need to be made for larger, soiled items. Bathing is possible providing the wound is protected with an occlusive, water-proof dressing.

Patients should be informed about arrangements for removing sutures. If another method of wound closure has been used, they need to be aware that removal will not be necessary.

Box 9.4   Guidelines for the prevention of surgical site infection

Preoperative recommendations

- Patients should be advised to take a shower or bath using soap (not antiseptic) the day before or on the day of surgery.
- Decolonisation with nasal mupirocin and chlorhexidine body washing should be undertaken for patients testing positive for methicillin-resistant *S. aureus* (MRSA). Routine decolonisation can be undertaken for patients undergoing procedures where risk of *S. aureus* infection is considered to be significant.
- Depilation is not recommended. Hair covering the site of the planned incision should be removed with clippers.
- Patients should be dressed in theatre attire to allow access to the operative site and the placement of devices (e.g. intravenous cannulae), with emphasis on comfort and dignity.

Perioperative recommendations

- Staff must wear sterile operating gowns and sterile gloves. Double gloving is recommended when risk of perforation is high or in very high-risk situations.
- Hand jewellery, artificial nails and nail polish should not be worn.
- Staff movements in and out of the operating theatre should be kept to a minimum while an operation is in progress.
- Staff should cleanse hands with an aqueous antiseptic solution before the first procedure on the list, before each subsequent procedure and between procedures.
- The skin at the surgical site should be cleansed with antiseptic solution immediately before the incision is created.
- At the end of the procedure, the incision should be covered with a sterile dressing.

Postoperative recommendations

- Aseptic technique should be employed when the dressing is changed.
- Sterile normal saline should be used to cleanse wounds up to 48 hours postoperatively. Tap water may then be used for cleansing after 48 hours or if pus has been drained. It is safe for patients to shower 48 hours postoperatively if an occlusive dressing has been applied.

Source: Adapted from National Institute for Health and Care Excellence (2020).

numerous studies but with variable success. Johnson et al. (2016) demonstrated lower rates of SSI for patients undergoing surgery for gynaecological malignancy but Serra-Aracil (2011) did not report decreased infection 30 days after bowel surgery. Contradictory findings are not surprising given the different patient populations studied, differences in the interventions included in different bundles and the type of procedure evaluated. The ability of bundled interventions to reduce SSI is further complicated because adherence by staff is often poor (Leaper et al. 2015).

Surveillance of Surgical Site Infection

The work of Cruse (1973) prompted the creation of a surveillance programme for SSI in the US that has since provided a model for systems in other countries (Haley et al. 1985). The aim of national surveillance schemes for SSI is to improve the quality of patient care by encouraging health providers to compare their own rates of SSI over time against a national benchmark and use the data to review and support practice. Postdischarge follow-up of patients (e.g. by telephone, text message) is essential to the success of these schemes (Sykes et al. 2005). Under the national SSI Surveillance Service (SSISS) in England, data are collected for 17 categories of surgery (e.g. general surgery, cardiothoracic, neurosurgery, gynaecology, orthopaedics). The system was established in 1997 and is voluntary. Since 2004, NHS trusts undertaking orthopaedic procedures have been required to conduct surveillance for a minimum of three consecutive months every financial year for at least one of four categories: hip replacement, knee replacement, repair of fractured neck of femur, or reduction of long bone fracture. Some health providers undertake additional surveillance. The main constraint is availability of resources. The benefits of surveillance have been demonstrated in many countries (Bataille et al. 2021).

The outcomes of surveillance and comparisons are only meaningful if the same methods of data collection are used everywhere. In England, a protocol is in place to ensure that the same definitions of SSI are applied and data collection tools are standardised with error checking to promote accuracy. Providing these precautions are taken, surveillance allows organisations to monitor their own performance over time and compare it to others. Over the last 10 years, SSI rates in England have declined. This has been attributed to the action taken by clinicians in response to feedback. Box 9.5 demonstrates how additional surveillance enabled one NHS trust to reduce SSI for a commonly undertaken surgical procedure, improving quality of care.

Chronic Wounds

Chronic wounds are defined as those not healing within a predicted time-frame (Tapiwa Chamanga 2018). Tissue loss is extensive and healing is by secondary intention. Risk of infection is very high because exposure of the tissues is

Box 9.5   Impact of a midwifery-led prevalence programme for caesarean section surgical site infection rates

Caesarean section accounts for 29% of all deliveries in the UK. SSI following this procedure is painful, distressing, affects the mother's ability to look after and bond with the baby and is a drain on healthcare resources. Undertaking a point prevalence study demonstrated that 26% of women undergoing caesarean sections in one NHS trust developed SSI. Infections declined to 8% after theatre etiquette was improved (e.g. not entering theatre unnecessarily when operations were in progress, minimising the number of people present), adhering to guidelines for skin preparation and postoperative removal of wound dressings. Women were advised not to shave the bikini line from the 36th week of gestation and community midwives were supplied with standard dressings.

Source: Adapted from Baxter (2021).

protracted and large numbers of micro-organisms are present, interfering with the inflammatory response. The presence of enzymes, oxygen free radicals and inflammatory cells further delays healing (Brown 2018). The underlying disease process that resulted in wound formation may also disrupt healing (e.g. poor vasculation). Instead of regenerating, the tissues break down and dead cells and exudate (slough) accumulate. The presence of infection is indicated by large amounts of slough, slough recurring after debridement and the appearance of moist, friable, dark red granulation tissue, especially if the tissue bleeds easily and odour develops.

Identifying the cause of infection is difficult as numerous different types of bacteria retrieved from specimens are likely to grow on culture media in the laboratory. It is hard to determine which antimicrobial is appropriate. Effectiveness is likely to be reduced because antimicrobials are unable to penetrate slough.

Choice of Dressing

Dressings need to provide an optimal environment for healing regardless of the type of wound and whether healing is by primary or secondary intention. Some types of dressings are designed to control moisture levels (e.g. alginates, films, foams, hydrogels, hydrocolloids). There is some evidence that they are more effective than traditional dressing materials but evaluation is difficult because clinical trials often compare their performance to gauze which is no longer recommended. There is no evidence that antimicrobial dressings (e.g. dressings impregnated with iodine or silver) are more effective than standard dressings. Comprehensive information on advanced wound dressings is provided in the British National Formulary.

Selecting the most appropriate dressing and frequency of dressing changes depends on a range of factors related to the individual patient and their wound (Box 9.6). For chronic wounds, the expertise of a tissue viability nurse is beneficial.

Debridement may be necessary to remove necrotic tissue, which impedes healing and is an excellent medium for bacterial growth and multiplication. Debridement can be achieved by using dressings that have a natural debriding effect (e.g. alginates, hydrogels, hydrocolloids), surgically or with chemicals. In recent years, there has been renewed interest in maggot and larval therapy (Bonn 2000). The maggots are bred and kept under sterile conditions and a controlled number is applied to the wound surface for a predetermined period of time. The maggots release an enzyme to liquefy the necrotic tissue, which they ingest.

The need for debridement can be reduced by negative-pressure wound therapy. A foam dressing with a vacuum pump is placed over the wound to draw out excess exudate and debris while drawing the wound margins together. There is tentative evidence that it is effective (Guy and Grothier 2012).

Unnecessary dressing changes should be avoided when treating chronic wounds as occlusion helps to maintain optimal temperature for healing and the risks of cross-infection are reduced.

Box 9.6   Factors to be considered when selecting wound dressings
• Stage of wound healing
• Amount of exudate
• Presence of infection
• Odour
• Adhesiveness of the dressing and required ease of removal
• Irritation (e.g. caused by the adhesive)
• Absorption
• Frequency of dressing changes
• Ease of use
• Amount of pain experienced at dressing change
• Protection of surrounding tissues required
• Patient preference
Source: Adapted from National Institute for Health and Care Excellence (2016).

Suggested Activities

Exercise 9.1 Self-assessment

1 Explain when healing by primary intention and healing by secondary intention occur.

2 Complete the sentence: 'A surgical site infections is defined as . . .'

3 Which of the following cause surgical site infection?
   A *Escherichia coli*
   B *Staphylococcus aureus*
   C *Klebsiella* spp.
   D *Clostridioides difficile*

4 Which of the following are risk factors for surgical site infection?
   A Taking steroids
   B Recent vaccination
   C Having an existing urinary tract infection
   D Negative nitrogen balance

5 Which of the following are recommended to reduce surgical site infection in official guidelines?
   A Using a wound adhesive
   B Avoiding the insertion of wound drains
   C Preoperative showering with chlorhexidine
   D None of the above

6 A surgical wound should be occluded with a sterile dressing applied in the operating theatre and remain in place for at least 48 hours.
   True/False

7 Numerous studies have been undertaken to evaluate the effectiveness of bundles in reducing the risks of surgical site infection. Explain why the results of different studies have been contradictory.

8 Explain the purpose of national surveillance schemes for surgical site infections.

9 Which of the following should be considered when selecting wound dressings?
   A Stage of healing
   B Presence of infection

C Frequency of dressing changes
D All the above

10 Which of the following reduce the risk of exogenous infection when wounds are dressed?
A Hand hygiene before the old dressing is removed
B Hand hygiene when the procedure is complete
C Double gloving with sterile gloves
D Double gloving with non-sterile gloves

Exercise 9.2

Investigate policy and practice for wound management in your clinical setting. What arrangements are in place for surveillance and audit? Is any additional surveillance undertaken in addition to mandatory requirements? What is the reason underpinning this decision?

Exercise 9.3

Access the paper by Baxter (2021) in the reference list. It describes the steps taken to address the high rate of postoperative infections reported in a service following a specific type of surgical intervention. Read the paper and address the following questions.
A What are the study findings?
B Are they trustworthy?
C Would the findings be helpful to support local practice elsewhere?

References

Aghdassi, S.J.S., Schröder, C., and Gastmeier, P. (2021). Urgency of surgery as an indicator for the occurrence of surgical site infections: data from over 100,000 surgical procedures. *J. Hosp. Infect.* 110: 1–6. https://doi.org/10.1016/j.jhin.2020.12.017.

Anderson, D.J., Podgorny, K., Berríos-Torres, S.I. et al. (2014). Strategies to prevent surgical site infections in acute care hospitals: 2014 update. *Infect. Control Hosp. Epidemiol.* 35: 605–627. https://doi.org/10.1086/676022.

Andersson, A.E., Bergh, I., Karlsson, J., and Nilsson, K. (2010). Patients' experiences of acquiring a deep surgical site infection: an interview study. *Am. J. Infect. Control* 38: 711–717. https://doi.org/10.1016/j.ajic.2010.03.017.

Annaqeeb, M.K., Zhang, Y., Dziedzic, J.W. et al. (2021). Influence of surgical team activity on airborne bacterial distribution in the operating room with a mixing ventilation system: a case study at St. Olav's Hospital. *J. Hosp. Infect.* 116: 91–98. https://doi.org/10.1016/j.jhin.2021.08.009.

Badia, J.M., Casey, A.L., Petrosillo, N. et al. (2017). Impact of surgical site infection on healthcare costs and patient outcomes: a systematic review in six European countries. *J. Hosp. Infect.* 96: 1–15. https://doi.org/10.1016/j.jhin.2017.03.004.

Barbadoro, P., Marmorale, C., Recanatini, C. et al. (2016). May the drain be a way in for microbes in surgical infections? *Am. J. Infect. Control* 44: 283–288. https://doi.org/10.1016/j.ajic.2015.10.012.

Bataille, C., Venier, A.-G., Caire, F. et al. (2021). Benefits of a 14-year surgical site infections active surveillance programme in a French teaching hospital. *J. Hosp. Infect.* 117: 65–73. https://doi.org/10.1016/j.jhin.2021.08.001.

Baxter, E. (2021). A midwifery-led prevalence programme for caesarean section surgical site infections. *J. Hosp. Infect.* 109: 78–81. https://doi.org/10.1016/j.jhin.2020.12.008.

Beldi, G., Bisch-Knaden, S., Banz, V. et al. (2009). Impact of intraoperative behavior on surgical site infections. *Am. J. Surg.* 198: 157–162. https://doi.org/10.1016/j.amjsurg.2008.09.023.

Bischoff, P., Kubilay, N.Z., Allegranzi, B. et al. (2017). Effect of laminar airflow ventilation on surgical site infections: a systematic review and meta-analysis. *Lancet Infect. Dis.* 17: 553–561. https://doi.org/10.1016/S1473-3099(17)30059-2.

Bode, L.G.M., Kluytmans, J.A.J.W., Wertheim, H.F.L. et al. (2010). Preventing surgical-site infections in nasal carriers of *Staphylococcus aureus*. *N. Engl. J. Med.* 362: 9–17. https://doi.org/10.1056/NEJMoa0808939.

Bonn, D. (2000). Maggot therapy: an alternative for wound infection. *Lancet* 356: 1174. https://doi.org/10.1016/S0140-6736(05)72870-1.

Bratzler, D.W., Dellinger, E.P., Olsen, K.M. et al. (2013). Clinical practice guidelines for antimicrobial prophylaxis in surgery. *Am. J. Health-Syst. Pharm.* 70: 195–283. https://doi.org/10.2146/ajhp120568.

Brown, A. (2018). Diagnosing and managing infection in acute and chronic wounds. *Nurs. Times* 114: 36–41.

Caroff, D.A., Chan, C., Kleinman, K. et al. (2019). Association of open approach vs laparoscopic approach with risk of surgical site infection after colon surgery. *JAMA Netw. Open* 2: e1913570. https://doi.org/10.1001/jamanetworkopen.2019.13570.

Charnley, J. (1970). Operating-theatre ventilation. *Lancet* 295: 1053–1054. https://doi.org/10.1016/S0140-6736(70)91174-8.

Chetter, I.C., Oswald, A.V., Fletcher, M. et al. (2017). A survey of patients with surgical wounds healing by secondary intention; an assessment of prevalence, aetiology, duration and management. *J. Tissue Viability* 26: 103–107. https://doi.org/10.1016/j.jtv.2016.12.004.

Coello, R., Charlett, A., Wilson, J. et al. (2005). Adverse impact of surgical site infections in English hospitals. *J. Hosp. Infect.* 60: 93–103. https://doi.org/10.1016/j.jhin.2004.10.019.

Cruse, P.J.E. (1973). A five-year prospective study of 23,649 surgical wounds. *Arch. Surg.* 107: 206. https://doi.org/10.1001/archsurg.1973.01350200078018.

Cruse, P.J.E. and Foord, R. (1980). The epidemiology of wound infection: a 10-year prospective study of 62,939 wounds. *Surg. Clin. North Am.* 60: 27–40. https://doi.org/10.1016/S0039-6109(16)42031-1.

Darouiche, R.O., Wall, M.J., Itani, K.M.F. et al. (2010). Chlorhexidine-alcohol versus povidone-iodine for surgical-site antisepsis. *N. Engl. J. Med.* 362: 18–26. https://doi.org/10.1056/NEJMoa0810988.

David, T.S. and Vrahas, M.S. (2000). Perioperative lower urinary tract infections and deep sepsis in patients undergoing total joint arthroplasty. *J. Am. Acad. Orthop. Surg.* 8: 66–74. https://doi.org/10.5435/00124635-200001000-00007.

Edmiston, C.E., Griggs, R.K., Tanner, J. et al. (2016). Perioperative hair removal in the 21st century: utilizing an innovative vacuum-assisted technology to safely expedite hair removal before surgery. *Am. J. Infect. Control* 44: 1639–1644. https://doi.org/10.1016/j.ajic.2016.03.071.

Guy, H. and Grothier, L. (2012). Using negative pressure therapy in wound healing. *Nurs. Times* 108: 16.

Haley, R.W., Culver, D.H., White, J.W. et al. (1985). The efficacy of infection surveillance and control programs in preventing nosocomial infections in US hospitals. *Am. J. Epidemiol.* 121: 182–205. https://doi.org/10.1093/oxfordjournals.aje.a113990.

Hennessey, D.B., Burke, J.P., Ni-Dhonochu, T. et al. (2010). Preoperative hypoalbuminemia is an independent risk factor for the development of surgical site infection following gastrointestinal surgery: a multi-institutional study. *Ann. Surg.* 252: 325–329. https://doi.org/10.1097/SLA.0b013e3181e9819a.

Hoffman, P.N., Williams, J., Stacey, A. et al. (2002). Microbiological commissioning and monitoring of operating theatre suites. *J. Hosp. Infect.* 52: 1–28. https://doi.org/10.1053/jhin.2002.1237.

Humphreys, H., Marshall, R.J., Ricketts, V.E. et al. (1991). Theatre over-shoes do not reduce operating theatre floor bacterial counts. *J. Hosp. Infect.* 17: 117–123. https://doi.org/10.1016/0195-6701(91)90175-8.

Jenks, P.J., Laurent, M., McQuarry, S., and Watkins, R. (2014). Clinical and economic burden of surgical site infection (SSI) and predicted financial consequences of elimination of SSI from an English hospital. *J. Hosp. Infect.* 86: 24–33. https://doi.org/10.1016/j.jhin.2013.09.012.

Johnson, M.P., Kim, S.J., Langstraat, C.L. et al. (2016). Using bundled interventions to reduce surgical site infection after major gynecologic cancer surgery. *Obstet. Gynecol.* 127: 1135–1144. https://doi.org/10.1097/AOG.0000000000001449.

Korol, E., Johnston, K., Waser, N. et al. (2013). A systematic review of risk factors associated with surgical site infections among surgical patients. *PLoS One* 8: e83743. https://doi.org/10.1371/journal.pone.0083743.

Leaper, D.J., Tanner, J., Kiernan, M. et al. (2015). Surgical site infection: poor compliance with guidelines and care bundles: surgical site infection guideline compliance. *Int. Wound J.* 12: 357–362. https://doi.org/10.1111/iwj.12243.

Leong, G., Wilson, J., and Charlett, A. (2006). Duration of operation as a risk factor for surgical site infection: comparison of English and US data. *J. Hosp. Infect.* 63: 255–262. https://doi.org/10.1016/j.jhin.2006.02.007.

Lidwell, O.M., Lowbury, E.J., Whyte, W. et al. (1982). Effect of ultraclean air in operating rooms on deep sepsis in the joint after total hip or knee replacement: a randomised study. *BMJ.* 285: 10–14. https://doi.org/10.1136/bmj.285.6334.10.

Lipp, A. and Edwards, P. (2014). Disposable surgical face masks for preventing surgical wound infection in clean surgery. *Cochrane Database Syst. Rev* 2: CD002929. https://doi.org/10.1002/14651858.CD002929.pub2.

Mitchell, A., Spencer, M., and Edmiston, C. (2015). Role of healthcare apparel and other healthcare textiles in the transmission of pathogens: a review of the literature. *J. Hosp. Infect.* 90: 285–292. https://doi.org/10.1016/j.jhin.2015.02.017.

Moucha, C.S., Clyburn, T., Evans, R.P., and Prokuski, L. (2011). Modifiable risk factors for surgical site infection. *J. Bone Joint Surg. Am.* 93: 398–404.

National Institute for Health and Care Excellence (2016). Chronic wounds: advanced wound dressings and antimicrobial dressings. www.nice.org.uk/advice/esmpb2/chapter/key-points-from-the-evidence

National Institute for Health and Care Excellence. (2020). Surgical site infections: prevention and treatment. www.nice.org.uk/guidance/ng125

NICE (2019). Surgical site infections: prevention and treatment NICE guideline [NG125]Published: 11 April 2019 Last updated: 19 August 2020. https://www.nice.org.uk/guidance/ng125/chapter/recommendations#preoperativephase.

Nolan, M.B., Martin, D.P., Thompson, R. et al. (2017). Association between smoking status, preoperative exhaled carbon monoxide levels, and postoperative surgical site infection in patients undergoing elective surgery. *JAMA Surg.* 152: 476. https://doi.org/10.1001/jamasurg.2016.5704.

Obara, H., Takeuchi, M., Kawakubo, H. et al. (2020). Aqueous olanexidine versus aqueous povidone-iodine for surgical skin antisepsis on the incidence of surgical site infections after clean-contaminated surgery: a multicentre, prospective, blinded-endpoint, randomised controlled trial. *Lancet Infect. Dis.* 20: 1281–1289. https://doi.org/10.1016/S1473-3099(20)30225-5.

Parvizi, J., Barnes, S., Shohat, N., and Edmiston, C.E. (2017). Environment of care: is it time to reassess microbial contamination of the operating room air as a risk factor for surgical site infection in total joint arthroplasty? *Am. J. Infect. Control* 45: 1267–1272. https://doi.org/10.1016/j.ajic.2017.06.027.

Paulson, E.C., Thompson, E., and Mahmoud, N. (2017). Surgical site infection and colorectal surgical procedures: a prospective analysis of risk factors. *Surg. Infect.* 18: 520–526. https://doi.org/10.1089/sur.2016.258.

Reichel, M., Heisig, P., and Kampf, G. (2011). Identification of variables for aerobic bacterial density at clinically relevant skin sites. *J. Hosp. Infect.* 78: 5–10. https://doi.org/10.1016/j.jhin.2011.01.017.

Reiffel, A.J., Barie, P.S., and Spector, J.A. (2013). A multi-disciplinary review of the potential association between closed-suction drains and surgical site infection. *Surg. Infect.* 14: 244–269. https://doi.org/10.1089/sur.2011.126.

Ridgeway, S., Wilson, J., Charlet, A. et al. (2005). Infection of the surgical site after arthroplasty of the hip. *J. Bone Joint Surg. Br.* 87-B: 844–850. https://doi.org/10.1302/0301-620X.87B6.15121.

Seamon, M.J., Wobb, J., Gaughan, J.P. et al. (2012). The effects of intraoperative hypothermia on surgical site infection: an analysis of 524 trauma laparotomies. *Ann. Surg.* 255: 789–795. https://doi.org/10.1097/SLA.0b013e31824b7e35.

Serra-Aracil, X. (2011). Surgical site infection in elective operations for colorectal Cancer after the application of preventive measures. *Arch. Surg.* 146: 606. https://doi.org/10.1001/archsurg.2011.90.

Stacey, A. and Humphreys, H. (2002). A UK historical perspective on operating theatre ventilation. *J. Hosp. Infect.* 52: 77–80. https://doi.org/10.1053/jhin.2002.1276.

Sykes, P.K., Brodribb, R.K., McLaws, M.-L., and McGregor, A. (2005). When continuous surgical site infection surveillance is interrupted: the Royal Hobart Hospital experience. *Am. J. Infect. Control* 33: 422–427. https://doi.org/10.1016/j.ajic.2005.04.244.

Tanner, J. and Khan, D. (2008). Surgical site infection, preoperative body washing and hair removal. *J. Perioper. Pract.* 18: 232–243. https://doi.org/10.1177/175045890801800602.

Tanner, J. and Parkinson, H. (2006). Double gloving to reduce surgical cross-infection. *Cochrane Database Syst. Rev.* 3: CD003087. https://doi.org/10.1002/14651858.CD003087.pub2.

Tanner, J., Norrie, P., and Melen, K. (2011). Preoperative hair removal to reduce surgical site infection. *Cochrane Database Syst. Rev.* 11: CD004122. https://doi.org/10.1002/14651858.CD004122.pub4.

Tanner, J., Padley, W., Davey, S. et al. (2013). Patient narratives of surgical site infection: implications for practice. *J. Hosp. Infect.* 83: 41–45. https://doi.org/10.1016/j.jhin.2012.07.025.

Tanner, J., Dumville, J.C., Norman, G., and Fortnam, M. (2016). Surgical hand antisepsis to reduce surgical site infection. *Cochrane Database Syst. Rev.* 1: CD004288. https://doi.org/10.1002/14651858.CD004288.pub3.

Tapiwa Chamanga, E. (2018). Clinical management of non-healing wounds. *Nurs. Stand.* 32: 48–63. https://doi.org/10.7748/ns.2018.e10829.

Tavolacci, M.P., Pitrou, I., Merle, V. et al. (2006). Surgical hand rubbing compared with surgical hand scrubbing: comparison of efficacy and costs. *J. Hosp. Infect.* 63: 55–59. https://doi.org/10.1016/j.jhin.2005.11.012.

Troughton, R., Mariano, V., Campbell, A. et al. (2019). Understanding determinants of infection control practices in surgery: the role of shared ownership and team hierarchy. *Antimicrob. Resist. Infect. Control* 8: 116. https://doi.org/10.1186/s13756-019-0565-8.

Tuuli, M.G., Liu, J., Stout, M.J. et al. (2016). A randomized trial comparing skin antiseptic agents at cesarean delivery. *N. Engl. J. Med.* 374: 647–655. https://doi.org/10.1056/NEJMoa1511048.

Waisbren, E., Rosen, H., Bader, A.M. et al. (2010). Percent body fat and prediction of surgical site infection. *J. Am. Coll. Surg.* 210: 381–389. https://doi.org/10.1016/j.jamcollsurg.2010.01.004.

Ward, V.P., Charlett, A., Fagan, J., and Crawshaw, S.C. (2008). Enhanced surgical site infection surveillance following caesarean section: experience of a multicentre collaborative post-discharge system. *J. Hosp. Infect.* 70: 166–173. https://doi.org/10.1016/j.jhin.2008.06.002.

Webster, J. and Osborne, S. (2015). Preoperative bathing or showering with skin antiseptics to prevent surgical site infection. *Cochrane Database Syst. Rev.* 2: CD004985. https://doi.org/10.1002/14651858.CD004985.pub5.

WHO (2018). Global guidelines for the prevention of surgical site infection, second edition. Geneva: World Health Organization; 2018. Licence: CC BY-NC-SA 3.0 IGO. https://www.who.int/teams/integrated-health-services/infection-prevention-control/surgical-site-infection.

Whyte, W., Hodgson, R., and Tinkler, J. (1982). The importance of airborne bacterial contamination of wounds. *J. Hosp. Infect.* 3: 123–135. https://doi.org/10.1016/0195-6701(82)90004-4.

Whyte, W., Hamblen, D.L., Kelly, I.G. et al. (1990). An investigation of occlusive polyester surgical clothing. *J. Hosp. Infect.* 15: 363–374. https://doi.org/10.1016/0195-6701(90)90093-4.

World Health Organization (2018). *Global Guidelines for the Prevention of Surgical Site Infection*, 2e. Geneva, Switzerland: World Health Organization.

Zhang, Y., Zheng, Q.-J., Wang, S. et al. (2015). Diabetes mellitus is associated with increased risk of surgical site infections: a meta-analysis of prospective cohort studies. *Am. J. Infect. Control* 43: 810–815. https://doi.org/10.1016/j.ajic.2015.04.003.

10

Respiratory Infections

Infections of the Respiratory Tract

The respiratory tract is protected by the coughing and sneezing reflexes. Within the nose, the nasal conchae increase the surface area of the mucosae and cause inspired air to eddy, trapping small particles as it travels over them. Lymphoid tissue in the pharyngeal, palatine and lingual tonsils operates as a further defence. The entire respiratory tree, except for the alveoli, is lined with mucus-secreting epithelium. The mucus traps foreign substances and is carried upwards to the pharynx by the action of the cilia and swallowed. Smoking paralyses the action of the cilia, eventually destroying them, explaining why people who smoke heavily are at particular risk of lower respiratory tract infections (Figure 10.1).

Respiratory infections are very common in the community and premises where healthcare is delivered. There are two broad categories.

- *Upper respiratory tract infections* (URTIs), involving the respiratory passages from the nostrils to the larynx. These are usually minor, often caused by viruses, contracted in the community and usually resolve without treatment.
- *Lower respiratory tract infections* involving the bronchi and alveoli. These are serious and often life-threatening.

Pneumonia

Pneumonia causes inflammation of the parenchymal (functional) tissue of the lung. It is responsible for most deaths caused by infection of the respiratory tract, particularly in older people and infants. Pneumonia can be acquired in hospital or the community. It results in the alveoli filling with pus, impairing gaseous exchange and reducing oxygenation, a condition are described as 'consolidation'.

Infection Prevention and Control in Healthcare Settings,
First Edition. Edward Pursell and Dinah Gould.
© 2023 John Wiley & Sons Ltd. Published 2023 by John Wiley & Sons Ltd.

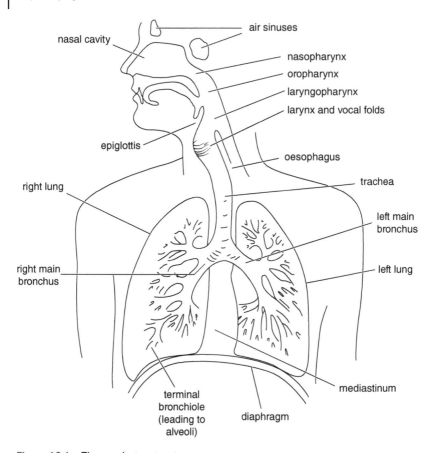

Figure 10.1 The respiratory tract.

In bronchopneumonia, consolidation is widely distributed. In lobar pneumonia, consolidation is localised.

Diagnosis of pneumonia is not straightforward and varies between centres (Browne et al. 2014). Initial diagnosis is based on clinical presentation: the appearance of greenish-yellow mucus that is often blood-stained, fever, pyrexia, shortness of breath and chest pain. Diagnosis is confirmed by microbial sampling of the sputum and chest x-ray. Bronchoscopy and bronchoalveolar lavage can be used to obtain sputum if insufficient is generated by expectoration. These are invasive procedures associated with complications, including further introduction of infection. For some pathogens, specific diagnostic tests are available. For example, pneumonia caused by *Streptococcus pneumoniae* can be confirmed by a test to detect pneumococcal antigens in the urine.

Treatment is with oral or intravenous antimicrobials.

Hospital-acquired Pneumonia

Hospital-acquired pneumonia (HAP) is defined as pneumonia manifesting at least 48 hours after admission. Early-onset HAP (occurring within four days of admission) is usually caused by the same types of pathogens as those responsible for community-acquired pneumonia (CAP). Late-onset HAP (occurring at least five days after admission) is usually caused by hospital pathogens and carries a higher mortality rate (see Table 10.1).

There are two types of HAP.

- Ventilator-associated pneumonia (VAP).
- Non-ventilator-associated pneumonia (nVAP).

Both require the prescription of broad-spectrum antibiotics which may act as a driver for antimicrobial resistance (Burton et al. 2016).

Ventilator-associated Pneumonia

Ventilator-associated pneumonia is HAP developing in patients who are being mechanically ventilated. Mechanical ventilation is a life-saving intervention undertaken to support patients who are critically ill. There is high risk of respiratory infection arising from loss of the protective coughing and sneezing reflexes and the presence of invasive devices.

In health, the bronchioles and alveoli are kept free of pathogens by the mucociliary escalator. The upper respiratory passages harbour large numbers of bacteria, including potential pathogens, and these can be transferred to the lower airways during the invasive procedures associated with mechanical ventilation (e.g. intubation, endotracheal suction) (Figure 10.2). Additional risk factors for VAP include obesity, impaired consciousness, a history of smoking, underlying respiratory disease and recent surgery.

Ventilator-associated pneumonia affects 10–20% of all intensive care patients, is the most common healthcare-associated infection reported in intensive care units and increases the costs of healthcare. It is associated with a 2–7% increase in risk of mortality although precise mortality rate is hard to estimate as these patients are already very ill (Hellyer et al. 2016). Mortality is higher for VAP than

Table 10.1 Bacteria most commonly responsible for healthcare-associated pneumonia.

Staphylococcus aureus
Pseudomonas aeruginosa
Acinetobacter baumannii
Escherichia coli
Klebsiella spp.

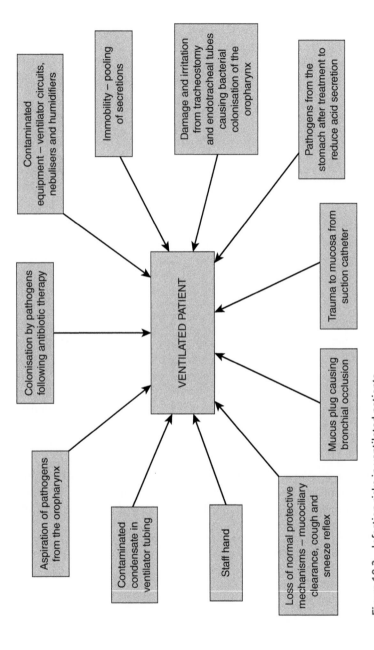

Figure 10.2 Infection risks in ventilated patients.

for CAP and it is not always easily diagnosed (Browne et al. 2014). Ventilated patients require daily monitoring to detect evidence of infection (Kalanuria et al. 2014).

Mechanisms of Contamination

Sources of pathogens responsible for VAP are:

- the oropharynx
- subglottic secretions
- the sinuses
- the stomach
- contaminated equipment.

Aspiration of Pathogens from the Oropharynx

This is the major source of bacterial VAP (Ewan et al. 2018). Many healthy people aspirate their oral secretions during sleep but they are dealt with by the body's immune defences. In ventilated patients, the risk of aspiration is increased by the presence of endotracheal and tracheostomy tubes and because the patient is sedated, has been anaesthetised or is being nursed supine.

Colonisation of the Oropharynx Colonisation of the oropharynx is usually caused by Gram-negative bacilli. They replace the normal flora after the patient has received antimicrobials (Johanson 1972).

Subglottic Secretions Contaminated secretions entering the trachea from the mouth and oropharynx seep downwards through the space between the outer wall of the endotracheal tube and the tracheal wall. The endotracheal tube should provide an airtight seal sufficient to occlude this space, but leakage is possible during periodic deflation of the cuff and because secretions accumulate in longitudinal folds in the cuff wall. It is estimated that subglottic secretions accumulate in 77% of patients intubated for longer than three days (Spray et al. 1976). Low-pressure, high-volume endotracheal tube cuffs do not eliminate pooling, but are associated with lower risk of infection (Lacherade et al. 2018).

Colonisation of the Stomach The stomach becomes heavily colonised with potential pathogens during mechanical ventilation (Torres et al. 1993). In health, ingested bacteria present in food are destroyed by hydrochloric acid which has a pH of 2. Colonisation of the stomach occurs if the patient is receiving drugs to neutralise gastric acid (e.g. antacids) or suppress its secretion (H_2-receptor antagonists, e.g. cimetidine). These drugs are commonly prescribed for critically ill patients to reduce the risk of stress-related peptic ulceration (Craven et al. 1986).

The oropharynx becomes colonised and the contaminated secretions are then aspirated into the respiratory passages.

Nasogastric Tubes   The presence of a nasogastric tube encourages gastric reflux, enabling the stomach contents to enter the oropharynx, followed by aspiration.

Endotracheal and Tracheostomy Tubes   Endotracheal and tracheostomy tubes rapidly become covered in biofilms, harbouring large numbers of bacteria protected from the immune defences.

Nebulisers   Nebulisers create aerosols of minute droplets able to penetrate deeply into the narrowest airways, carrying potential pathogens with them (Botman and de Krieger 1987).

Humidification   The ventilator circuit needs to be humidified to prevent the airways becoming dehydrated. The water in the reservoir of the humidifier leads to condensate forming on the lumen of the ventilator tubing. Both sources of water are a potential source of pathogens (Craven et al. 1984). The use of heat-moisture-exchange (HME) filters reduces the risk of contamination and helps to recycle the moisture in exhaled air without generating condensate.

Tracheobronchial Suction   Tracheobronchial suction is intended to prevent the contamination of secretions pooling in the respiratory tract but poor technique can introduce potential pathogens (Florentini 1992). Mucous membranes are more easily traumatised than skin. Consequently, abrasions from the suction catheter further increase the risk of infection.

Preventing Ventilator-associated Pneumonia

Ventilator-associated pneumonia can be avoided by using alternatives to mechanical ventilation and by reducing the duration of mechanical ventilation when no alternative exists. Spontaneous breathing can be encouraged through the use of standardised weaning protocols (Blackwood et al. 2011). Non-invasive intermittent positive-pressure breathing (IPPB) is an alternative to mechanical ventilation and is more suitable for patients with existing pulmonary disease (Burns et al. 2009), including COVID-19 (Burns et al. 2020). Box 10.1 outlines key infection prevention measures which can be used when mechanical ventilation is unavoidable.

Risks of Lower Respiratory Tract Infection in Postoperative Patients

Postoperative patients are at particular risk of lower respiratory tract infection, especially after major procedures requiring sedation and ventilation (Johnson et al. 2007). Risk is increased if they are too frightened to move and reluctant to

Box 10.1   Strategies to Prevent Ventilator-Associated Pneumonia

- Perform hand hygiene before and after every contact with intubated patients.
- Use a new pair of non-sterile disposable gloves for all routine contacts with respiratory equipment.
- Use HME filters to protect the breathing circuit.
- Drain condensate from the ventilator tubing.
- Drain subglottic secretions.
- Use disposable equipment (e.g. humidifiers, nebulisers), replace every 24 hours and between patients.
- Replace oxygen masks and tubing between patients.
- Store all respiratory equipment clean and dry.
- Perform tracheobronchial suction with a gloved hand and using a sterile suction catheter.

Source: Adapted from Caroff et al. (2016).

Numerous guidelines to prevent VAP have been developed based on care bundles, in which each component is designed to reduce a major source of risk (Hellyer et al. 2016). Key interventions include:

- reducing risks associated with the endotracheal tube and other instruments
- elevating the head of the bed to 30–45° to prevent the aspiration of gastric contents
- improving subglottic secretion drainage with low-pressure, high-volume endotracheal tube cuffs
- avoiding unnecessary manipulation of the circuit. Handling encourages potentially contaminated secretions to enter the lumen of the endotracheal tube, allowing bacteria to enter the lower airways.

A number of additional strategies to reduce risk of VAP exist but are not usually included in bundles, either because the evidence is considered too weak or because their use has disadvantages.

- Oral hygiene is important to promote patient comfort but its efficacy in reducing VAP has not been established.
- Using oral chlorhexidine to decontaminate the oropharynx. However, mortality may actually be increased by this, perhaps because of aspiration as well as disruption to microbiotica (Bouadma and Klompas 2018).
- Routinely changing the ventilator circuit. The ventilator is protected by filters between the machine and the breathing circuit and is not a source of micro-organisms. Frequent changing is unnecessary and has cost implications. The circuit should be changed between patients and if it becomes faulty or visibly soiled.
- Routine use of prophylaxis to reduce risk of gastric ulceration. Risk of bleeding should be assessed for the individual patient before proton pump inhibitors are prescribed. Overall improvements in care appear to have reduced the incidence of bleeding in recent years.

expectorate because pain control is poor. Immobility may result in one or more of the airways becoming occluded with a plug of tenacious mucus, leading to the pooling of secretions in the air passages distal to the obstruction. The airways collapse when the air within the alveoli is absorbed and gaseous exchange in the affected area ceases. The tissue is still perfused, but the blood reaching it no longer receives oxygen and cannot be relieved of carbon dioxide. Any bacteria present multiply, giving rise to infection. The larger the mucus plug, the greater the problem because more airways are involved. An extensive area of the lung may be affected, leading to collapse (atelectasis).

If infection occurs, the mucus plug may have to be removed by bronchoscopy and aspiration if physiotherapy is insufficient to dislodge it. Antibiotics are of secondary importance to mechanical removal. Good nursing care and physiotherapy are required to prevent postoperative respiratory tract infection (Box 10.2).

Non-ventilator-associated Pneumonia

Non-ventilatory-associated pneumonia has received far less attention than VAP but this situation is now changing as it has become apparent that it is more common than previously suspected (Wolk 2021). Surveillance is hampered because at present there is no standard means of identifying cases. Prevention focuses on oral care, increasing mobility and managing dysphagia but the success of these strategies remains to be established (Mitchell et al. 2019).

Community-Acquired Pneumonia

Community-acquired pneumonia is usually caused by bacteria (Table 10.2) but can also be caused by viruses, fungi and mycoplasmas. Some cases of CAP can be managed at home but admission is often necessary to administer antimicrobials,

---

Box 10.2 Preventing Postoperative Respiratory Tract Infection

- Teach patients deep breathing exercises and the importance of early preoperative ambulation. Those with abdominal and sternal wounds should be shown how to support the incision during deep breathing and coughing.
- Disinfect anaesthetic equipment between patients, taking care to avoid recontamination when it is reassembled.
- Ensure that pain control is effective to encourage physiotherapy and early ambulation.
- Encourage patients to sit upright to prevent stasis of respiratory secretions.
- Maintain good hydration to decrease the risk of respiratory secretions becoming viscous and difficult to dislodge.

Table 10.2 Micro-organisms commonly responsible for community-acquired pneumonia.

Streptococcus pneumoniae
Mycoplasma pneumoniae
Haemophilus influenzae
Legionella pneumophila
Staphylococcus aureus

---

deliver supportive treatment and provide physiotherapy (percussion, breathing exercises, postural drainage). The incidence of CAP is increasing. The main risk factors are age, smoking and co-morbidities (Brown 2012).

Respiratory Pathogens

Streptococcus pneumoniae

Streptococcus pneumoniae is the most common cause of CAP. It is an encapsulated Gram-positive coccus transmitted via aerosols, droplets and direct contact with respiratory secretions. Transmission increases with close contact and prolonged close contact. *S. pneumoniae* is also responsible for other infections. Some are mild (e.g. otitis media, sinusitis), but severe, invasive infections may also result (e.g. meningitis, septicaemia) (Desai et al. 2016). Over 75% of cases occur in older age groups and men are more often affected than women. Invasive pneumococcal disease (IPD) most commonly occurs at the extremes of life and in any population, young children operate as the main reservoirs of infection. *S. pneumoniae* pneumonia is most common in people with pre-existing co-morbidities (e.g. diabetes, cardiovascular, hepatic and splenic disease) and often arises as a complication of another respiratory infection. Costs to health services are considerable (Campling et al. 2019). Mortality for those admitted to hospital with CAP is 5–15% and over 30% for those admitted to intensive care (Ladhani et al. 2018).

Vaccination was introduced in the UK in 2003. The pneumococcal vaccine is part of the childhood immunisation programme and is offered to adults when they reach 65 years of age. It is also recommended for people who have had splenectomy, those with dysfunction of the spleen and other chronic conditions.

Legionella pneumophila

Legionella pneumophila is a tiny, motile, Gram-negative bacillus found in soil and water. It multiplies between 20 °C and 40 °C and is responsible for legionnaires' disease. Legionnaires' disease is not uncommon but patients are slow to seroconvert and the bacteria are difficult to detect and isolate (Cunha et al. 2016).

The first recorded outbreak occurred in 1976 among delegates attending a convention of the American Legion in Philadelphia (Fraser et al. 1977). Epidemics have since been reported in many countries, mainly in hotels and hospitals. The largest outbreak in the UK occurred in Stafford District General Hospital in 1985. The ventilation system was faulty, leading to contamination of the water supply, and there were 28 deaths (O'Mahony et al. 1990). Approximately 300 cases of pneumonia caused by *L. pneumophila* are reported annually in the UK every year. Most occur in people who have been infected overseas but outbreaks originating in the UK are occasionally reported.

Epidemiological links between *Legionella* infection and contaminated hospital water are well documented and usually associated with faulty air conditioning, faulty ventilation systems or water from cooling towers (Vincent-Houdek 1993). *Legionella* has been isolated from shower units, nebulisers, humidifiers, cold and hot water circuits, water tanks and calorifiers (Liu et al. 1993). Transmission is via contaminated aerosols from humidifiers and respiratory equipment but not from showers (Woo et al. 1986). Inhalation either leads to subclinical or mild infection not involving the lungs (Pontiac fever) or fulminant pneumonia, which can be fatal. Isolation is not necessary as person-to-person spread has never been documented. Individuals who are immunocompromised are at particular risk (Vincent-Houdek 1993).

Control measures involve maintaining the hot water temperature at 60 °C and chlorinating incoming water. It is vital to maintain water systems in good working order, closing down redundant parts of the circuit that cannot be maintained at an adequate temperature and monitoring the speed of flow. Water containers and humidifiers should be cleaned and descaled at regular intervals and kept dry if the system is shut. The value of bacteriological sampling in routine prevention is debated (Liu et al. 1993).

In the UK, the treatment of choice is erythromycin with the addition of rifampicin for severe infection. Quinolone or doxycycline are also sometimes prescribed.

Mycobacterial Infections

Many species of mycobacteria exist. They inhabit soil and water and some cause animal disease transmissible to the human host. *Mycobacterium avium* occasionally causes opportunistic infections in people who are immunocompromised. *M. leprae* causes leprosy.

Tuberculosis

Mycobacterium tuberculosis is a Gram-positive species often described as the 'acid-fast' bacillus because it does not react to Gram's stain. It can infect animals but transmission is possible only between human hosts. Tuberculosis (TB) causes a chronic, progressive, serious infection but is curable and preventable. 'Consumption' was a major cause of morbidity and mortality throughout the pre-industrial era. Improvements in living conditions and the availability of antibiotics decreased prevalence in high-income countries until the 1980s but there has since been a resurgence in many countries, including the UK and US.

Transmission is via aerosols which carry the mycobacteria deep into the alveoli. Prolonged contact with an infected person increases the risk of transmission because the risk of inhalation increases with exposure. Members of the same household are at very high risk of infection. Infection contracted after brief exposure (e.g. on public transport) is rare and usually the result of super-spreading.

Mycobacteria have tough, waxy walls able to resist the humoral immune response of the host. The organisms multiply slowly and when phagocytosed are able to resist destruction. They grow inside macrophages and when these cells die, they escape and continue to multiply in the extracellular tissues of the host. Mycobacteria can remain dormant for long periods if the extracellular environment is unfavourable, resulting in the formation of a calcified lesion. This condition is described as latent TB. Patients are usually unaware that they are infected unless the lesion is revealed by chest x-ray.

The initial lesion develops in the lung at the site where the mycobacteria settled. In 90% of cases, they are contained by the host immune system but reactivation is possible and often occurs years after the original exposure in response to a change in health (e.g. developing another chronic disease, immunosuppressive therapy). The result is postprimary (secondary) TB (Hunter 2011). Postprimary TB does not confer immunity. Reinfection is possible and is very common in parts of the world where the prevalence of TB is high.

In postprimary TB, the mycobacteria multiply in large numbers, resulting in extensive tissue damage and the formation of cavities in the lungs. 'Open TB' occurs if a bronchus is eroded. The mycobacteria can be expelled during coughing and can infect other people. Patients become increasingly ill and without treatment will eventually die through loss of functional lung tissue, haemorrhage or secondary infection. Extrapulmonary TB develops if the mycobacteria spread from infected lymph nodes to the bloodstream or to other organs. In miliary TB, they travel in the bloodstream, giving rise to small foci throughout the body. The term *miliary* is derived from the appearance of the foci which are said to resemble millet seeds. Extrapulmonary TB can affect the lymph nodes, bones and joints, gastrointestinal system, bladder, reproductive system and central nervous system.

Tuberculosis mostly affects adults but all age groups are at risk. Outbreaks have been reported from closed and semi-closed environments, including hospitals, sometimes involving health workers (Haley et al. 1989). Infections are most common in the immunocompromised, especially those with HIV disease and diabetes. Other risk factors include undernutrition, smoking and high alcohol intake.

Symptoms of active disease develop slowly over weeks or months and initially may be mild, leading to delay seeking healthcare, placing other people at risk. Individuals with postprimary TB are likely to experience cough with sputum sometimes containing blood, fever, night sweats, appetite and weight loss, chest pains and fatigue. Symptoms of extrapulmonary TB may include persistently enlarged lymph nodes, abdominal pain, pain or loss of movement in an affected bone or joint and headaches and confusion if the central nervous system is involved.

Diagnosing TB is not always straightforward, particularly in children. It is based on clinical presentation, the results of chest x-ray and microbiological examination of the sputum. Mycobacteria grow very slowly in culture and early morning specimens are most likely to give the best results because the bacteria will be present in respiratory secretions that have pooled overnight. Nebulised sputum or gastric washings may be obtained from patients with dry cough. The use of rapid near-patient testing is recommended where available as it allows swift diagnosis, rapid treatment and prompt introduction of public health measures (Escombe et al. 2008). Microscopy and culture are still necessary to identify antibiotic-resistant mycobacteria, including multidrug-resistant tuberculosis (MDR-TB).

Diagnosis of extrapulmonary TB diagnosis requires CT scans, MRI scans or ultrasound scan of the affected part of the body or endoscopy. Latent TB is identified by the interferon gamma release assay (IGRA) blood test or Mantoux test. A small, hard red lesion appearing on the skin of the forearm 48–72 hours after the injection of a small amount of tuberculin is positive. Individuals who have been vaccinated may have a mild skin reaction to the Mantoux test but that does not mean that they have latent TB.

Tuberculosis is challenging to treat because the mycobacteria are protected by the macrophages and lung cavities. Patients with active disease usually receive a combination of four different anti-TB drugs (isoniazid, rifampicin, pyrazinamide, ethambutol) for 12 months. At least two drugs are given together and the drugs are changed after a few months to reduce the risk of antimicrobial resistance. Patients with pulmonary disease remain contagious for 2–3 weeks after treatment has commenced and should receive health education to reduce risks of transmission (Box 10.3). In hospital, isolation precautions are required. Patients 65 and over may experience severe side-effects from anti-TB drugs and require careful monitoring, especially if they develop other health conditions. Patients with extrapulmonary TB are often prescribed corticosteroids to reduce inflammation. Latent TB is usually treated with isoniazid for six months to prevent the infection becoming active (Getahun et al. 2015).

Box 10.3   Advice to Patients with Pulmonary Tuberculosis to Reduce Risks of Transmission during Early Treatment

- Stay away from work/school until advised that it is safe to return.
- Cover your mouth with a disposable tissue when coughing, sneezing or laughing.
- Place used tissues in a plastic bag and seal it before disposal.
- Open windows to ensure good ventilation.
- Avoid sleeping in the same room as other people. They could be exposed to the risk of infection if you cough or sneeze while asleep.

Most patients do not require hospital admission but outreach working by specialist teams is beneficial to encourage adherence to treatment to (Munro et al. 2007) which is often poor and associated with complex attitudes related to the nature of the disease, the length of time necessary for symptoms to resolve, complexity of the regimen and side-effects (Izzard et al. 2021).

Global Burden of Tuberculosis

Globally, the burden of TB is immense. Over 95% of cases and deaths are in low-income countries, with most new cases reported from India, Indonesia, China, Philippines, Pakistan, Nigeria, Bangladesh and South Africa. The WHO estimates that approximately 25% of the global population has latent TB. Of these, 5–10% are at risk of developing active infection. The WHO has set targets for reducing the global burden of TB.

Multidrug-resistant Tuberculosis

Resistance to anti-TB drugs arises through mutations on the bacterial chromosome, not by a transmissible agent (e.g. plasmid). Mutations occur spontaneously and are uncommon but if the mycobacterial population is exposed to a single antibiotic, any organisms already resistant continue to thrive but will be destroyed if a second antibiotic is administered at the same time. This is the theory underpinning combination therapy. MDR-TB develops if mycobacteria already resistant to one drug become resistant to another. If MDR-TB has developed in one patient, it is transmissible to others. Prevalence is greatest in low-income countries where access to drugs is poor, compounding the problems of resistance acquired through non-adherence to treatment. MDR-TB is a public health crisis globally. Cure is possible with second-line drugs but they must be taken for up to two years and treatment outcomes are less favourable.

In the UK MDR-TB is rare (1% of cases); 7% of cases are resistant to isoniazid only. Most cases of MDR-TB occur in people originating from countries where prevalence is high.

The more recent identification of bacterial strains able to cause extensively drug-resistant tuberculosis (XDR-TB) is extremely worrying, as treatment options are very limited. XDR-TB is a global issue with cases in many countries on most continents. In 2021, a new definition for XDT-TB was agreed. It is now characterised by the drug resistance pattern of MDR-TB with additional resistance to fluoroquinolone antibacterial drugs and at least one of the most potent second line anti-TB drugs, known as group A drugs, which (levofloxacin, moxifloxacin, bedaquiline, and linezolid) (World Health Organization 2021).

In hospital, patients with suspected or confirmed MDR-TB should be admitted to a single room with negative-pressure ventilation and the door kept closed. FFP3 masks should be worn and if the patient needs to leave the room, they should wear an FFP3 mask. Visitors should be restricted to those who had close contact with the patient before admission.

Public Health Measures for Tuberculosis

Surveillance for TB is well established in the UK and other high-income countries. Early diagnosis and immediate commencement of treatment are essential for control. Rapid diagnosis benefits the individual and is important in reducing risks to others. Transmission usually occurs between the onset of cough and the commencement of treatment (Storla et al. 2008). Contact tracing is important (Fox et al. 2013). When a patient is diagnosed with TB, their treatment team assesses which other people might be at risk of infection: household members, work colleagues and social contacts. Those at risk are followed up and advised about testing and treatment if infected. The Bacillus Calmette–Guérin vaccine (BCG) has not been given routinely to children in the UK since 2005 but is offered when an individual child is considered to be at risk. Vaccination is 70–80% effective in children but less effective in adults.

Acute Bronchitis

Acute bronchitis is a self-limiting infection causing inflammation of the lower airways without involvement of the parenchyma of the lung. There is no universally accepted diagnosis. Illness can last for 21 days or longer. The predominant symptom is coughing. Acute bronchitis is usually a community-acquired infection following URTI. Some children are prone to bronchitis. It appears to be related to poor living conditions (overcrowding, poor hygiene, poor nutrition) and is exacerbated by maternal smoking, especially during pregnancy. Individuals who have experienced childhood bronchitis are at risk of developing further symptoms during their teenage years if they smoke.

Upper Respiratory Tract Infections

Upper respiratory tract infections involve the nasal passages, pharynx, tonsils and epiglottis (see Figure 10.1). Most are minor infections acquired in the community and are caused by viruses. URTIs account for a high proportion of days lost from work and school and their impact on the health of individuals and the social and economic consequences should not be dismissed. The consequences are occasionally more serious for the very young and older adults.

Coughs and Colds

Coughs and colds are usually caused by rhinoviruses. Over 200 different types exist. Consequently, an individual recently recovered from one cold may succumb to another caused by a different rhinovirus. Rhinoviruses survive in the inanimate environment if they are protected by mucus. Frequently handled items (e.g. doorknobs, light switches, crockery) become contaminated readily and the viruses can be transferred to a new host, reaching the eyes or nose when the face is touched (Hendley et al. 1973). The nasal discharge associated with colds contains virus particles, dead cells from the nasal mucosa and bacteria of the same type present in health. General hygiene and hand hygiene are important to prevent rhinovirus infection. Other viruses occasionally responsible for 'colds' are shown in Table 10.3.

Colds are a nuisance and can cause problems in those with pre-existing respiratory difficulties, especially older adults. There is no evidence that developing an URTI is related to becoming wet or 'chilled'. The high prevalence of colds in the

Table 10.3 Viruses responsible for colds.

Rhinoviruses
Parainfluenza virus
Reoviruses
Coxsackie viruses
Adenoviruses
Respiratory syncytial virus (RSV)
Coronaviruses
Echoviruses

UK has been attributed to the damp climate but they also occur in hot, dry countries. In babies and young children, URTIs can interfere with feeding and may be associated with acute otitis media (AOM) or involvement of the lower airways. The community nurse's advice is helpful. They can provide reassurance to parents and recognise when medical intervention is necessary (Taylor 1988) (Box 10.4). Bacterial invasion of the damaged epithelium is rare and antimicrobials are seldom required.

Acute Otitis Media and Otitis Media

Acute otitis media is inflammation of the middle ear. It is a common childhood complaint. Symptoms include pain, pyrexia and discharge from the ear (otorrhoea). The child is likely to rub the ear and is fretful and irritable. The middle ear is lined with respiratory mucosa and often becomes inflamed. Purulent fluid collects in the middle ear, causing the tympanic membrane to bulge and change in appearance, increasing pressure and pain. Perforation may occur under pressure to release bloodstained mucopurulent discharge.

Antimicrobials should not be routinely prescribed for AOM but if parents are concerned, delayed treatment is an option; if the child's condition has not improved after 72 hours, treatment can then be administered (Scottish Intercollegiate Guidelines Network 2003). A short initial course of antibiotics (e.g. amoxicillin) may be beneficial in children under two years of age or with severe disease. Analgesics (paracetamol) that also reduce temperature are useful. When

---

Box 10.4   Managing Upper Respiratory Tract Infections in Children

- Antipyretics can reduce pyrexia. Paracetamol dose calculated according to body weight is safe and has analgesic properties. Aspirin and aspirin-containing preparations should not be given to children under the age of 16 years as they have been associated with encephalopathy and hepatitis (Reye syndrome).
- Decongestant drops may be helpful before a feed to allow the infant to breathe when swallowing frequently.
- Antihistamines may be useful in cases of allergy when the nasal mucosa is swollen but they do not speed recovery. They cause drowsiness which may be a nuisance in older children.
- Antitussive medicines suppress coughing and may be helpful if the household has been disturbed at night or the child is distressed.
- Antibiotics should only be prescribed in the event of bacterial infection (e.g. streptococcal throat infection).

frequent attacks of AOM occur, referral to an ear and throat specialist should be advised (Scottish Intercollegiate Guidelines Network 2003).

Otitis media with effusion (OME) ('glue ear') is the term used to describe inflammation accompanied by the collection of viscous fluid inside the middle ear. OME usually resolves spontaneously and should not be treated with antibiotics (Scottish Intercollegiate Guidelines Network 2003). Children with OME should be carefully monitored so hearing loss and problems with speech and language, development, behaviour and difficulties at school can be detected. In some cases, the fluid is aspirated from the middle ear and grommets (plastic aeration tubes) are inserted through the tympanic membrane into the middle ear.

Croup

Croup (laryngeal spasm) is a complication of a viral infection affecting the larynx and trachea. The child develops a blocked nose followed by noisy, harsh-sounding inspiration (stridor). Croup is a very common condition. It is usually short-lived and resolves spontaneously but is very distressing for the child and frightening for parents (Bjornson and Johnson 2013). At one time, treatment involved using steam to liquefy secretions and relieve obstruction. The modern alternative is a steamy bathroom.

Most children recover without treatment but croup remains a worrying condition because:

- children occasionally develop airway obstruction and exhaustion leading to emergency admission to ensure that the airways remain patent
- rarely, acute epiglottitis supervenes and emergency treatment is necessary. Acute epiglottitis is usually caused by *Haemophilus influenzae*
- children occasionally experience repeated attacks of croup. In this situation, allergy should be suspected.

Respiratory Syncytial Virus

Respiratory syncytial virus (RSV) causes acute respiratory infection in infants, young children and adults who are immunocompromised, resulting in significant health burden (French et al. 2016). Infection is more likely to be severe in babies under the age of six months. Bronchiolitis (inflammation of the bronchioles) and pneumonia may result and death is not uncommon. In older children, RSV infection is usually milder. By the age of four years, most children show serological evidence of previous infection, but this does not necessarily result in lasting immunity. Outbreaks of RSV have been documented in the community and may occur in hospital, especially among very sick children, contributing to morbidity and mortality. Virus particles are present in nasal secretions and nosocomial transmission is possible via hands (Isaacs et al. 1991).

Pertussis

Pertussis (whooping cough) is caused by the Gram-negative bacterium *Bordetella pertussis*. The bacteria do not appear to be carried in a healthy throat (Weiss and Hewlett 1986). Non-specific symptoms without the typical cough develop within 5–7 days. The child appears to have a cold but is highly infectious, releasing a large number of bacteria from the nasopharynx. The later paroxysmal phase is characterised by coughing ending in a characteristic 'whoop', sometimes with vomiting. Pertussis is particularly severe in infants under six months of age and is sometimes life-threatening (Bedford and Elliman 2006). Vaccination is an important public health measure.

Diphtheria

Diphtheria is caused by the Gram-positive bacillus *Corynebacterium diphtheriae*. Childhood vaccination has been very successful and cases are extremely rare in the UK. Travellers to Eastern Europe, the former Soviet Union and low-income countries may be exposed to the organism. Infection results in an acute respiratory illness characterised by the formation of a tenacious 'membrane' (comprising leucocytes, bacteria and respiratory epithelial cells) within the upper respiratory tract. This membrane can cause laryngeal obstruction, leading to death unless emergency tracheostomy is undertaken to maintain a patent airway. *C. diphtheriae* releases an exotoxin causing severe complications (e.g. myocarditis, peripheral neuropathy). Diphtheria is a notifiable disease to allow contact tracing (Box 10.5).

Influenza

Influenza is caused by RNA viruses belonging to the family of orthomyxoviruses. They have an affinity for mucoproteins on the surface of human and other mammalian cells. There are three types of influenza virus: A, B and C. The surface of each is coated with a number of specific antigens (V, H, N) to which the host responds by secreting the corresponding antibody. Standard nomenclature is employed to classify the different strains according to their surface antigens. For influenza A, the type that causes most disease in humans, the key antigens are the H (Hemagglutinin) and N (Neuraminidase) antigens. Thus Influenza H1 N1, as type 1 of each, and H3N2 has Hemagglutinin 3 and Neuraminidase 2.

Box 10.5   Management of Patients and Contacts with Diphtheria

- Inform the proper officer of the relevant public health authority that a case of diphtheria has been identified.
- Isolate patients.
- Use personal protective clothing (gloves, aprons, masks).
- Treat the patient with penicillin and diphtheria antitoxin.
- Treat contacts with erythromycin and immunisation with diphtheria toxoid.
- Pay meticulous attention to oral hygiene and pain relief.
- Monitor vital signs, including respiration.
- Cardiac monitoring if myocardial involvement is suspected.

Influenza is transmitted via infected nasopharyngeal secretions, resulting in an acute infection with fever, headache, anorexia, myalgia, profound malaise and relatively minor respiratory symptoms. The antiviral drugs oseltamivir and zanamivir can be used within 48 hours of the onset of symptoms to shorten the duration of illness for specified groups, for postexposure prophylaxis to those at high risk and in outbreaks.

Influenza is an unpleasant, debilitating illness, disrupting work or school. The consequences can be grave for older adults and those in poor health. Pneumonia can result if the traumatised respiratory epithelium is colonised by potential pathogens (e.g. *Staphylococcus aureus, H. influenzae*).

Influenza viruses are widespread globally, resulting in epidemics every few years in the winter (Paules and Fauci 2019). Spread across the community is most common for type A, which is the most virulent. Type C is least likely to cause epidemics. Super-spreading, in which a few highly infectious individuals are responsible for a disproportionately large number of infections, has been reported (Lau et al. 2013).

Globally, pandemics have been recorded but are difficult to predict. In 1918, 20 million people died from influenza and, unusually, most were young adults. In the 1950s, a pandemic of Asian flu resulted in a high incidence of infection but a lower rate of mortality. Most major outbreaks represent the emergence of new variants of influenza virus with different surface antigens (antigenic drift). The population has no immunity against the new antigens so infection becomes rife. Antigenic drift is most marked with type A.

The existence of the three different strains of the virus, differences in the surface antigens displayed by members of the same strain and the phenomenon of antigenic drift mean that the control of influenza is challenging. No single vaccine provides lasting immunity. Instead, annual vaccination is necessary as each new strain emerges. In the UK, children and particular groups at risk are offered vaccination (Table 10.4).

Table 10.4   Target groups offered influenza vaccination in the United Kingdom.

- People aged 65 and older
- Patients with chronic respiratory disease, including those with asthma who require use of a nebuliser
- Patients with chronic heart disease
- Patients with chronic renal disease
- Patients with diabetes
- Patients with immunosuppressive conditions
- Staff engaged in health and social care

The control of nosocomial outbreaks of influenza is challenging. Vaccinating health workers reduces risk to patients and helps avoid service disruption (Carman et al. 2000).

The influenza vaccine, prepared from inactivated, highly purified viruses, is cheap and safe with few side-effects. Immunisation is available in health centres, pharmacies and from occupational health departments for eligible health workers. Practice nurses and pharmacists play an important role encouraging uptake which historically has been poor. Reasons for not receiving vaccination for influenza are related to the belief that it is not very effective because it must be repeated annually and the associated inconvenience of attending for vaccination each year. Outbreaks in hospitals and nursing homes frequently result in service disruption through staff sickness.

'Swine Flu'

'Swine flu' was the popular name given to the virus responsible for the influenza pandemic occurring in 2009–2010. It was first reported in Mexico and was so named because it is similar to the virus affecting pigs. Rapid transmission occurred internationally because this was a new infection for which existing immunity was lacking. The infection was not more serious than other types of influenza and most cases were mild, although there were some reports of serious illness, mainly in the immunocompromised and pregnant women. The WHO declared the pandemic officially over in August 2010. Infection is now prevented as part of the annual influenza vaccination.

Avian Influenza

Avian influenza ('bird flu') is a highly contagious disease of birds caused by influenza A viruses (Campbell 2006). In birds, it can present as a mild illness with low mortality or as a severe illness with a very high mortality rate. The H5N1 strain is a particular threat because it can remain viable in bird droppings for long periods and is able to spread among birds and from birds to other animals through ingestion and inhalation. Migratory birds often carry H5N1 asymptomatically but domestic flocks of poultry appear especially susceptible to rapid, fatal epidemics. The widespread occurrence of H5N1 has prompted concern that it could give rise to a novel human influenza illness with pandemic potential, although so far it appears to have infected mostly people in close contact with birds.

Guidelines for the management of pandemics have been developed (UK Government Departments 2017). Drugs having the greatest potential for treatment are oseltamivir and zanamivir.

Suggested Activities

Exercise 10.1 Self-assessment

1 Pneumonia is responsible for most deaths caused by respiratory tract infection. True/False

2 Complete the sentence: 'There are two types of hospital acquired pneumonia (HAP). These are called . . .'

3 Which of the following can result in pneumonia in patients who are mechanically ventilated?
   A Aspiration of pathogens from the mouth
   B Colonisation of the stomach
   C Contaminated suction catheters
   D All the above

4 *Escherichia coli* is the pathogen most often causing community-acquired pneumonia. True/False

5 Explain why isolation precautions are not considered necessary for patients with infection caused by *Legionella pneumophila*.

6 Infections caused by *Mycobacterium tuberculosis* are:
   A Always highly resistant to the commonly used antimicrobials
   B Particularly severe for people who live with HIV disease
   C Restricted to the lungs
   D Prevented by routine vaccination in high-income countries

7 Influenza viruses are:
   A DNA viruses
   B Coated with specific antigens
   C Capable of antigenic drift
   D Capable of causing severe infection in particular groups

8 What does the acronym AGP stand for?

9 Which of the following groups benefit from influenza vaccination?
   A School-age children
   B Patients with diabetes
   C Patients undergoing renal dialysis
   D None of the above

10 Pertussis (whooping cough) is caused by the Gram-positive bacterium *Bordetalla pertussis*.
    True/False

Exercise 10.2

Choose a respiratory pathogen that has caused problems/has the potential to cause problems in your own clinical setting.

- What are the problems/potential problems?
- Apply the chain of infection to suggest solutions.
- Identify lessons for future clinical practice, policy and education in your organisation.

Exercise 10.3

Obtain the paper by Browne et al. (2014) from the reading list at the end of this chapter. It describes an online survey undertaken to explore how VAP is diagnosed and managed in different centres. Read the paper and address the following questions.
   A What are the study findings?
   B Do you believe them?
   C Can this study be used to improve local practice?

References

Bedford, H. and Elliman, D. (2006). Prevention, diagnosis and management of pertussis. *Nurs. Times* 102: 42–44.

Bjornson, C.L. and Johnson, D.W. (2013). Croup in children. *Can. Med. Assoc. J.* 185: 1317–1323. https://doi.org/10.1503/cmaj.121645.

Blackwood, B., Alderdice, F., Burns, K. et al. (2011). Use of weaning protocols for reducing duration of mechanical ventilation in critically ill adult patients: cochrane systematic review and meta-analysis. *BMJ.* 342: c7237. https://doi.org/10.1136/bmj.c7237.

Botman, M.J. and de Krieger, R.A. (1987). Contamination of small-volume medication nebulizers and its association with oropharyngeal colonization. *J. Hosp. Infect.* 10: 204–208. https://doi.org/10.1016/0195-6701(87)90148-4.

Bouadma, L. and Klompas, M. (2018). Oral care with chlorhexidine: beware! *Intens. Care Med.* 44: 1153–1155. https://doi.org/10.1007/s00134-018-5221-x.

Brown, J.S. (2012). Community-acquired pneumonia. *Clin. Med.* 12: 538–543. https://doi.org/10.7861/clinmedicine.12-6-538.

Browne, E., Hellyer, T.P., Baudouin, S.V. et al. (2014). A national survey of the diagnosis and management of suspected ventilator-associated pneumonia. *BMJ Open Respir. Res.* 1: e000066. https://doi.org/10.1136/bmjresp-2014-000066.

Burns, K.E.A., Adhikari, N.K.J., Keenan, S.P., and Meade, M. (2009). Use of non-invasive ventilation to wean critically ill adults off invasive ventilation: meta-analysis and systematic review. *BMJ.* 338: b1574–b1574. https://doi.org/10.1136/bmj.b1574.

Burns, G.P., Lane, N.D., Tedd, H.M. et al. (2020). Improved survival following ward-based non-invasive pressure support for severe hypoxia in a cohort of frail patients with COVID-19: retrospective analysis from a UK teaching hospital. *BMJ Open Respir. Res.* 7: e000621. https://doi.org/10.1136/bmjresp-2020-000621.

Burton, L.A., Price, R., Barr, K.E. et al. (2016). Hospital-acquired pneumonia incidence and diagnosis in older patients. *Age Ageing* 45: 171–174. https://doi.org/10.1093/ageing/afv168.

Campbell, S. (2006). Avian influenza: are you prepared? *Nurs. Stand.* 21: 51–56. https://doi.org/10.7748/ns2006.10.21.5.51.c6372.

Campling, J., Jones, D., Chalmers, J.D. et al. (2019). The impact of certain underlying comorbidities on the risk of developing hospitalised pneumonia in England. *Pneumonia* 11: 4. https://doi.org/10.1186/s41479-019-0063-z.

Carman, W.F., Elder, A.G., Wallace, L.A. et al. (2000). Effects of influenza vaccination of health-care workers on mortality of elderly people in long-term care: a randomised controlled trial. *Lancet* 355: 93–97. https://doi.org/10.1016/S0140-6736(99)05190-9.

Caroff, D.A., Li, L., Muscedere, J., and Klompas, M. (2016). Subglottic secretion drainage and objective outcomes: a systematic review and meta-analysis. *Crit. Care Med.* 44: 830–840. https://doi.org/10.1097/CCM.0000000000001414.

Craven, D.E., Goularte, T.A., and Make, B.J. (1984). Contaminated condensate in mechanical ventilator circuits. A risk factor for nosocomial pneumonia? *Am. Rev. Respir. Dis.* 129: 625–628.

Craven, D.E., Kunches, L.M., Kilinsky, V. et al. (1986). Risk factors for pneumonia and fatality in patients receiving continuous mechanical ventilation. *Am. Rev. Respir. Dis.* 133: 792–796.

Cunha, B.A., Burillo, A., and Bouza, E. (2016). Legionnaires' disease. *Lancet* 387: 376–385. https://doi.org/10.1016/S0140-6736(15)60078-2.

Desai, S., Policarpio, M.E., Wong, K. et al. (2016). The epidemiology of invasive pneumococcal disease in older adults from 2007 to 2014 in Ontario, Canada:

a population-based study. *CMAJ Open* 4: E545–E550. https://doi.org/10.9778/cmajo.20160035.

Escombe, A.R., Moore, D.A.J., Gilman, R.H. et al. (2008). The infectiousness of tuberculosis patients coinfected with HIV. *PLoS Med.* 5: e188. https://doi.org/10.1371/journal.pmed.0050188.

Ewan, V.C., Reid, W.D.K., Shirley, M. et al. (2018). Oropharyngeal microbiota in frail older patients unaffected by time in hospital. *Front. Cell. Infect. Microbiol.* 8: 42. https://doi.org/10.3389/fcimb.2018.00042.

Florentini, A. (1992). Potential hazards of tracheobronchial suctioning. *Intens. Crit. Care Nurs.* 8: 217–226. https://doi.org/10.1016/0964-3397(92)90053-M.

Fox, G.J., Barry, S.E., Britton, W.J., and Marks, G.B. (2013). Contact investigation for tuberculosis: a systematic review and meta-analysis. *Eur. Respir. J.* 41: 140–156. https://doi.org/10.1183/09031936.00070812.

Fraser, D.W., Tsai, T.R., Orenstein, W. et al. (1977). Legionnaires' disease: description of an epidemic of pneumonia. *N. Engl. J. Med.* 297: 1189–1197. https://doi.org/10.1056/NEJM197712012972201.

French, C.E., McKenzie, B.C., Coope, C. et al. (2016). Risk of nosocomial respiratory syncytial virus infection and effectiveness of control measures to prevent transmission events: a systematic review. *Influenza Other Respir. Viruses* 10: 268–290. https://doi.org/10.1111/irv.12379.

Getahun, H., Matteelli, A., Chaisson, R.E., and Raviglione, M. (2015). Latent *mycobacterium tuberculosis* infection. *N. Engl. J. Med.* 372: 2127–2135. https://doi.org/10.1056/NEJMra1405427.

Haley, C.E., McDonald, R.C., Rossi, L. et al. (1989). Tuberculosis epidemic among hospital personnel. *Infect. Control Hosp. Epidemiol.* 10: 204–210. https://doi.org/10.2307/30144334.

Hellyer, T.P., Ewan, V., Wilson, P., and Simpson, A.J. (2016). The Intensive Care Society recommended bundle of interventions for the prevention of ventilator-associated pneumonia. *J. Intens. Care Soc.* 17: 238–243. https://doi.org/10.1177/1751143716644461.

Hendley, J.O., Wenzel, R.P., and Gwaltney, J.M. (1973). Transmission of rhinovirus colds by self-inoculation. *N. Engl. J. Med.* 288: 1361–1364. https://doi.org/10.1056/NEJM197306282882601.

Hunter, R.L. (2011). Pathology of post primary tuberculosis of the lung: an illustrated critical review. *Tuberculosis* 91: 497–509. https://doi.org/10.1016/j.tube.2011.03.007.

Isaacs, D., Dickson, H., O'Callaghan, C. et al. (1991). Handwashing and cohorting in prevention of hospital acquired infections with respiratory syncytial virus. *Arch. Dis. Child.* 66: 227–231. https://doi.org/10.1136/adc.66.2.227.

Izzard, A., Wilders, S., Smith, C. et al. (2021). Improved treatment completion for tuberculosis patients: the case for a dedicated social care team. *J. Infect.* 82: e1–e3. https://doi.org/10.1016/j.jinf.2020.12.019.

Johanson, W.G. (1972). Nosocomial respiratory infections with gram-negative bacilli: the significance of colonization of the respiratory tract. *Ann. Intern. Med.* 77: 701. https://doi.org/10.7326/0003-4819-77-5-701.

Johnson, R.G., Arozullah, A.M., Neumayer, L. et al. (2007). Multivariable predictors of postoperative respiratory failure after general and vascular surgery: results from the patient safety in surgery study. *J. Am. Coll. Surg.* 204: 1188–1198. https://doi.org/10.1016/j.jamcollsurg.2007.02.070.

Kalanuria, A., Zai, W., and Mirski, M. (2014). Ventilator-associated pneumonia in the ICU. *Crit. Care* 18: 208. https://doi.org/10.1186/cc13775.

Lacherade, J.-C., Azais, M.-A., Pouplet, C., and Colin, G. (2018). Subglottic secretion drainage for ventilator-associated pneumonia prevention: an underused efficient measure. *Ann. Transl. Med.* 6: 422–422. https://doi.org/10.21037/atm.2018.10.40.

Ladhani, S.N., Collins, S., Djennad, A. et al. (2018). Rapid increase in non-vaccine serotypes causing invasive pneumococcal disease in England and Wales, 2000–17: a prospective national observational cohort study. *Lancet Infect. Dis.* 18: 441–451. https://doi.org/10.1016/S1473-3099(18)30052-5.

Lau, L.L.H., Ip, D.K.M., Nishiura, H. et al. (2013). Heterogeneity in viral shedding among individuals with medically attended influenza A virus infection. *J. Infect. Dis.* 207: 1281–1285. https://doi.org/10.1093/infdis/jit034.

Liu, W.K., Healing, D.E., Yeomans, J.T., and Elliott, T.S.J. (1993). Monitoring of hospital water supplies for Legionella. *J. Hosp. Infect.* 24: 1–9. https://doi.org/10.1016/0195-6701(93)90084-D.

Mitchell, B.G., Russo, P.L., Cheng, A.C. et al. (2019). Strategies to reduce non-ventilator-associated hospital-acquired pneumonia: a systematic review. *Infect. Dis. Health* 24: 229–239. https://doi.org/10.1016/j.idh.2019.06.002.

Munro, S.A., Lewin, S.A., Smith, H.J. et al. (2007). Patient adherence to tuberculosis treatment: a systematic review of qualitative research. *PLoS Med.* 4: e238. https://doi.org/10.1371/journal.pmed.0040238.

O'Mahony, M.C., Stanwell-Smith, R.E., Tillett, H.E. et al. (1990). The Stafford outbreak of Legionnaires' disease. *Epidemiol. Infect.* 104: 361–380. https://doi.org/10.1017/S0950268800047385.

Paules, C.I. and Fauci, A.S. (2019). Influenza vaccines: good, but we can do better. *J. Infect. Dis.* 219: S1–S4. https://doi.org/10.1093/infdis/jiy633.

Scottish Intercollegiate Guidelines Network (2003). *Diagnosis and Management of Childhood Otitis Media in Primary Care: A National Clinical Guideline.* Edinburgh: SIGN.

Spray, S.B., Zuidema, G.D., and Cameron, J.L. (1976). Aspiration pneumonia. *Am. J. Surg.* 131: 701–703. https://doi.org/10.1016/0002-9610(76)90181-1.

Storla, D.G., Yimer, S., and Bjune, G.A. (2008). A systematic review of delay in the diagnosis and treatment of tuberculosis. *BMC Pub. Health* 8: 15. https://doi.org/10.1186/1471-2458-8-15.

Taylor, B. (1988). Coughs and colds in children. *Health Visit.* 612: 313–315.

Torres, A., El-Ebiary, M., González, J. et al. (1993). Gastric and pharyngeal flora in nosocomial pneumonia acquired during mechanical ventilation. *Am. Rev. Respir. Dis.* 148: 352–357. https://doi.org/10.1164/ajrccm/148.2.352.

UK Government Departments (2017). Pandemic flu. www.gov.uk/guidance/pandemic-flu

Vincent-Houdek, M. (1993). Legionella monitoring: a continuing story of nosocomial infection prevention. *J. Hosp. Infect.* 25: 117–124. https://doi.org/10.1016/0195-6701(93)90102-6.

Weiss, A.A. and Hewlett, E.L. (1986). Virulence factors of *Bordetella pertussis*. *Annu. Rev. Microbiol.* 40: 661–686. https://doi.org/10.1146/annurev.mi.40.100186.003305.

Wolk, D.M. (2021). Non-ventilator-associated hospital-acquired pneumonia: implications for the clinical laboratory. *Clin. Microbiol. Newslett.* 43: 53–60. https://doi.org/10.1016/j.clinmicnews.2021.03.003.

Woo, A.H., Yu, V.L., and Goetz, A. (1986). Potential in-hospital modes of transmission of *Legionella pneumophila*. Demonstration experiments for dissemination by showers, humidifiers, and rinsing of ventilation bag apparatus. *Am. J. Med.* 80: 567–573. https://doi.org/10.1016/0002-9343(86)90809-0.

World Health Organization (2021). WHO announces updated definitions of extensively drug-resistant tuberculosis. www.who.int/news/item/27-01-2021-who-announces-updated-definitions-of-extensively-drug-resistant-tuberculosis

11

Infections Associated with Intravascular Devices

Intravascular devices are indwelling instruments used to obtain venous or arterial access. Peripheral lines are used to access small blood vessels. Central venous catheters (CVCs) are inserted into large vessels. Intravascular devices are used extensively in hospital to:

- administer fluids, medication, blood products and nutrients
- facilitate haemodynamic monitoring (e.g. central venous pressure)
- permit frequent blood sampling.

Infection Risks Associated with Intravascular Devices

Infection is a risk with any intravascular device because insertion breaches the skin, which is the body's major barrier against pathogens. Contamination of the blood has very serious consequences because it is usually sterile. Bacteraemia (the presence of bacteria in the blood) may be transient or lead to septicaemia (multiplication of bacteria in the blood) and overwhelming sepsis. Septicaemia results in fever, chills, rigors and hypertension. Circulating micro-organisms can become lodged in tissues in other parts of the body, causing secondary infection (e.g. osteomyelitis, endocarditis) through haematogenous seeding. Risk of infection is much higher for central venous catheters than peripheral vascular catheters (PVCs). Mortality for patients with catheter-related bloodstream infections (CR-BSI) is 15%.

Sources of Infection Associated with Intravascular Devices

The routes allowing pathogenic invasion are shown in Figure 11.1.

Micro-organisms can gain access via four possible routes (Zingg and Pittet 2009).

Infection Prevention and Control in Healthcare Settings,
First Edition. Edward Purssell and Dinah Gould.
© 2023 John Wiley & Sons Ltd. Published 2023 by John Wiley & Sons Ltd.

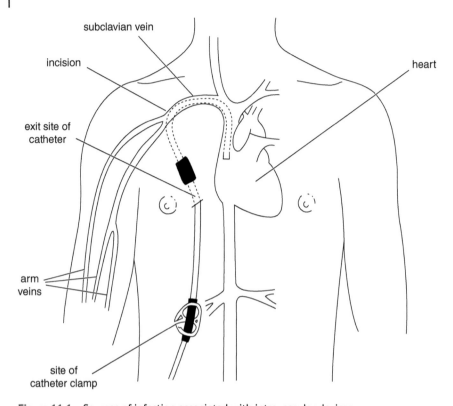

Figure 11.1 Sources of infection associated with intravascular devices.

- Along the inside of the vein from the cannula insertion point or between the outside of the device and the vein. These are described as the *intraluminal* and *extraluminal* routes respectively. Migration can occur when the device is introduced or when it is manipulated.
- Along the vein from a contaminated catheter hub (injection access port). This is a major entry route as the hub is frequently manipulated and decontamination is often overlooked (Moureau and Flynn 2015).
- From another infected source, often the urinary or respiratory tract. Pathogens may be carried from another site via the bloodstream and settle onto the device as they are carried past.
- From contaminated infusate. Contamination during commercial production is unlikely because stringent quality control measures are employed. It usually occurs in clinical settings via the hands of health workers.

The source of a bloodstream infection has key implications for clinical practice (Box 11.1)

Box 11.1 Classifying bloodstream infections and applications to practice
• Primary bloodstream infections are directly related to the presence of an intravascular device. Strategies to prevent and control these infections focus on how the device is managed.
• Secondary bloodstream infections are seeded from another site of infection elsewhere in the body. They are avoided by strategies to prevent and control infection at these other sites (e.g. good practice managing urinary catheters).

Collectively, bloodstream infections account for only 7.3% of healthcare-associated infections (HCAIs) in the UK but individually they are the most expensive to treat (National Institute for Health and Care Excellence 2013). Sixty percent of bloodstream infections reported in hospital are related to the use of an intravascular device and of these, 80% are associated with a CVC. Morbidity and mortality are high for this group (Guembe et al. 2015) but as these patients are already very sick, in many cases it is not possible to determine whether the infection was directly responsible for death (O'Grady et al. 2011).

The consequences of developing a bloodstream infection for the patient and costs to the health service have prompted numerous studies to improve practice for patients in intensive care units (Bion et al. 2013; Pronovost et al. 2006, 2010). Their findings indicate wide variation in practice between different organisations and considerable scope for improving practice. Nevertheless, some aspects of infection prevention and control have received surprisingly little research and there are many unanswered questions concerning management.

Pathogens Causing Infections Associated with Intravascular Devices

The pathogens most commonly responsible for infections associated with intravascular devices are shown in Table 11.1. Staphylococcal infections usually originate from the patient's skin or health workers' hands. Gram-negative infections are more likely to originate from the hospital environment.

Pathogenesis

The first step towards infection is colonisation of the catheter (Cercenado 1990). Bacteria adhere to the surface and a biofilm forms within 24 hours. As it develops, the organisms become incorporated into the biofilm and are protected from the host defences, multiplying in sufficient numbers to establish infection (Raad 1998).

Table 11.1 Pathogens most commonly responsible for infections associated with intravascular devices.

Gram-positive bacteria	Gram-negative bacteria	Fungi
Staphylococcus aureus	*Escherichia coli*	*Candida* spp.
Staphylococcus epidermidis		*Pseudomonas* spp.
		Burkholderia cepacia
		Enterobacter spp.

Biofilms may eventually harbour large communities of different organisms with different antimicrobial susceptibility. A device that has become infected must be removed because the biofilm protects the bacteria from the action of antimicrobials used to treat the infection.

Diagnosis of Intravascular Device-related Bloodstream Infection

Traditionally, bloodstream infections have been diagnosed on the basis of a positive blood culture coupled with the signs and symptoms of infection. Two blood cultures are obtained – one from a peripheral vein, the other from the catheter. Infection is indicated if both test positive for the same organism. A swab should also be taken from the exit site of the device if there are signs of inflammation.

Diagnosis is not always straightforward because many patients are immunocompromised and do not develop the signs and symptoms of infection and false-negative results are common because patients may already be receiving antimicrobials (Safdar et al. 2005). If the catheter has been removed, the catheter tip can be cultured. This approach is inexact (sometimes described as semi-quantitative) because accidental contamination is possible during removal. The recovery of more than 15 organisms is taken as an indication that the catheter is the source of infection.

The present unsatisfactory approaches to diagnosis are being superseded by molecular diagnostics.

Treatment

If an intravenous catheter appears to be infected, it must be removed and the tip sent for culture. Broad-spectrum antimicrobial therapy usually begins at once because bloodstream infections are so serious.

Types of Intravascular Device

Peripheral Vascular Catheters

Peripheral vascular catheters are used to administer fluids and medication. They are intended for short-term intravenous therapy (up to 90 hours) and are not suitable for administering vesicant or highly irritating drugs (e.g. chemotherapeutic agents). PVCs are sited for 30–80% of inpatients at some point during their stay (Zhang et al. 2016). PVCs are short devices, 7.5 cm long or less. They are inserted into a vein in the patient's hand, arm or occasionally foot with the tip terminating a short distance into the vein.

Despite widespread use, PVCs are often misused. They are frequently inserted unnecessarily and left in place when no longer needed or no longer function properly (Zingg and Pittet 2009). Examples of malfunction include leakage, occlusion and extravasation of the infusate into the tissues, resulting in mechanical phlebitis (inflammation of the vein).

The incidence of bloodstream infection reported for PVCs is 0.2–0.7 per 1000 days of intravenous device use (Maki et al. 1977). This is much lower than infection rates associated with CVCs but still represents considerable morbidity and patient distress because the number of PVCs inserted is so high (Mermel 1995).

Phlebitis

Phlebitis is the most common complication associated with the use of PVCs. It is caused by the device or the infusate irritating the endothelial wall of the vein and is often accompanied by the formation of a blood clot (thrombophlebitis). Estimated rates range widely (2–80%), probably reflecting differences in practice and reporting; there is no internationally agree definition. Numerous scales have been developed to quantify severity but are of doubtful value as none have been validated (Ray-Barruel et al. 2014). Phlebitis is not indicative of infection but is uncomfortable and patients may assume that infection is developing because the symptoms of inflammation and infection are similar (Table 11.2).

Risk factors for phlebitis include inadequate skin antisepsis when the device is inserted, inadequate training for health workers and dressings failing to protect

Table 11.2 Signs and symptoms of phlebitis.

Erythema over the insertion point of the cannula
Tenderness
Pain
Swelling
Warmth

the insertion point from contamination, often because they have become dislodged (Alexandrou et al. 2018). Extended dwell time, antimicrobial administration, use of irritant infusates, female gender, insertion into the forearm and prior existence of infection are further predisposing factors (Lv and Zhang 2020).

The value of replacing peripheral devices routinely to avoid complications is debatable as they are not designed to be used for longer than 72–96 hours, use is frequently abandoned early before therapy is complete (Marsh et al. 2015) and replacement is not accompanied by decreased infection rates (Rickard et al. 2012). Recommendations to prevent mechanical phlebitis and infection are shown in Box 11.2.

The risk of infection for peripheral venous cannulation appears to be greater if phlebitis has occurred and is usually caused by migration of bacteria from the insertion point. Localised cutaneous infection may also develop at the point where the cannula enters the skin, resulting in erythema and the appearance of pus. Cannulae should be removed if phlebitis develops.

Catheter hubs are frequently manipulated and become heavily contaminated but the most effective method of cleansing remains to be determined (Moureau and Flynn 2015). UK guidelines recommend scrubbing with 2% chlorhexidine based on expert opinion (Loveday et al. 2014).

Box 11.2 Preventing mechanical phlebitis and infection associated with peripheral intravascular devices

- Provide training for all staff responsible for siting intravascular devices and caring for patients with devices in place.
- Use the smallest gauge cannula compatible with patient need.
- Undertake hand hygiene and adopt aseptic technique to insert and manipulate the device.
- Disinfect the skin (2% chlorhexidine in 70% isopropanyl) before insertion.
- Avoid siting the device in the forearm (devices at this site often become dislodged or do not function effectively).
- Secure the device firmly in place to avoid mechanical irritation caused by friction.
- Treat the insertion point like a wound: apply a sterile, occlusive dressing that will allow inspection of the insertion site. Replace dressings if they become loose or contaminated.
- Avoid use when potentially irritant infusates and drugs will be administered.
- Monitor dwell time and remove when the device is no longer needed or after 90 hours.
- Maintain records of when and why the device was inserted and other key information.

Midline Catheters

Midline catheters are 7.5–20 cm in length. They are inserted into the antecubital vein in the upper arm. The tip does not reach the central veins in the thorax. Midline catheters are used to permit venous access for up to four weeks. They are not suitable for administering vesicant or highly irritant drugs (Alexandrou et al. 2011) but otherwise are safe and effective (Mermel 1995). The number of bloodstream infections is 0.2 per 1000 days of intravascular device use (Maki et al. 1977). Midline catheters can be valuable for patients who need therapy for up to four weeks in cases where peripheral access is poor but their use has largely been superseded by peripherally inserted central catheters (PICCs), which have the added benefits of central tip location and are designed for long-term use.

Central Venous Catheters

Central venous catheters are used to administer large volumes of intravenous fluids, medication or blood products when administration over a long period is anticipated; administer medication that would be highly irritating to peripheral veins; permit long-term access to the central venous system for repeated procedures (e.g. blood sampling); and when peripheral venous access is impossible or poor. They are inserted via the subclavian, jugular or femoral veins and terminate in the great veins of the thorax. Subclavian insertion is associated with lower risk of infection. Risk of contamination at the femoral vein site is high, while devices inserted into the jugular vein are easily dislodged and contamination is possible, probably from the adjacently situated otolarynx. Risk of phlebitis is less than with PVCs.

Centrally Inserted Central Venous Catheters
Three types are available.

- Non-tunnelled catheters
- Skin-tunnelled catheters
- Implantable ports

These devices are usually multilumen (have numerous channels). Each lumen allows independent access to the venous circulation, permitting incompatible drugs and fluids to be administered via the same line.

Non-tunnelled CVCs
Non-tunnelled CVCs are multilumen devices intended for short-term venous access for patients in acute settings. They are usually inserted via the subclavian, jugular or femoral veins and are fastened to the patient's skin with non-dissolving sutures.

Skin-tunnelled Catheters

Skin-tunnelled catheters (e.g. Hickman lines, Broviac lines) are large-bore silicone catheters used when longer-term vascular access is required and are often employed to deliver blood products, chemotherapy or total parenteral nutrition (TPN). One end of the catheter is introduced into a vein (usually the cephalic, subclavian, internal or external jugular vein) and threaded into the superior vena cava. The other end is tunnelled under the skin and pulled out to form an exit site away from the point of insertion. This helps reduce the risk of pathogens on the skin gaining access to the bloodstream.

Most tunnelled CVCs have a fibrous cuff positioned beneath the skin about 1.5 cm from the exit site. Initially, the cuff is held in place with sutures but the patient's tissues grow around the cuff and it can be removed 7–21 days later. The cuff acts as a mechanical barrier to bacteria and risk of infection is less than with non-tunnelled catheters. Complications include occlusion; mechanical phlebitis and deep venous thrombosis.

Implantable Ports

Implantable ports (e.g. Port-a-Caths®) comprise a catheter attached to a reservoir implanted into a surgically created pocket in the chest wall or upper arm. A needle is inserted into the port to allow access to the reservoir. Implantable ports are intended for long-term use, often for patients managed in the community. They interfere less with daily activities than other types of CVCs and reduce risks of infection but insertion and removal are more challenging than for other types of CVC. Insertion is by needle and there is risk of needlestick injury to health workers.

Peripherally Inserted Catheters

Peripherally inserted catheters (PICCs) are fine-bore CVCs introduced into a peripheral vein (usually the basilic or cephalic vein) and threaded towards the heart. They are used for patients requiring intravenous therapy long term (up to six months). PICC lines are used to deliver parenteral nutrition, antimicrobial drugs, chemotherapy and when multiple blood transfusions are necessary. They are not secured by a cuff and must be sealed by a clamp or alternative device. Associated complications include displacement, occlusion, mechanical phlebitis and deep venous thrombosis but risks of infection are lower than for other types of CVC.

Haemodynamic Monitoring Systems

Haemodynamic monitoring systems are used to monitor blood pressure inside the veins, heart and arteries, measure blood flow and blood oxygen saturation for very sick patients in the intensive care unit, patients undergoing major surgery and for some diagnostic procedures. Associated risks are serious: haematoma formation, arteriovenous fistula, stenosis of a vessel and blood loss (O'Horo et al. 2014).

Pulmonary Artery Catheters
Pulmonary artery catheters (Swan–Ganz) are used to manage very sick patients who are haemodynamically unstable. Insertion can traumatise the heart valves and cardiac endothelium, leading to endocarditis.

Haemodialysis Catheters
Haemodialysis catheters used during sort term renal dialysis are placed in one of the great veins. There are two lumens, one carrying blood from the patient to the dialysis machine, the other returning it. These devices are not intended for long-term haemodialysis because they are associated with a very high risk of infection (Hoen et al. 1998). For patients needing haemodialysis long term, a cuffed tunnelled catheter is used to reduce risks of infection.

Umbilical Catheters
Umbilical catheters are used in neonatal care to permit repeated blood sampling and haemodynamic monitoring. The catheter enters via the umbilical vein, passes through the hepatic vein and into the inferior vena cava. Umbilical catheters should not be used for longer than 14 days because infection risk from the heavily colonised umbilical stump is high.

Risk Factors for Infection Associated with Intravascular Devices

Risks are influenced by a number of factors.

- Type of intravascular device (Maki et al. 1977) (Table 11.3).
- Catheter material. Biofilm formation and colonisation progress more rapidly over rough than smooth surfaces. Catheters manufactured from smooth, inert materials (e.g. Teflon˚, silicone, polyurethane) are less likely to become colonised than those made of polyvinyl chloride (Sheth et al. 1983). Catheters intended for longer-term use are made of silicone or Teflon because they are less irritant to the venous endothelium, further helping to reduce risks of infection (Toltzis and Goldmann 1990).
- Dwell time. The longer that the catheter remains in place, the greater the risk of contamination (Raad et al. 1993).

Table 11.3 Bloodstream infections associated with different types of central venous catheters (CVC) and other intravascular devices.

Device	Bloodstream infection per 1000 days of use
Non-cuffed CVC	1
Non-tunnelled CVC	2.7
Umbilical CVC	2.7
Tunnelled CVC	1.7
Arterial catheter (haemodynamic monitoring)	1.7
Pulmonary artery catheters (Swan–Ganz)	3.7
Haemodialysis catheters	4.8

Source: Adapted from Maki et al. (2006).

- The patient's condition. Risk of infection is highest among those who are immunocompromised and those requiring parenteral nutrition or drugs administered via the intravascular route (e.g. antimicrobials, cytotoxic therapy).

Preventing Infection Associated with Central Venous Catheters

Numerous guidelines have been developed to recommend good practice when CVCs are inserted and manipulated (O'Grady et al. 2011). Although there are gaps in the evidence available and many of the recommendations are based on expert opinion, advice is consistent.

- CVCs are best introduced in the upper extremities because skin over the femoral vein is more likely to be heavily contaminated.
- Hand hygiene is essential before and after inserting the device and whenever the intravascular system is accessed.
- Aseptic technique is essential when the device is inserted and when the system is accessed. The use of sterile gloves, gowns and drapes (full barrier precautions) is recommended.
- Before the device is inserted, the patient's skin should be disinfected with 2% chlorhexidine gluconate in 70% alcohol. If the patient is allergic to these antiseptics, an alternative should be used (e.g. povidone iodine).
- The insertion point should be covered with a sterile, transparent semipermanent membrane dressing. If this is not practical (e.g. bleeding, heavy perspiration), sterile gauze can be used.

- The skin should be disinfected with 2% chlorhexidine gluconate in 70% alcohol or an alternative at every dressing change.
- Dressings at CVC entry sites should be changed every two days. Those covering tunnelled or implanted devices can be changed after seven days unless they become dislodged or contaminated.
- Catheter hubs, connector ports and administration sets should be managed aseptically to avoid contamination.
- Administration sets can be left in place for 72 hours unless they become disconnected or infection is suspected.
- The use of multidose vials should be avoided when drugs are administered to reduce risks of contamination.
- In-line filters can remove particulate material but there is no evidence that they reduce infection risks.
- Devices should be removed as soon as they are no longer required.

Standardised and Bundled Interventions

There is evidence that a standardised approach to the insertion of CVCs can reduce CR-BSIs (Bion et al. 2013; Pronovost et al. 2006, 2010). These studies have been highly influential and have directed policy and practice internationally (Box 11.3) but implementation has been better in some units than others and is likely to be influenced by a range of factors, especially the leadership style of senior staff and health workers' motivation (Dixon-Woods et al. 2011).

Box 11.3   Research evaluating the impact of bundled interventions to reduce catheter-related bloodstream infections

Pronovost et al. (2006) based their intervention bundle on hand hygiene, adopting full barrier precautions when CVCs were inserted, disinfecting the skin with chlorhexidine, avoiding the femoral site and removing catheters as soon as they were no longer required. Simultaneously, an educational programme for staff was introduced. The bundle was implemented in 103 intensive care units in the US and data were collected for 375 757 catheter-days. Infection rate declined from 7.7 per 1000 catheter-days at baseline to 1.4 per 1000 catheter-days 18 months later (Pronovost et al. 2010). Substantial reductions in infections related to the use of CVCs have since been reported in intensive care units in England where a similar bundle has been implemented (Bion et al. 2013).

Box 11.4   Advantages reported following the introduction of a dedicated vascular access team

Ability to standardise care
Improved quality of patient care
Improved patient outcomes
Greater patient satisfaction
Decreased costsv
Decreased CVC infection rates

Source: Savage et al. (2019); Whalen et al. (2017).

Vascular Access Teams

Many health providers have now introduced dedicated vascular access teams to promote a standardised approach to managing CVCs. Evaluations have been positive and in some centres fewer infections have been reported (Box 11.4).

Care of Patients with Indwelling Intravascular Devices Outside Hospital

Today, many patients requiring chemotherapy and long-term total parenteral therapy are managed at home. They require support from specialist nursing teams and must be taught how to manage the device before they leave hospital. Ability to recognise the signs and symptoms of infection and knowing where to seek help are essential. Comprehensive guidelines for management have been developed in conjunction with patients and other stakeholders (Chapman et al. 2019).

Suggested Activities

Exercise 11.1 Self-assessment

1   Distinguish between bacteraemia and septicaemia.

2   Complete the sentence: 'Secondary bloodstream infections are . . .'

3   Which of the following are commonly associated with bacterial bloodstream infections?
   A *Treponema pallidum*
   B *Staphylococcus aureus*
   C *Staphylococcus epidermidis*
   D Human immunodeficiency virus

4 Biofilm formation is an early important step in the development of blood-stream infection associated with intravascular devices.
True/False

5 Phlebitis is always an indicator of infection of the blood vessels.
True/False

6 A previously healthy patient who has developed a bloodstream infection is likely to have:
A Pyrexia
B Chills
C Seeding of the infection from another body site
D A positive blood culture

7 Which of the following is associated with the highest risk of bloodstream infection?
A Peripheral catheter
B Tunnelled device
C Haemodialysis catheter
D Swan–Ganz catheter

8 Care bundles can reduce the risk of bloodstream infection in patients with central venous devices.
True/False

9 Care bundles can reduce the risk of bloodstream infection in patients with peripheral intravascular devices.
True/False

10 Which of the following have been reported after the introduction of vascular access teams?
A Standardised care
B Improved patient satisfaction
C Improved quality of care
D None of the above

Exercise 11.2

Investigate the use of intravascular devices in your clinical setting. Based on the information contained in this chapter, do you think that good practice and surveillance are achieved? Identify any improvements that could be introduced and how the impact of these changes could be monitored.

Exercise 11.3

Access the paper by Bion et al. (2013) in the reference list at the end of this chapter. What levels of evidence are used to underpin the recommendations suggested to reduce bloodstream infections?
  A Summarise the study findings.
  B Do you believe them?
  C Would they be helpful to support local practice?

References

Alexandrou, E., Ramjan, L.M., Spencer, T. et al. (2011). The use of midline catheters in the adult acute care setting – clinical implications and recommendations for practice. *J. Assoc. Vascul. Acc.* 16: 35–41. https://doi.org/10.2309/java.16-1-5.

Alexandrou, E., Ray-Barruel, G., Carr, P.J. et al. (2018). Use of short peripheral intravenous catheters: characteristics, management, and outcomes worldwide. *J. Hosp. Med.* 13: https://doi.org/10.12788/jhm.3039.

Bion, J., Richardson, A., Hibbert, P. et al. (2013). 'Matching Michigan': a 2-year stepped interventional programme to minimise central venous catheter-blood stream infections in intensive care units in England. *BMJ Qual. Saf.* 22: 110–123. https://doi.org/10.1136/bmjqs-2012-001325.

Cercenado, E. (1990). A conservative procedure for the diagnosis of catheter-related infections. *Arch. Intern. Med.* 150: 1417. https://doi.org/10.1001/archinte.1990.00390190077011.

Chapman, A.L.N., Patel, S., Horner, C. et al. (2019). Updated good practice recommendations for outpatient parenteral antimicrobial therapy (OPAT) in adults and children in the UK. *JAC-Antimicrobial. Resist.* 1: dlz026. https://doi.org/10.1093/jacamr/dlz026.

Dixon-Woods, M., Bosk, C.L., Aveling, E.L. et al. (2011). Explaining Michigan: developing an ex post theory of a quality improvement program. *Milbank. Quart.* 89: 167–205. https://doi.org/10.1111/j.1468-0009.2011.00625.x.

Guembe, M., Pérez-Granda, M.J., Capdevila, J.A. et al. (2015). Nationwide study on the use of intravascular catheters in internal medicine departments. *J. Hosp. Infect.* 90: 135–141. https://doi.org/10.1016/j.jhin.2015.01.024.

Hoen, B., Paul-Dauphin, A., Hestin, D., and Kessler, M. (1998). EPIBACDIAL: a multicenter prospective study of risk factors for bacteremia in chronic hemodialysis patients. *JASN* 9: 869–876. https://doi.org/10.1681/ASN.V95869.

Loveday, H.P., Wilson, J.A., Pratt, R.J. et al. (2014). epic3: National Evidence-Based Guidelines for preventing healthcare-associated infections in NHS hospitals in

England. *J. Hosp. Infect.* 86: S1–S70. https://doi.org/10.1016/S0195-6701(13) 60012-2.

Lv, L. and Zhang, J. (2020). The incidence and risk of infusion phlebitis with peripheral intravenous catheters: a meta-analysis. *J. Vasc. Access.* 21: 342–349. https://doi.org/10.1177/1129729819877323.

Maki, D.G., Weise, C.E., and Sarafin, H.W. (1977). A semiquantitative culture method for identifying intravenous-catheter-related infection. *N. Engl. J. Med.* 296: 1305–1309. https://doi.org/10.1056/NEJM197706092962301.

Maki, D.G., Kluger, D.M., and Crnich, C.J. (2006). The risk of bloodstream infection in adults with different intravascular devices: a systematic review of 200 published prospective studies. *Mayo Clin. Proc.* 81: 1159–1171. https://doi. org/10.4065/81.9.1159.

Marsh, N., Webster, J., Mihala, G., and Rickard, C.M. (2015). Devices and dressings to secure peripheral venous catheters to prevent complications. *Cochrane Database Syst. Rev.* 6: CD011070. https://doi.org/10.1002/14651858.CD011070. pub2.

Mermel, L.A. (1995). The risk of midline catheterization in hospitalized patients: a prospective study. *Ann. Intern. Med.* 123: 841. https://doi.org/10.7326/0003-4819-12 3-11-199512010-00005.

Moureau, N.L. and Flynn, J. (2015). Disinfection of needleless connector hubs: clinical evidence systematic review. *Nurs. Res. Pract.* 2015: 1–20. https://doi. org/10.1155/2015/796762.

National Institute for Health and Care Excellence (2013). Intravenous fluid therapy in adults in hospital. www.nice.org.uk/guidance/cg174

O'Grady, N.P., Alexander, M., Burns, L.A. et al. (2011). Guidelines for the prevention of intravascular catheter-related infections. *Clin. Infect. Dis.* 52: e162–e193. https:// doi.org/10.1093/cid/cir257.

O'Horo, J.C., Maki, D.G., Krupp, A.E., and Safdar, N. (2014). Arterial catheters as a source of bloodstream infection: a systematic review and meta-analysis. *Crit. Care. Med.* 42: 1334–1339. https://doi.org/10.1097/CCM.0000000000000166.

Pronovost, P., Needham, D., Berenholtz, S. et al. (2006). An intervention to decrease catheter-related bloodstream infections in the ICU. *N. Engl. J. Med.* 355: 2725–2732. https://doi.org/10.1056/NEJMoa061115.

Pronovost, P.J., Goeschel, C.A., Colantuoni, E. et al. (2010). Sustaining reductions in catheter related bloodstream infections in Michigan intensive care units: observational study. *BMJ* 340: c309–c309. https://doi.org/10.1136/bmj.c309.

Raad, I. (1998). Intravascular-catheter-related infections. *Lancet.* 351: 893–898. https://doi.org/10.1016/S0140-6736(97)10006-X.

Raad, I., Umphrey, J., Khan, A. et al. (1993). The duration of placement as a predictor of peripheral and pulmonary arterial catheter infections. *J. Hosp. Infect.* 23: 17–26. https://doi.org/10.1016/0195-6701(93)90126-K.

Ray-Barruel, G., Polit, D.F., Murfield, J.E., and Rickard, C.M. (2014). Infusion phlebitis assessment measures: a systematic review. *J. Eval. Clin. Pract.* 20: 191–202. https://doi.org/10.1111/jep.12107.

Rickard, C.M., Webster, J., Wallis, M.C. et al. (2012). Routine versus clinically indicated replacement of peripheral intravenous catheters: a randomised controlled equivalence trial. *Lancet.* 380: 1066–1074. https://doi.org/10.1016/S0140-6736(12)61082-4.

Safdar, N., Fine, J.P., and Maki, D.G. (2005). Meta-analysis: methods for diagnosing intravascular device-related bloodstream infection. *Ann. Intern. Med.* 142: 451. https://doi.org/10.7326/0003-4819-142-6-200503150-00011.

Savage, T.J., Lynch, A.D., and Oddera, S.E. (2019). Implementation of a vascular access team to reduce central line usage and prevent central line-associated bloodstream infections. *J, Infusion Nurs.* 42: 193–196. https://doi.org/10.1097/NAN.0000000000000328.

Sheth, N.K., Franson, T.R., Rose, H.D. et al. (1983). Colonization of bacteria on polyvinyl chloride and Teflon intravascular catheters in hospitalized patients. *J. Clin. Microbiol.* 18: 1061–1063. https://doi.org/10.1128/jcm.18.5.1061-1063.1983.

Toltzis, P. and Goldmann, D.A. (1990). Current issues in central venous catheter infection. *Annu. Rev. Med.* 41: 169–176. https://doi.org/10.1146/annurev.me.41.020190.001125.

Whalen, M., Maliszewski, B., and Baptiste, D.-L. (2017). Establishing a dedicated difficult vascular access team in the emergency department: a needs assessment. *J. Infusion Nurs.* 40: 149–154. https://doi.org/10.1097/NAN.0000000000000218.

Zhang, L., Cao, S., Marsh, N. et al. (2016). Infection risks associated with peripheral vascular catheters. *J. Infect. Prevent.* 17: 207–213. https://doi.org/10.1177/1757177416655472.

Zingg, W. and Pittet, D. (2009). Peripheral venous catheters: an under-evaluated problem. *Int. J. Antimicrob. Agents* 34: S38–S42. https://doi.org/10.1016/S0924-8579(09)70565-5.

12

Gastrointestinal Infections

Food-borne and water-borne infections are major causes of morbidity and mortality globally. Outbreaks are commonly reported. In hospitals and nursing homes, they disrupt normal services and sometimes lead to service closures. All food contains micro-organisms and some raw foods are highly contaminated (Jørgensen et al. 2017). Two types of illness can result.

- Enteric infection (gastroenteritis)
- Food-borne intoxication

Enteric Infection

Enteric infection (gastroenteritis) is caused by:

- ingesting contaminated food or water
- contact with contaminated vomit and faeces
- transmission via the hands of health workers who have handled vomit or excreta without adequate hand hygiene
- person-to-person spread in the case of some enteric pathogens (e.g. *Salmonella*).

There is an incubation period while the bacteria establish themselves inside the host and multiply. Consequently, the signs and symptoms of enteric illness do not appear until several days later. Patients are infectious and precautions must be taken when excreta and vomitus are handled. Most bacteria, including those commonly responsible for enteric infection, multiply readily between 20 °C and 40 °C in a moist environment. Multiplication occurs much more slowly under refrigeration (5–10 °C) and below 0 °C food can be stored for long periods as few

Infection Prevention and Control in Healthcare Settings,
First Edition. Edward Purssell and Dinah Gould.
© 2023 John Wiley & Sons Ltd. Published 2023 by John Wiley & Sons Ltd.

bacteria are able to multiply. Heating food to 60 °C destroys most bacteria responsible for enteric infection unless it is very heavily contaminated but this is impractical for some dishes (e.g. custards, lightly boiled eggs).

Food-borne Intoxication

Food-borne intoxication is caused by ingesting food containing toxins released by micro-organisms. No incubation period is necessary and symptoms are experienced suddenly, often within a few hours. Patients with food-borne intoxication are not infectious. The toxins are heat stable and not destroyed by cooking, pasteurisation or other heat treatments.

Signs and Symptoms of Food-borne Illness

The signs and symptoms of enteric infection and intoxication are the same (Table 12.1).

Pathogens Causing Enteric Infection and Intoxication

The pathogens associated with enteric infection and intoxication are shown in Table 12.2.

Epidemiology

Food-borne illness is a major health problem, especially in low-income countries, but the burden of disease is significant everywhere. Poor hygiene in kitchens and cross-contamination between raw and cooked food are often to blame, either in

Table 12.1   Signs and symptoms of enteric infection and intoxication.

Nausea
Vomiting
Diarrhoea
Dehydration
Cramping abdominal pain
Malaise
Pyrexia

Table 12.2   Enteric infection and intoxication.

Infections	Intoxications
Salmonella	*Staphylococcus aureus*
Shigella	*Bacillus cereus*
Campylobacter	*Clostridium perfringens*
Listeria	*Clostridium botulinum*
Escherichia coli	

mass catering or domestic premises. In the UK, 17 million cases of community-acquired enteric illnesses are reported annually (Tam et al. 2012) and every year one in five people is affected. Outbreaks occur when two or more people experience similar illness after eating the same food. They are a common occurrence and require investigation by the public health authorities. According to the World Health Organization, 420 000 people die each year from eating contaminated food (World Health Organization n.d.a). Many sporadic cases of gastrointestinal infection also occur annually.

Risk Factors

Notified cases of food-borne illness underestimate the total number occurring because outbreaks are much more likely to be reported and investigated than sporadic cases. The main risk factors are:

- preparing food in advance
- inadequate cooking
- inadequate cooling
- improper storage
- reheating.

Faults during food production and processing, transport and storage before reaching the consumer further contribute to increased risk. Contamination is possible at source or at any stage in food production, transport or storage. Manufacturers use different preventive strategies. Eliminating contamination before storage is achieved by canning, freezing and the much older method of salting. Freezing maintains the bacteria at temperatures too low for multiplication and is acknowledged as one of the safest methods of preserving food, although *Salmonella* already present can survive until it is thawed, then multiply. In theory, food can remain frozen safely for years provided the equipment is in good working order, but the colour and texture of some items may deteriorate. Vacuum packing is widely used to prevent botulism.

Inadequate chilling during storage is a major contributory factor in many cases of food-borne illness and is overcome by refrigeration because bacteria multiply very slowly at 5–10 °C.

Risk factors fall into two broad categories.

- Intrinsic factors reflecting the immune status of the individual.
- Extrinsic factors reflecting lifestyle choices affecting food choice and preparation.

Intrinsic Factors

The following groups are at particular risk.

- The very young. An immature immune system results in high susceptibility to infection. Specialist community public health nurses (health visitors) play an important role educating the public about the importance of hygiene, especially when infant feeds are prepared. The incidence of gastroenteritis is higher for bottle-fed babies. Vomiting and diarrhoea are very common, resulting either because feeds are too concentrated or because of infective gastroenteritis. Today, children with chronic illness are often managed at home. Those requiring enteral nutrition are at risk if feeds become contaminated during storage or administration (Anderton et al. 1993).
- Older adults. Fewer organisms are necessary to produce an infective dose and diarrhoea and vomiting are more likely to result in dehydration and electrolyte imbalance.
- People with severe illnesses, especially the immunocompromised.

Extrinsic Factors

Groups at high risk include the following.

- Individuals unable or reluctant to leave the home to purchase fresh food through frailty, decreased mobility or mental health problems.
- Individuals with limited financial means unable to afford good-quality produce. If they lack transport, they may rely on local shops where turnover is slower and perishable items remain longer on the shelves. They are also less likely to discard suspect items because they cannot afford waste. Lack of refrigeration can be a problem in bed-and-breakfast accommodation where families with young children are housed by the social services.
- People who frequently eat out or rely on pre-prepared food.
- People travelling to countries with low standards of hygiene.
- People dependent on mass catering (e.g. schools, prisons, nursing homes, hospitals).

Investigating Outbreaks of Food-borne Illness

Outbreaks must be thoroughly investigated by the public health authorities. In hospital, the infection prevention team should be notified if food-borne illness is suspected. They will contact the local public health department as necessary and the consultant in communicable disease control (CCDC) may need to be informed. The action taken if more than one patient or health worker is affected is shown in Box 12.1.

In the community, outbreaks of food-borne illness are reported to the public health department. The CCDC assumes responsibility for undertaking investigations, providing advice and monitoring. The information is used to inform future public health campaigns and health promotion. Local authorities are responsible for reporting outbreaks of food-borne illness to the Food Standards Agency.

Outbreaks of Food-borne Illness Not Related to Gastrointestinal Illness

Sometimes cases of gastrointestinal illnesses are related to a common factor not associated with food (Table 12.3). These cases should also be reported.

Box 12.1   Required Action when Food-Borne Illness is Suspected

Hospitals

- Inform the infection prevention team and medical team in charge of the affected patients.
- Obtain stool specimens.
- Wash and dry hands thoroughly after all contact with affected patients and the near-patient environment.
- Transfer patients to single rooms with en-suite facilities if possible.
- Use protective personal equipment when handling body fluids.
- Advise affected staff not to return to work until free of symptoms.

Nursing homes

- Inform general practitioners responsible for the residents and the CCDC.
- Obtain stool specimens from affected individuals.
- Wash and dry hands thoroughly after all contact with affected residents and their close environment.
- Use protective personal equipment when handling body fluids.
- Advise affected staff not to return to work until free of symptoms.

Table 12.3   Outbreaks caused by enteric pathogens not related to food.

Exposure to recreational events outdoors involving contact with a contaminated environment (e.g. mud)

Contact with animals or their faeces

Outbreaks of verocytotoxin-producing *E. coli* (VTEC) arising through person-to-person contact

---

Preventing Food-borne Infection

Food-borne infection is preventable (Barrie 1996). Good practice includes:

- complying with the legal requirements for catering
- protecting food from contamination at all stages from production to consumption
- ensuring that all food handlers receive training in food and personal hygiene
- educating the public about food hygiene.

Legal Requirements

In the UK, the Food Standards Agency protects consumers' interests, gives advice about food safety and monitors the enforcement of legislation. The Food Safety Act 1990, the Food Hygiene Act 2013 and the Food Hygiene Regulations 2006 are intended to ensure that premises where food is prepared are safe and properly maintained. All premises used to prepare, store or serve food must be registered with the local authority and may be inspected by the Environmental Health Officers (EHOs) they employ. EHOs can inspect premises and obtain samples of food and are empowered to issue warnings and improvement notices detailing actions necessary within a given period or to close premises. They are also able to prosecute individuals responsible for breaching the regulations. Similar arrangements are in place in Europe (European Commission 2006).

Principles of Food Safety

The principles of food safety are the same in restaurants, domestic and commercial premises and in hospitals and nursing homes (Box 12.2). Healthcare practitioners (e.g. community nurses and specialist community public health nurses) and social care practitioners play an important role in the promotion of food safety.

The responsibilities of food handlers in healthcare premises vary according to the nature of the service. In large hospitals, they may only be required to hand out trays with ready-prepared meals or serve snacks from ward and satellite kitchens but in small nursing homes, they may participate in all stages of food preparation.

Box 12.2   Principles of Food Safety

Purchasing

Avoid products that do not look fresh, cans that are misshapen or pierced, cracked eggs and cartons with bulging lids (sign of fermentation).

Storage

Keep all surfaces and refrigerators scrupulously clean.
Keep kitchen cloths clean and dry. Use disposables or change daily.
Store food below 8 °C or above 63 °C.
Maintain heated trolleys used to transport food at 63 °C.
Place food in the refrigerator as soon as possible after purchase and not more than 1.5 hours later.
Keep refrigerators at 1–4 °C.
Cover all stored food to reduce risks of cross-contamination.
Store raw and cooked items separately.
Place raw food at the bottom of the refrigerator where it will not drip onto other items, especially those consumed raw.
Store items intended for human and animal consumption apart.
Monitor items and discard if not used. Sell-by dates are a suggestion only, irrespective of the date on the package.
Never put food into refrigerators used to store specimens, blood or drugs.

Preparation

Wash and dry hands thoroughly before touching food and after handling raw items.
Occlude cuts and sores on the hands with waterproof dressings.
Keep hair tied away from the face.
Use separate chopping boards and utensils for cooked and raw food and wash with detergent after use.
Wash fruit and vegetables in cold, running water.
Adhere to recommended cooking times (e.g. for pre-prepared items).
Dismantle blenders and food processors after use. Wash and dry all the parts thoroughly.

Cooking and reheating

Thaw frozen food thoroughly before cooking.
Ensure that ovens reach the required temperature before cooking time begins.
Some enteric pathogens (e.g. *Campylobacter, Salmonella*) deep in the carcasses of poultry might not otherwise be destroyed.

Stir liquids to avoid 'cold spots' around the sides of the saucepan.
Ensure that meat, poultry and fish are cooked thoroughly.
Cool food rapidly and place in the refrigerator unless it is to be consumed immediately.
If food is to be kept hot before serving, hold it at 63 °C or above.
Never refreeze food that has thawed unless it has been cooked.
Take special care with microwave ovens. 'Cold spots' can develop where heat fails to penetrate. Always follow the manufacturer's guidelines for equipment and food. Heating time should be adjusted if the machine is at a lower wattage, stirring halfway for microwaves without a turntable.
In healthcare premises, report all gastrointestinal illness in staff to the occupational health department or to a manager in smaller organisations which do not have their own occupational health department.

Under food hygiene legislation, all must receive training and managers are responsible for ensuring that they comply with legal requirements.

Cook-Chill

Cook–chill involves bulk precooking followed by rapid cooling to 0–3 °C. The items are reheated immediately before serving, usually in a microwave oven. Cook–chill is used commercially to prepare convenience foods and has been introduced in many hospitals and community-based meal provision services for the housebound. Meals should not be stored for longer than five days and should be reheated at 70 °C for at least two minutes. Cook–chill products are safe in mass catering providing the correct controls are in place during preparation, storage and plating (Shanaghy et al. 1993).

In a typical hospital system, food is prepared in a central kitchen, portioned, chilled, held under refrigeration for a maximum of five days, served onto cold plates and distributed to the wards in refrigerated trolleys before reheating. In a traditional system of bacteriological monitoring, audit involves taking samples at any stage in this process. A more comprehensive method of quality control is offered by the Hazard Analysis Critical Control Point (HACCP) system (Richards et al. 1993). A flow chart is constructed to depict all stages in production from the arrival of raw articles to the meal reaching the consumer. A number of critical points are selected at which monitoring is considered vital and sampling is performed with every batch. HACCP has improved food quality in hospitals by encouraging guidelines for good practice to be implemented and refined (Shanaghy et al. 1993).

Enteric Infections

Campylobacter

Campylobacter jejuni and *C. coli* are Gram-negative, highly motile bacteria. *Campylobacter* was not recognised as a human pathogen until the 1970s. The number of reported cases has since increased every year and it is now one of the most common causes of enteric infection (Kaakoush et al. 2015). Health workers are more likely to see patients with *Campylobacter* than many other enteric pathogens because the symptoms of severe abdominal pain and bloodstained diarrhoea are likely to prompt the victim to seek help. The incubation period is 2–10 days and illness lasts 10–14 days.

Campylobacter is widespread in the environment and has been isolated from sewage, untreated water, raw or undercooked poultry and unpasteurised milk (Silva et al. 2011). The bacteria do not multiply below 30 °C and are unlikely to grow on food at room temperature. Cross-contamination occurs between stored items which can then operate as vehicles for infection. Death is unusual but morbidity is considerable and it has been suggested that *Campylobacter* infection might be linked to the later development of Guillain–Barré syndrome.

Campylobacter appears to be less infectious than many other bacteria causing enteric infection. Person-to-person spread is rare, with only occasional reports among members of the same household (usually children during the acute diarrhoeal phase). Outbreaks are uncommon. Infection has resulted from handling family pets carrying the bacteria. Vertical transmission from mother to foetus has also been documented.

The illness is usually self-limiting but is treatable with erythromycin or aminoglycosides.

Salmonella

Salmonella is a Gram-negative, motile bacillus able to thrive under aerobic and anaerobic conditions. There are over 2500 different serotypes. The optimum temperature for growth is 37 °C, but salmonellae can multiply between 7 °C and 48 °C. They are readily destroyed by heat but withstand freezing and drying, especially if protected by protein in the food. The bacteria have been isolated from the fingers after washing and drying (Pether and Gilbert 1971). Many wild and domestic animals carry salmonellae and some cases have resulted after handling cats, dogs or exotic pets (e.g. reptiles). Traditionally, salmonellosis has been associated with eating raw and undercooked eggs but the consumption of many other types of food, including meat, especially poultry, salads and dairy products, has caused infection.

Salmonella has an incubation period of 12–72 hours in the human host. Symptoms appear up to seven days after ingestion. The illness lasts 2–5 days and is more severe in older people and the very young. Although the acute stage of infection is usually over quickly, bacteria can be shed in the faeces of asymptomatic carriers for up to three months. Diagnosis is by stool culture; bacteria are not usually present in the blood.

Management involves fluid replacement and supportive care. Antibiotics prolong carriage, but if infection is severe with complications (e.g. septicaemia or damage to the intestinal mucosa resulting in malabsorption and nutrient loss), ciprofloxacin is prescribed to reduce the duration of diarrhoea and vomiting and eliminate the bacteria from the stools (Ahmad et al. 1991). Trimethoprim may be used to treat invasive *Salmonella* infection.

Major outbreaks are associated with mass food production. In 2021, the European Centre for Disease Control (2021) reported cases of *Salmonella enteritidis* in 11 countries across Europe associated with eating pre-prepared chicken products. Over 200 people developed symptoms and a large number of cases were reported in the UK. Whole-genome sequencing indicated that all the cases had originated from the same source in Poland with evidence of person-to-person spread, illustrating the complexity of contemporary food preparation and distribution chains.

Nosocomial Salmonellosis

At one time, nosocomial salmonellosis was common. The most notorious outbreak occurred at the Stanley Royd Hospital in Wakefield, Yorkshire, in 1984. It involved over 400 patients and staff who had consumed food from the same kitchen. Nineteen frail elderly people died. The outbreak prompted a public enquiry with recommendations for the investigation, control and prevention of future outbreaks, emphasising improving kitchen facilities and practices. Until 1987, hospital kitchens were protected from prosecution by EHOs (Crown Immunity). As a result of the Stanley Royd outbreak, hospital authorities and NHS trusts whose catering departments fail to comply with requirements have since been liable to prosecution in the same way as commercial premises. The Stanley Royd incident drew attention to standards of long-term hospital care more generally, particularly the unsuitability of much of the hospital estate at the time and need for urgent improvement (Wallis 2016).

Nosocomial outbreaks caused by salmonellae are less common today as a result of improved food handling and hand hygiene but are still occasionally reported (Lee and Greig 2013). Transmission is by person-to-person spread as well as by consuming contaminated food. Occasionally, contaminated endoscopes have been implicated in transmission (Robertson et al. 2017). Salmonellae survive well in moist environments and it may be impossible to trace the source of infection.

The Enteric Fevers

The enteric fevers are caused by *Salmonella enterica* serovar Typhi and *S. enterica* serovar Paratyphi. Transmission is via contaminated water. The global burden of disease is substantial and antimicrobial resistance is a major concern (World Health Organization n.d.b). The incubation period is about 14 days. Typhoid is usually a severe illness (Box 12.3). Fever may continue for weeks and septicaemia develops about 10 days after the onset of infection, accompanied by the appearance of bacteria in the blood, urine and stools. Once the acute phase of infection is over, asymptomatic infection may continue for months, sometimes years. The usual seat of infection is the gallbladder but other organs, including the liver, may be involved. Paratyphoid fever is generally milder and of shorter duration.

Box 12.3 Typhoid

Onset of disease

- Fever: the temperature rises in a typical 'stepladder' fashion
- Slow pulse relative to the increase in body temperature
- Malaise
- Headache
- Muscular aches
- Constipation

End of first week/second week

- Rose-coloured rash ('rose spots') on the abdomen and back
- Profuse 'pea soup' diarrhoea, often bloodstained
- Abdominal distension
- Enlarged spleen
- Cough
- Apathy
- Elevated temperature

End of second week/third week

- Delirium
- Drowsiness (progressing to altered consciousness and death if untreated)
- Elevated temperature

Potential complications manifesting in the third week

- Toxaemia leading to myocarditis pneumonia and cholecystitis
- Intestinal haemorrhage
- Bowel perforation

The enteric fevers are common in low-income countries where sanitation and clean water are lacking but may affect travellers (Xavier 2006).

Salmonella enterica can be transmitted by the faecal–oral route and is highly infectious. Consumption of food washed in contaminated water can also lead to infection. Outbreaks are frequently reported, especially from Asia and Africa (Appiah et al. 2020). Diagnosis is by stool or blood culture and an agglutination test for antibodies (Widal reaction). Public health measures include eliminating the source of infection, providing safe water supplies, food preparation and pasteurising milk. Travellers to regions where typhoid is endemic can receive active immunisation.

Treatment is with chloramphenicol, ciprofloxacin, cefotaxime or azithromycin, depending on severity, the region of origin and the antimicrobial resistance of the strain causing infection. Supportive measures include correcting fluid and electrolyte imbalance.

Cholera

Vibrio cholerae is an aerobic, Gram-negative vibrio causing acute enteric infection. It occurs in regions lacking clean water and sanitation and is endemic throughout Asia, Africa and Central and South America. Transmission is by the faecal–oral route (Hainsworth 2004). The infective dose is high; large numbers of vibrios must be ingested to cause symptoms and consequently, person-to-person transmission is rare. Contaminated water is usually responsible for outbreaks, which often follow natural disasters that result in water supplies becoming disrupted. Chronic carriage is unusual although the contacts of acutely infected patients may carry vibrios asymptomatically for a few days. Although once widespread in the UK, cholera has long since been eradicated (Box 12.4).

The incubation period of cholera ranges from a few hours to five days. Many infections are mild and severe life-threatening illness occurs in only 5–10% of cases. The bacteria release an enterotoxin which alters the metabolism of the cells in the gastrointestinal mucosa. They release large volumes of fluid rapidly,

---

Box 12.4   The Broad Street Pump Incident

During the nineteenth century, cholera was endemic in the UK and a leading cause of mortality. In 1854 Dr John Snow traced an outbreak in London to a public water pump in Broad Street, Soho. At Snow's instigation, the pump handle was removed and the outbreak was controlled. Snow's work has been recognised as a very early example of an epidemiological investigation and he became known as the 'father of epidemiology'.

resulting in copious diarrhoea and vomiting. Adults lose up to a litre of fluid in one hour. Stools and vomitus are watery and specked with small white flocculi consisting of fragments of intestinal epithelium ('rice water stools'). Without treatment, massive dehydration, circulatory collapse and renal failure develop and mortality is high. Diagnosis is by microscopy and confirmed by faecal culture.

Treatment with tetracyclines can reduce diarrhoea and the duration of vibrio excretion. Vibrios are developing resistance to tetracycline so trimethoprim may be given instead. Fluid and electrolyte replacement (oral rehydration solution or intravenous fluid replacement) is essential. Public health measures include providing clean water supplies and sanitation, promoting food safety and scrupulous personal hygiene.

Shigella sonnei

Shigella sonnei is a Gram-negative bacillus causing dysentery, commonly occurring in low- and middle-income countries (Tickell et al. 2017). Infection causes acute inflammation of the large bowel and loose stools containing blood, pus and mucus. There are four species causing disease of variable severity (Table 12.4). *S. sonnei* causes the mildest symptoms. It is the species most often reported in the UK and is spread by the faecal–oral route. Outbreaks are most often reported in nurseries. Infection prevention and control measures include good standards of personal hygiene, especially hand hygiene. Chronic carriage is rare but individuals recovering from acute infection may continue to shed bacteria for several weeks.

Escherichia coli

Escherichia coli is a Gram-negative bacterium commensal in the human bowel. Colonisation occurs within a few weeks of birth and benefits the host because it reduces the risk of overgrowth by other potential pathogens. Some serotypes cause food-borne infection. These are related to a wide range of contaminated

Table 12.4   Shigella species.

Species	Geographical distribution	Presentation
Shigella dysenteriae	Tropical and subtropical	Severe
Shigella flexneri	Tropical and subtropical	Moderate
Shigella boydii	Tropical and subtropical	Moderate
Shigella sonnei	Temperate	Mild

foods (Yang et al. 2017). Cases related to vegetables are increasing although in many outbreaks, meat and dairy products have been implicated.

Serotypes fall into four groups depending on their virulence factors and the way they interact with the intestinal mucosa. The most serious infections are caused by serotypes that release shiga toxins. These are heat labile and can be destroyed by heating food to 70 °C or higher. The four groups are:

- enteropathic *E. coli* (EPEC)
- enteroinvasive *E. coli* (EIEC)
- enterotoxigenic *E. coli* (ETEC)
- enterohaemorrhagic *E. coli* (EHEC).

Enteropathic *E. coli*

Enteropathic *E. coli* is a major cause of severe diarrhoea in infants in low-income countries. Most outbreaks have been reported from hospitals or nurseries and in each case traced to a food handler or water contaminated with human sewage (Doyle 1990). This serotype is highly pathogenic because the bacteria adhere to the intestinal mucosa tightly, destroying the microvilli and disrupting absorption.

Enteroinvasive *E. coli*

Enteroinvasive *E. coli* was first described in the 1940s (Doyle 1990) and has since caused numerous outbreaks. The usual sources are food handlers or contaminated water but person-to-person spread is possible. EIEC causes invasive dysentery and bloodstained diarrhoea.

Enterotoxigenic *E. coli*

Enterotoxigenic *E. coli* causes traveller's diarrhoea in those visiting countries with poor standards of hygiene. Infection is uncommon in the UK except in those recently returned from overseas but is a major cause of enteric infection in all age groups in low-income countries. Outbreaks are usually traced to a human source. The bacteria invade the intestinal mucosa to produce watery diarrhoea without blood staining. Recovery is usually complete.

Enterohaemorrhagic *E. coli*

Enterohaemorrhagic *E. coli* is responsible for a wide range of illnesses, from mild diarrhoea to severe abdominal pain with haemorrhagic colitis. Symptoms are the result of an enterotoxin called verocytotoxin, which is produced when the bacteria adhere to the intestinal wall. The bacterium is known as verocytotoxin-producing *E. coli* (VTEC) or *E. coli* O157. It is extremely virulent and relatively low numbers cause symptoms (Williams and Ellison 1998). Infection with *E. coli* O157 can

---

Box 12.5 Outbreak of *E. coli* O157:H7 in Lanarkshire

In 1996, a serious outbreak of *E. coli* O157:H7 occurred in Lanarkshire, central Scotland, resulting in 20 deaths, all in people over 65 years. The source of infection was traced to a butcher's shop which had supplied contaminated meat and meat products to business outlets and households. Tracing the source was complicated because the products had been widely distributed. Recommendations for food handling, training, minimising contamination, regulations and enforcement and managing outbreaks have since been published by the Pennington Group, which was established by the government to investigate all aspects of the outbreak.

Source: Adapted from Williams and Ellison (1998).

---

cause thrombocytopenia and haemolytic uraemia. Both are serious conditions requiring hospitalisation. Outbreaks have been reported in the USA, Canada and the UK in households, nurseries, schools, residential homes and hospitals (Box 12.5).

Person-to-person spread occurs via the faecal–oral route and asymptomatic carriage is possible. Outbreaks have been linked to the consumption of many types of meat, especially undercooked beef products, cold cooked meats, meat pies and hamburgers, unpasteurised milk and milk products, faecally contaminated water and vegetables washed in it. Dairy cattle can operate as reservoirs.

The illness is usually self-limiting and most people recover within eight days but a small number of those infected (mainly infants, children and older people) develop haemolytic uraemic syndrome (HUS). This is a form of renal failure with a mortality of 17%. Survivors may have residual renal problems.

Many animals carry *E. coli*. Visits to farms for educational or recreational purposes carry a risk of infection with zoonoses, including *E. coli* O157. Infection is possible through contact with animals or faeces. Visitors to open farms and 'petting' zoos should receive the information shown in Box 12.6. Children are at particular risk because they frequently touch their mouths (e.g. nail biting, chewing pens, sucking thumbs).

Listeria monocytogenes

Listeria monocytogenes is a facultative Gram-positive, non-sporing bacillus present in soil and water and on vegetation. It was identified as an animal pathogen early in the twentieth century but its ability to cause human disease was not recognised until the 1980s. Most people develop immunity through exposure to bacteria in the environment and some become asymptomatic carriers.

Box 12.6   Preventing Enteric Infection from Animal Contact at Visitor Attractions

- The risk of zoonotic infection occurs through contact with animals and their environment.
- Visitors should be informed where and when they will have access to hand washing facilities. Alcohol-based hand hygiene products are not suitable on farms because hands are likely to be physically soiled.
- Ensure that hands are thoroughly washed after cleaning shoes, wheels of pushchairs, etc.
- Avoid purchasing or eating food until after leaving animal contact areas and hand washing facilities.
- Staff working in venues where animals will be handled should be aware of the associated risks and importance of hand washing.

Source: Adapted from Health and Safety Executive (n.d.).

Infection is usually mild and causes influenza-like symptoms (Levy 1989). The incubation period is 7–70 days and usually follows the consumption of unpasteurised milk and cheeses (e.g. Brie, Camembert, blue vein cheese), chilled cold meats, pâté, undercooked chicken, prepared salads (e.g. coleslaw) and cook–chill products. Hard cheeses (e.g. Cheddar), processed and cottage cheese are safe, as are pasteurised milk and milk powder because they are heated during production. Listeria grows at temperatures as low as 2 °C and multiplies in refrigerated food.

Outbreaks are seasonal and usually occur in the autumn. Food probably becomes contaminated from environmental sources during production. Occasional cases have been linked to exposure to sheep at lambing time. In pregnant women, bacteria cross the placenta and can cause spontaneous miscarriage, stillbirth or the delivery of an acutely ill baby (Buchanan et al. 2017). Neonatal listeriosis (during the first 28 days) is classified as early (within 2–3 days of delivery) or late (five days or more) onset. In early-onset cases, the infant develops septicaemia with a mortality rate of 40–50%. With late-onset listeriosis, meningitis is the most common presentation. Neonatal mortality is 25% but maternal recovery occurs spontaneously without treatment after delivery.

In adults, diagnosis is by blood or cerebrospinal fluid culture. In cases of suspected neonatal infection, swabs are obtained from the eyes, ears and placenta. Severe listeriosis is also possible for immunocompromised patients. Adults are treated with high doses of ampicillin. Infants are given gentamicin for at least two weeks. Meningitis is treated with amoxicillin or gentamicin.

Food Intoxication

Staphylococcus aureus

Staphylococcus aureus is the most common cause of food intoxication globally (Fetsch and Johler 2018). It is not reportable in the UK so its incidence is unknown and is thought to vary, depending on eating habits. Gastrointestinal symptoms are caused by ingesting heat-stable enterotoxins. The amount necessary to cause symptoms is unknown but is thought to be as little as $1\,\mu g/100\,g$ of food. Vomiting and diarrhoea usually develop within 2–6 hours, depending on the amount consumed. The cause of symptoms is poorly understood; it is thought that the toxin irritates receptors in the gut wall, relaying impulses to the vomiting centres in the brain. Typical episodes last 2–3 days.

The source of staphylococcal food intoxication is always another person and usually the result of poor hand hygiene. Risk is increased if the food handler has a septic lesion not covered by a waterproof dressing. Staphylococci multiply in the warm, damp conditions frequently provided by inadequately refrigerated food display counters in shops, restaurants and fast-food outlets, releasing large amounts of toxin. Intoxication is often linked to salty foods (e.g. ham) and sugary products. The salt or sugar discourages the growth of other bacteria, enabling large numbers of staphylococci to flourish unchecked. Other foods incriminated include fish, poultry, cakes with cream or custard fillings and salads. Cross-contamination between items stored close together is possible. Box 12.7 describes a typical outbreak and the investigation subsequently undertaken.

Box 12.7   Investigating An Outbreak of Food-Borne Illness caused by Staphylococcal Intoxication

Twenty-four members of a sports team developed vomiting, diarrhoea and abdominal pain within three hours of eating a meal in a restaurant in Umbria and 11 required emergency care. Eighteen other people eating in the same restaurant on the same day were unaffected. The public health authorities used a questionnaire to obtain food histories from affected and unaffected diners. Food samples were obtained and tested. Samples were taken from the waiters and cooks and the kitchen environment was swabbed. Staphylococcal enterotoxins were identified from a Chantilly cream dessert (consisting predominantly of cream and sugar) which had been stored outside the refrigerator for five hours. Five members of staff tested positive for the same bacteria and toxin.

Source: Adapted from Ercoli et al. (2017).

Clostridia

Clostridia are anaerobic, Gram-positive, spore-forming bacteria. They inhabit soil and play an important role in the decomposition of dead organisms. Some commensal species inhabiting the human gut release toxins after the bacteria have been ingested.

Clostridioides difficile

Clostridioides difficile is discussed in Chapter 7.

Clostridium perfringens

Clostridium perfringens is one of the most common causes of food-borne illness worldwide and has been associated with numerous outbreaks, usually associated with mass catering. The bacteria multiply rapidly between 37 °C and 41 °C. They produce 16 different toxins, which cause symptoms within 5–24 hours of ingestion. The tough spores withstand cooking but germinate when the food, often meat or gravy, is inadequately reheated. The source of an outbreak is often difficult to establish because *C. perfringens* is widespread in the environment in soil and water and is often present in the human gut, especially among long-stay patients/residents (Box 12.8).

C. perfringens is also the causative organism of gas gangrene.

Clostridium botulinum

Botulism was first described during the early nineteenth century. It is a paralytic illness resulting from the consumption of food contaminated with neurotoxins

---

Box 12.8   Investigating an Outbreak of Food-Borne Illness Caused by *Clostridium perfringens*

The source of clostridial food-borne illness in a nursing home in the UK was traced to a mince and vegetable pie and gravy. Fifteen residents aged 74–99 developed symptoms a few hours after the meal and were ill for an average of two days. Investigation by the public health authorities revealed poor kitchen practice. The mince had been cooked, cooled, reheated and served again over several days and used to make the gravy which was served with a number of different dishes. Investigation revealed lack of formal training for kitchen staff and poor record keeping concerning menu choices and what food residents had eaten. After the investigation, the nursing home was charged and fined for serving unsafe food and for poor hygienic practices. Measures were put in place to improve food standards and staff training.

Source: Adapted from Acheson et al. (2016).

released by *C. botulinum*. Symptoms develop within 2–6 hours, causing a very serious illness with a mortality rate of 5–10%. The muscles supplied by the cranial nerves are usually affected first, leading to visual disturbance, difficulty with speech and swallowing, followed by paralysis. Symptoms are variable and this, coupled with the rarity of the disease, makes diagnosis difficult. It is not always possible to detect the toxin in faeces, blood or gastric washings. Diagnosis is confirmed by detecting the toxin in stool samples. Treatment is with botulinum antitoxin to neutralise circulating toxin, accompanied with supportive therapy and symptomatic treatment.

Most cases of botulism have been associated with preserved meat, fish or vegetables because the bacteria and spores survive under anaerobic conditions that exclude competing bacteria. The toxin is destroyed by heating at 80 °C for 30 minutes but eliminating spores involves heating to 121 °C for at least 2.5 minutes. This is possible on a commercial scale but difficult to achieve domestically, with clear implications for those who preserve their own produce. The increased availability of frozen food, vacuum packing and improved distribution of fresh produce have reduced the incidence of botulism.

The largest outbreak reported in the UK involved 27 people who had eaten the same brand of hazelnut yoghurt. There was one death. The source was traced to a blown can of hazelnut conserve and unopened cartons of the yoghurt. Investigation revealed that the process used to make the hazelnut conserve had not destroyed the spores. The outbreak was controlled by halting production of the yoghurt, withdrawing it from sale, recalling the cans of conserve and warning the public to avoid consumption of all hazelnut yoghurts (O'Mahony et al. 1990).

Bacillus cereus

Bacillus cereus is a Gram-positive rod present in soil. It frequently contaminates rice, other starchy foods, meat, fish and dairy products and has been estimated to cause 1–12% of all food-borne diseases worldwide. Under-reporting probably occurs because most cases are mild and self-limiting but occasionally more serious illness results (López et al. 2015). The spores are not destroyed by boiling and germinate if the food is stored overnight without adequate refrigeration. The bacteria multiply and release toxins not destroyed if reheating is gentle (e.g. to prepare 'special fried rice' in Chinese restaurants).

Gastric Infection Caused by Viruses

Outbreaks of diarrhoea and vomiting caused by viruses are common in hospitals and the community. Although electron microscopy can be used to diagnose these infections, it is not always attempted as they are often mild and self-limiting.

Norovirus

Norovirus is the most common cause of gastroenteritis worldwide (Lopman et al. 2016). It occurs in the community and is responsible for outbreaks in hospitals and nursing homes. It is spread by contact with faeces and in air-borne particles of vomit and by ingesting contaminated food (see Chapter 7).

Hepatitis A Virus

Hepatitis A virus (HAV) is an RNA virus causing liver inflammation. Small clusters of infection have been reported in families and institutions. Larger outbreaks are often linked to the consumption of contaminated water, milk and food. Symptoms include malaise, nausea, vomiting, abdominal pain and jaundice. The incubation period is 15–50 days, with a mean of 28 days. Subclinical infection is common and gives lasting immunity in areas where sanitation is poor. The high standard of living in the UK has reduced exposure and increased the risk of infection in adulthood.

Vaccination is recommended for the following groups:

- people visiting countries where hepatitis A is common
- injecting drug users
- people whose sexual behaviour places them at risk (men who have sex with men)
- people whose work places them at risk (e.g. contact with raw sewage)
- people with a history of liver disease.

There is no specific treatment.

Hepatitis E Virus

Hepatitis E virus (HEV) is a calicivirus spread by the faecal–oral route. HEV is a major cause of epidemic, water-borne hepatitis worldwide in countries where sanitation is poor, especially in Asia. Most infections occur in young people. The incubation period is 2–10 weeks. Most people recover well but HEV occasionally causes fulminant (severe, sudden) liver disease. Symptoms are otherwise similar to hepatitis A.

Rotavirus

Rotavirus is an RNA virus and is the most common cause of infectious gastroenteritis for babies and young children in high-income countries (Frühwirth et al. 2001). Vaccination is offered routinely in the UK. Cases sometimes show seasonal clustering, although they can occur at any time. Adults can become infected but the illness is usually mild and self-limiting except for those who are immunocompromised. In low-income countries, rotavirus infection is much more serious and infant mortality through dehydration commonly occurs (Crawford et al. 2017). Dissemination appears to depend on direct contact between individuals. The mainstay of prevention is good hygiene, especially hand hygiene.

Gastric Infections Caused by Protozoa

Giardia intestinalis

Giardia intestinalis (also known as *G. duodenalis* and *G. lamblia*) is an obligate, cyst-forming protozoal parasite. Infection results when the cysts are ingested. Prevalence of symptomatic cases is low in the UK although asymptomatic carriage appears to be more widespread than previously estimated (Waldram et al. 2017). Most cases arise in parts of the world where hygiene is poor but outbreaks are occasionally reported in high-income countries. A large outbreak of giardiasis was reported in Belgium resulting from contamination of the water supply (Braeye et al. 2015).

Transmission is by the faecal–oral route when contaminated water is consumed or used to wash food served raw. *G. intestinalis* does not multiply in food. Person-to-person spread is possible. Household pets and livestock may carry *G. intestinalis* and zoonotic transmission is possible. The incubation period is 1–3 weeks and unless treated, illness persists for 4–6 weeks. The protozoa inhabit the small bowel and the main symptom is offensive diarrhoea with cramping abdominal pain, sometimes accompanied by malabsorption and weight loss. Asymptomatic carriage is common. Cysts can withstand chlorination at concentrations used to disinfect water and may survive for over two weeks in damp, cool environments. They are destroyed by heat and prolonged freezing but ice cubes in drinks have been associated with infection. The infectious dose is possibly no more than 10 cysts. Treatment is with metronidazole.

Cryptosporidium spp.

Infection with *Cryptosporidium* is responsible for 4000 cases of diagnosed illness in England and Wales annually. The incubation period is 3–10 days. Symptoms include watery diarrhoea, abdominal pain and vomiting lasting up to six days in otherwise healthy people. Risk factors include ingestion of contaminated water and food, contact with farm animals and person-to-person spread. No drug is currently effective against *Cryptosporidium*, but infection is usually self-limiting in otherwise healthy people. Outbreaks represent approximately 10% of cases and one large outbreak in England and Scotland was traced to the ingestion of contaminated salad leaves (McKerr et al. 2015). Transmission between members of the same household probably accounts for a high proportion of cases and has been underestimated in the past (McKerr et al. 2021).

Chronic cryptosporidiosis is one of the hallmarks defining HIV disease.

Entamoeba histolytica

Entamoeba histolytica is an amoeba causing infection when the cysts are ingested in food and is usually the result of poor hygiene. The incubation period ranges from two weeks to several years (Todd et al. 2018). Infection results in blood-stained, mucoid diarrhoea. *Entamoeba* is endemic in poor communities in tropical and temperate countries but outbreaks in high-income countries are rare. Treatment is with metronidazole.

Suggested Activities

Exercise 12.1 Self-assessment

1   Which of the following can cause enteric infection?
    A *Bacillus cereus*
    B *Staphylococcus epidermidis*
    C Norovirus
    D Enterohaemorrhagic *E. coli*

2   Complete the following sentence: 'The signs and symptoms of *Staphylococcus aureus* food-borne illness appear rapidly because . . .'

3   Which of the following groups are at particular risk of food-borne illness?
    A Infants
    B Patients receiving cancer chemotherapy
    C People who eat hazelnuts as a staple part of the diet
    D All the above

4   What immediate action would you take if three ward patients or nursing home residents developed diarrhoea and vomiting within the same 24-hour period?

5   Food-borne illness is caused exclusively by Gram-negative bacteria.
    True/False

6 Which of the following form spores?
   A *Staphylococcus aureus*
   B *Clostridium perfringens*
   C *Bacillus cereus*
   D *Giardia intestinalis*

7 What advice would you give to people responsible for preparing meals?
   A Store food at 0 °C or above 63 °C
   B Store food below 8 °C or above 63 °C
   C Store food below 8 °C or above 70 °C
   D None of the above

8 Which of the following would you advise a pregnant woman to avoid?
   A Full cream milk
   B Brie
   C Hazelnuts
   D Cottage cheese

9 What diagnostic test is used for typhoid?

10 Vaccination is possible for which of the following?
   A Rotavirus
   B *Cryptosporidium*
   C *Campylobacter*
   D Botulism

Exercise 12.2

Who is responsible for food preparation and handling in your workplace? Investigate the arrangements in place for food handlers and records kept of training. Are these arrangements adequate? Suggest any improvements that could be made to improve training or record keeping.

Exercise 12.3

Obtain the paper by Ercoli et al. (2017) appearing in the reference list.

- What kind of study is reported in this paper?
- Does the investigation provide definitive evidence that the outbreak originated from the source reported?
- What recommendations would you suggest to prevent another incident of this nature?

References

Acheson, P., Bell, V., Gibson, J. et al. (2016). Enforcement of science – using a *Clostridium perfringens* outbreak investigation to take legal action. *J. Public Health* 38: 511–515. https://doi.org/10.1093/pubmed/fdv060.

Ahmad, F., Prescott, R.W.G., Acquilla, S., and Lightfoot, N.F. (1991). Management of a Salmonella outbreak in a geriatric hospital by ciprofloxacin therapy. *J. Hosp. Infect.* 18: 79–81. https://doi.org/10.1016/0195-6701(91)90098-S.

Anderton, A., Nwoguh, C.E., McKune, I. et al. (1993). A comparative study of the numbers of bacteria present in enteral feeds prepared and administered in hospital and the home. *J. Hosp. Infect.* 23: 43–49. https://doi.org/10.1016/0195-6701(93)90129-N.

Appiah, G.D., Chung, A., Bentsi-Enchill, A.D. et al. (2020). Typhoid outbreaks, 1989–2018: implications for prevention and control. *Am. J. Trop. Med. Hyg.* 102: 1296–1305. https://doi.org/10.4269/ajtmh.19-0624.

Barrie, D. (1996). The provision of food and catering services in hospital. *J. Hosp. Infect.* 33: 13–33. https://doi.org/10.1016/S0195-6701(96)90026-2.

Braeye, T., De Schrijver, K., Wollants, E. et al. (2015). A large community outbreak of gastroenteritis associated with consumption of drinking water contaminated by river water, Belgium, 2010. *Epidemiol. Infect.* 143: 711–719. https://doi.org/10.1017/S0950268814001629.

Buchanan, R.L., Gorris, L.G.M., Hayman, M.M. et al. (2017). A review of *Listeria monocytogenes*: an update on outbreaks, virulence, dose-response, ecology, and risk assessments. *Food Control* 75: 1–13. https://doi.org/10.1016/j.foodcont.2016.12.016.

Crawford, S.E., Ramani, S., Tate, J.E. et al. (2017). Rotavirus infection. *Nat. Rev. Dis. Primers* 3: 17083. https://doi.org/10.1038/nrdp.2017.83.

Doyle, M.P. (1990). Pathogenic *Escherichia coli*, *Yersinia enterocolitica*, and *Vibrio parahaemolyticus*. *Lancet* 336: 1111–1115. https://doi.org/10.1016/0140-6736(90)92582-3.

Ercoli, L., Gallina, S., Nia, Y. et al. (2017). Investigation of a staphylococcal food poisoning outbreak from a Chantilly cream dessert, in Umbria (Italy). *Foodborne Pathog. Dis.* 14: 407–413. https://doi.org/10.1089/fpd.2016.2267.

European Centre for Disease Prevention and Control, European Food Safety Authority (2021). Multi-country outbreak of Salmonella Enteritidis sequence type (ST)11 infections linked to poultry products in the EU/EEA and the United Kingdom. www.ecdc.europa.eu/en/publications-data/salmonella-enteritidis-multi-country-poultry-joint-outbreak-risk-assessment

European Commission (2006). Food hygiene. https://ec.europa.eu/food/safety/bio logical-safety/food-hygiene_en

Fetsch, A. and Johler, S. (2018). *Staphylococcus aureus* as a foodborne pathogen. *Curr. Clin. Microbiol. Rep.* 5: 88–96. https://doi.org/10.1007/s40588-018-0094-x.

Frühwirth, M., Heininger, U., Ehlken, B. et al. (2001). International variation in disease burden of rotavirus gastroenteritis in children with community- and nosocomially acquired infection. *Pediatr. Infect. Dis. J.* 784–791. https://doi.org/10.1097/00006454-200108000-00013.

Hainsworth, T. (2004). The value of cholera vaccination in promoting travel health. *Nurs. Times* 100: 30–31.

Health and Safety Executive (n.d.) Preventing or controlling ill health from animal contact at visitor attractions or open farms. www.hse.gov.uk/agriculture/topics/visitor-attractions.htm

Jørgensen, F., Sadler-Reeves, L., Shore, J. et al. (2017). An assessment of the microbiological quality of lightly cooked food (including sous-vide) at the point of consumption in England. *Epidemiol. Infect.* 145: 1500–1509. https://doi.org/10.1017/S0950268817000048.

Kaakoush, N.O., Castaño-Rodríguez, N., Mitchell, H.M., and Man, S.M. (2015). Global epidemiology of Campylobacter infection. *Clin. Microbiol. Rev.* 28: 687–720. https://doi.org/10.1128/CMR.00006-15.

Lee, M.B. and Greig, J.D. (2013). A review of nosocomial Salmonella outbreaks: infection control interventions found effective. *Public Health* 127: 199–206. https://doi.org/10.1016/j.puhe.2012.12.013.

Levy, J. (1989). Listeria and food poisoning – a growing concern. *Matern. Child Health* 14: 380–383.

López, A.C., Minnaard, J., Pérez, P.F., and Alippi, A.M. (2015). A case of intoxication due to a highly cytotoxic *Bacillus cereus* strain isolated from cooked chicken. *Food Microbiol.* 46: 195–199. https://doi.org/10.1016/j.fm.2014.08.005.

Lopman, B.A., Steele, D., Kirkwood, C.D., and Parashar, U.D. (2016). The vast and varied global burden of norovirus: prospects for prevention and control. *PLoS Med.* 13: e1001999. https://doi.org/10.1371/journal.pmed.1001999.

McKerr, C., Adak, G.K., Nichols, G. et al. (2015). An outbreak of *Cryptosporidium parvum* across England & Scotland associated with consumption of fresh pre-cut salad leaves, May 2012. *PLoS One* 10: e0125955. https://doi.org/10.1371/journal.pone.0125955.

McKerr, C., Chalmers, R.M., Elwin, K. et al. (2022). Cross-sectional household transmission study of Cryptosporidium shows that *C. Hominis* infections are a key risk factor for spread. *BMC Infect. Dis* 22: 114. https://doi.org/10.21203/rs.3.rs-659412/v1.

O'Mahony, M., Mitchell, E., Gilbert, R.J. et al. (1990). An outbreak of foodborne botulism associated with contaminated hazelnut yoghurt. *Epidemiol. Infect.* 104: 389–395. https://doi.org/10.1017/S0950268800047403.

Pether, J.V.S. and Gilbert, R.J. (1971). The survival of salmonellas on finger-tips and transfer of the organisms to foods. *Epidemiol. Infect.* 69: 673–681. https://doi.org/10.1017/S002217240002194X.

Richards, J., Parr, E., and Riseborough, P. (1993). Hospital food hygiene: the application of hazard analysis critical control points to conventional hospital catering. *J. Hosp. Infect.* 24: 273–282. https://doi.org/10.1016/0195-6701(93)90059-9.

Robertson, P., Smith, A., Anderson, M. et al. (2017). Transmission of *Salmonella enteritidis* after endoscopic retrograde cholangiopancreatography because of inadequate endoscope decontamination. *Am. J. Infect. Control* 45: 440–442. https://doi.org/10.1016/j.ajic.2016.11.024.

Shanaghy, N., Murphy, F., and Kennedy, K. (1993). Improvements in the microbiological quality of food samples from a hospital cook-chill system since the introduction of HACCP. *J. Hosp. Infect.* 23: 305–314. https://doi.org/10.1016/0195-6701(93)90148-S.

Silva, J., Leite, D., Fernandes, M. et al. (2011). *Campylobacter spp.* as a foodborne pathogen: a review. *Front. Microbiol.* 2: 200. https://doi.org/10.3389/fmicb.2011.00200.

Tam, C.C., Rodrigues, L.C., Viviani, L. et al. (2012). Longitudinal study of infectious intestinal disease in the UK (IID2 study): incidence in the community and presenting to general practice. *Gut* 61: 69–77. https://doi.org/10.1136/gut.2011.238386.

Tickell, K.D., Brander, R.L., Atlas, H.E. et al. (2017). Identification and management of Shigella infection in children with diarrhoea: a systematic review and meta-analysis. *Lancet Glob. Health* 5: e1235–e1248. https://doi.org/10.1016/S2214-109X(17)30392-3.

Todd, W., Lockwood, D., and Sundar, S. (2018). *Davidson's Principles and Practice of Medicine*, 23e. Edinburgh: Churchill Livingstone/Elsevier.

Waldram, A., Vivancos, R., Hartley, C., and Lamden, K. (2017). Prevalence of Giardia infection in households of Giardia cases and risk factors for household transmission. *BMC Infect. Dis.* 17: 486. https://doi.org/10.1186/s12879-017-2586-3.

Wallis, J. (2016). In the shadow of the asylum: the Stanley Royd Salmonella outbreak of 1984. *Med. Humanities* 42: 11–16. https://doi.org/10.1136/medhum-2015-010671.

Williams, P. and Ellison, J. (1998). Food fears. *Nurs. Times* 94: 72–74.

World Health Organization (n.d.a). Food safety. www.who.int/news-room/fact-sheets/detail/food-safety

World Health Organization (n.d.b). Typhoid. www.who.int/news-room/fact-sheets/detail/typhoid

Xavier, G. (2006). Management of typhoid and paratyphoid fevers. *Nurs. Times* 102: 49–51.

Yang, S.-C., Lin, C.-H., Aljuffali, I.A., and Fang, J.-Y. (2017). Current pathogenic *Escherichia coli* foodborne outbreak cases and therapy development. *Arch. Microbiol.* 199: 811–825. https://doi.org/10.1007/s00203-017-1393-y.

13

Infection from Blood and Body Fluids

Occupational Health Risks Associated with Blood-borne Infections

Infection caused by blood-borne viruses (BBVs) is an occupational health risk for health workers (Elseviers et al. 2014). Risk arises through exposure to blood and other body fluids and from sharps injuries (e.g. needles, scalpels, lancets, broken glass). Nurses and doctors are the groups most at risk and injuries are frequently associated with the use of hollow-bore needles which are more likely to transmit infection than solid items (e.g. sutures) (Ward and Hartle 2015).

Two types of exposure are possible.

- *Percutaneous (puncture) injuries*: the skin is pierced by a needle or other sharp object (e.g. scalpel). Bites and scratches are also classified as percutaneous injuries.
- *Mucocutaneous (splash) injuries*: involve the mucous membranes (mouth, eyes, nose) or contamination of non-intact skin with a patient's blood or other body fluids.

Table 13.1 lists activities most likely to result in sharps injury.

Viruses Transmitted in Blood and Body Fluids

The most frequently encountered BBVs are the hepatitis viruses B and C and the human immunodeficiency virus (HIV). The hepatitis D virus (HDV, delta agent) is a defective virus also transmitted in blood and body fluids but replicates and causes infection only in the presence of hepatitis B virus (HBV). Exposure to patients with viral haemorrhagic fever (Ebola, Marburg and Lassa haemorrhagic fever [LHF]) occasionally occurs in high-income countries if health workers encounter infected patients recently arrived from regions where these viruses are endemic.

Infection Prevention and Control in Healthcare Settings,
First Edition. Edward Purssell and Dinah Gould.
© 2023 John Wiley & Sons Ltd. Published 2023 by John Wiley & Sons Ltd.

Table 13.1   Activities most likely to result in sharps injury.

Venepuncture
Resheathing needles
Not disposing of sharps promptly
Overfilling sharps disposal containers

Public Health Measures to Reduce Occupational Health Risks

In the UK and many other countries, the public health authorities monitor significant occupational exposures (SOEs) to BBVs among clinical and ancillary staff and report cases where seroconversion has occurred. Records are available from 1997 onwards in the UK. The aims of surveillance are listed in Table 13.2. It is estimated that 100 000 needlestick injuries occur in the NHS annually but as audit is not mandatory, it is likely that some incidents are omitted from official figures.

The risk of health workers acquiring a BBV from a patient depends on:

- prevalence of the virus in a specific clinical setting
- nature of the exposure: seroconversion is more likely if a deep injury has been sustained and the instrument was bloodstained
- experience: junior staff are more likely to sustain needlestick injuries than experienced health workers (Jagger et al. 1990). Sharps injuries are largely preventable and risk can be reduced by staff training (Castella et al. 2003).

Risk of Seroconversion After Injury

The risk of seroconversion following exposure is very low (Elder and Paterson 2006). The only report of HIV seroconversion among health workers in the UK occurred in 1999 following percutaneous exposure from a hollow-bore needle. There appear

Table 13.2   The purpose of needlestick injury surveillance.

Primary aim

Determine the number of transmissions of HIV, HBV and HCV to health workers resulting in SOE.

Secondary aims

- Estimate risk of transmission of HIV, HBV and HCV to health workers as a consequence of SOE. These data are stratified by type of exposure (percutaneous or mucocutaneous).
- Describe the number and rate of SOEs over time.
- Estimate uptake of treatment, vaccination and postexposure prophylaxis (PEP).

to have been no recent HBV seroconversions. Since 2014, there have been two reports of confirmed hepatitis C virus (HCV) seroconversions, all arising from accidents related to the use of hollow-bore needles. Sharps injuries have been reported from all clinical settings where healthcare is delivered (Riddell et al. 2015).

Exposure-prone Procedures

Exposure-prone procedures (EPPs) are those in which there is a possibility that health workers' gloved hands might come into contact with sharp instruments or sharp tissues (e.g. bone) in a wound or body cavity where the hands are not always visible. If the health worker is carrying a BBV, there is a risk of transmission to the patient. EPPs should not be undertaken by health workers who test positive for HIV or HBV e antigen. Health workers with HCV should not undertake EPPs unless they respond to antiviral treatment.

Blood-borne Virus Infections

Human Immunodeficiency Virus

The human immunodeficiency virus is an RNA retrovirus that uses an enzyme called reverse transcriptase to convert its RNA into DNA. Many anti-HIV drugs operate by blocking the activity of reverse transcriptase. Tests for HIV measure the viral load in a sample of blood. HIV tests can be obtained from GPs, genitourinary medicine (GUM) clinics, NHS Direct, helplines/websites (e.g. Terence Higgins Trust) and private clinics. Self-test kits are also available. In the case of occupational exposure, testing is undertaken in the occupational health department. Seroconversion can take months so testing must be repeated if it is undertaken very soon after exposure.

Testing a sample of blood obtained by venepuncture is important to confirm the results of point-of-care and self-testing (Box 13.1). Those testing positive are referred to specialist HIV services.

HIV Transmission

Human immunodeficiency virus is transmitted sexually, perinatally and via blood and other body fluids. The virus has been isolated from blood, semen, vaginal secretions, breast milk, saliva and tears but the level in saliva and tears is probably too low to result in transmission (Lifson 1988).

The following groups are at high risk of contracting HIV.

- Patients with blood clotting disorders (e.g. haemophilia). Since 1987, blood products in the UK have been heat treated to destroy HIV, eliminating the risk

---

Box 13.1   Types of HIV tests

Molecular tests detect the virus present in the blood and viral load, generate results more quickly than other types of HIV tests and are the most accurate and expensive. They require a blood sample obtained through venepuncture.

Antigen–antibody tests detect the core HIV virus antigen p24. These tests are accurate and provide early results because p24 appears before antibodies are generated. They require a blood sample obtained through venepuncture or a finger-prick test.

HIV antibody tests detect HIV antibodies in blood or oral secretions. The results are not accurate until the immune system has had time to respond to the virus and has generated antibodies. Most inexpensive rapid tests and self-test kits detect HIV antibodies.

Point-of-care HIV testing is available using oral secretions or blood obtained from finger-prick and can detect antibodies. The result is available within a few minutes but must be repeated.

---

of new infections. Nevertheless, over 1200 people with haemophilia (about 30% of the total) in the UK are seropositive.

- People who engage in drug misuse and share contaminated injection equipment.
- Sexual transmission between adults. Risk is very high for men who have sex with men (MSM), especially those who are the receptive partner during anal intercourse. The rectal mucosa is more delicate than the vaginal mucosa, enabling the virus to gain access via tears and abrasions. It is possible for women to become infected and in some geographical regions both sexes are infected in equal numbers.
- Vertical transmission from infected mothers to infants.
- Iatrogenic transmission to health workers.

Public Health Measures for HIV

The most important method of preventing HIV transmission is by treating people with HIV, as the risk of transmission is related to viral load. Reducing viral load to 'undetectable' levels reduces the risk of transmission to almost zero and is often referred to as 'treatment as prevention'. It is also the rationale behind pre-exposure prophylaxis. For those who are exposed to HIV, postexposure prophylaxis should be offered. Other preventive strategies include the following.

- Promoting the use of barrier precautions (condoms) and emphasising the need for 'safe sex'. Explicit advice can be obtained from the Terence Higgins Trust.

- Screening all donated blood and heat-treating blood products.
- Discouraging members of the public who assess themselves at high risk from donating blood, semen or tissues. Organs cannot be used if the donor is antibody positive.
- Informing the public and health workers of the risks associated with blood and other body fluids and safe handling.
- Alerting the public to the dangers of sharing potentially contaminated items (e.g. razors, toothbrushes, sewing needles, scissors).
- Supplying needles and syringes to people who use intravenous drugs for recreational purposes. 'Needle exchange' schemes are well established but remain controversial.

The World Health Organization (WHO) recommends HIV postexposure prophylaxis if:

- exposure occurred within the past 72 hours
- the potentially exposed individual is not infected or not known to be infected with HIV
- mucous membrane or non-intact skin was significantly exposed to a potentially infectious body fluid
- the source is HIV infected or their HIV status is unknown (World Health Organization 2014).

Further information about HIV and its treatment is provided in Chapter 14.

Hepatitis

Hepatitis is a generic term for inflammation of the liver. It may be acute or chronic and is caused by a number of viruses, including several of the hepatitis viruses, rubella, cytomegalovirus and herpes simplex. This chapter outlines the hepatitis viruses B, C, D and other hepatitis viruses. Hepatitis A and hepatitis E are discussed in Chapter 12.

Hepatitis B

The HBV is a DNA virus (Figure 13.1). It is highly infectious and a serious occupational health risk to health workers. Transmission from health workers to patients is rare and only a few cases have been documented (Lewis et al. 2015).

The structure of the virus particle has been deduced by studying the surface antigens of the virus. The following terminology has been suggested by the WHO.

- Dane particle – the entire virus particle
- HBV – hepatitis B virus
- HBsAg – hepatitis B surface antigen

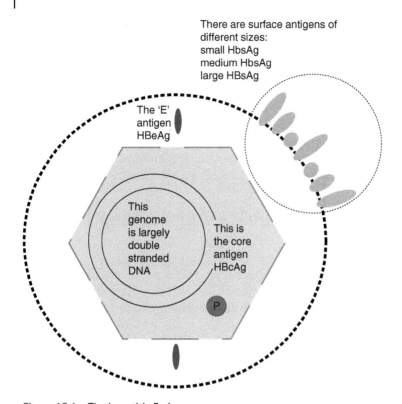

There are surface antigens of different sizes:
small HbsAg
medium HbsAg
large HBsAg

The 'E' antigen HBeAg

This genome is largely double stranded DNA

This is the core antigen HBcAg

P

Figure 13.1 The hepatitis B virus.

- HBcAg – hepatitis B core antigen
- HBeAg – the e antigen associated with the core of the virus
- Anti-HBs – antibody to hepatitis B surface antigen
- Anti-HBc – antibody to hepatitis B core antigen
- Anti-HBe – antibody to the e antigen

HBV is detected by identifying serological markers in the blood. Liver damage is assessed by ultrasound.

Infectious particles have been isolated from numerous body fluids, including saliva and semen. Resolution of HBV infection is considered to have occurred when HBsAg and anti-HB can no longer be detected. Those who test positive for HBsAg on at least two occasions six months apart are regarded as chronic carriers. Infectivity is closely associated with the presence of the e antigen, which indicates that active viral replication is occurring.

Hepatitis B has an incubation period of four weeks to six months and the infectious dose is very small (Venkatakrishnan and Zlotnick 2016). Individuals appear most infectious during the early, acute stages. Most adults (90–95%) recover fully from acute HBV infection but there is a risk of progression to chronic hepatitis. If chronic infection occurs, the liver becomes inflamed and the hepatocytes are destroyed.

Hepatitis B remains a global health problem although cases have fallen since vaccination was introduced in 1982. Treatment has also become more effective. About 2 billion people are infected and 350 million are chronic carriers (Liaw and Chu 2009). The symptoms of acute hepatitis tend to be non-specific (e.g. fever, anorexia, malaise) and are experienced by 30–40% of individuals. Jaundice does not always develop, or may be too mild to be noticeable. Between 50% and 60% of patients develop subclinical infection and remain asymptomatic despite serological evidence of exposure. These individuals are most likely to become chronic carriers and are the group at greatest risk of developing liver cirrhosis and hepatocellular cancer. These are rare but grave complications and treatment is not always successful (Main 1991).

Transmission of HBV occurs sexually (vaginal or anal intercourse), via percutaneous sharps injury, sharing infected needles, contamination of mucous membranes and during tattooing/body piercing where equipment is not sterile and precautions are not in place. The risk of infection after percutaneous exposure to the blood of a carrier for the e antigen is about 30% (Beltrami et al. 2000). Transmission is possible via minute abrasions on apparently intact skin, explaining why many people who develop infection or become carriers cannot recall injury.

Infants whose mothers developed acute HBV infection during the third trimester or who are highly infectious carriers are at risk of infection by vertical transmission during the perinatal period. The level of risk depends on how the virus was transmitted and is highest when transmitted vertically from mother to infant.

Groups at high risk of HBV infection include:

- intravenous drug users
- MSM
- sex workers
- health workers
- immigrants from geographical regions where HBV is endemic (e.g. Africa, South-East Asia, Far East)
- residents in institutions for people with learning difficulties
- prison inmates.

In the UK, HBV infection is a notifiable disease. Public health measures include:

- health promotion campaigns to highlight the risks of unsafe sexual practices and sharing equipment by those who inject drugs

- adhering to blood and body fluid precautions when healthcare is delivered
- screening all blood for transfusion for HBsAg and excluding carriers from donating
- using only virus-treated blood and blood products
- encouraging uptake of the vaccine by those at risk.

Immunisation has been available against HBV since 1982. The duration of immunity is 3–5 years. Protection is also provided against hepatitis D, which is only able to cause infection in the presence of HBV. Guidelines for the management of patients with hepatitis B are available from NICE and the British Association of Sexual Health and HIV (2017).

Hepatitis C

Hepatitis C is caused by an RNA flavivirus. It is endemic globally with a high prevalence in East Asia and Eastern Europe and is a major cause of ill health globally. Worldwide, over 170 million people are infected. HCV is transmitted predominantly via blood and body fluids. Intravenous drug users are most at risk. In the UK, donated blood has been screened for HCV since 1991. Before this, numerous cases of seroconversion occurred as a result of blood transfusion or receiving blood products. Patients undergoing renal dialysis are at higher risk than other patient groups and occasional nosocomial transmission has also been associated with use of contaminated equipment (e.g. endoscopes, vials) (Nguyen et al. 2016).

Sexual and maternal-to-child HCV transmission have been documented but breast feeding is considered safe as there have been no reported cases of infection via this route (Mast 2004). Health workers are at occupational risk through exposure to blood and body fluids. Most seroconversions result from unsafe practice when handling blood and other body fluids (Pozzetto 2014). HCV is more damaging than HBV. About 80% of those infected become chronic carriers and of these, 20% develop cirrhosis and 4% develop hepatocellular cancer although seroconversion may not occur until several months after exposure. Many people remain asymptomatic for up to 20 years apart from experiencing occasional non-specific ill health and are unaware that they are infected (Rogers and Campbell 2003).

The disease trajectory is variable and not always easy to predict but is exacerbated by alcohol consumption. Cirrhosis resulting from hepatitis C is fatal without liver transplantation. Guidelines for the treatment of hepatitis C are available from NICE and the British Association of Sexual Health and HIV.

Hepatitis D

Hepatitis D (delta virus) is an RNA virus able to cause infection only in the presence of active HBV infection. It is transmitted in the same way as HBV and the same groups are at risk. The incubation period is 30–50 days. Mortality from acute HDV infection is 2–20%. Infection is diagnosed by identifying the antigen (HDAg) in the blood. Routine testing is not undertaken, so prevalence is unknown. The virus appears to be most common in the countries of the former USSR, Middle East and Africa. Vaccination against HBV infection offers protection against both viruses.

The Viral Haemorrhagic Fevers

The viral haemorrhagic fevers (Ebola, LHF and Marburg) are transmitted in blood and other body fluids. They carry a high risk of mortality and present a serious occupational health risk to health workers in regions where these viruses are endemic. Most cases of viral haemorrhagic fever in high-income countries are reported in cities with good links to major airports. The incubation period is long (up to 21 days) and those arriving from overseas may not know that they have been exposed to infection or attribute non-specific symptoms of malaise and fever to malaria. The infection usually progresses rapidly with haemorrhage into the internal organs, the appearance of a bleeding rash and seizures. Even with intensive supportive treatment, mortality is very high. Stringent isolation in a specialist unit is required.

Health workers need to avoid contact with the patient's blood and body fluids and contaminated surfaces and materials. When in close contact (within 1 m) of patients, they should wear face protection, a fluid-resistant long-sleeved gown and gloves. These conditions are not easy to maintain in field hospitals.

Ebola Virus Disease

Ebola virus disease (EVD) is caused by a filovirus that interferes with blood clotting, leading to internal bleeding, inflammation and tissue damage. Mortality is estimated at 50%. EVD was first reported in 1976. The largest outbreak occurred in 2014–2016 in West Africa, commencing in Guinea before moving into Sierra Leone and Liberia (Coltart et al. 2017).

Bats are believed to be the natural hosts and it is thought that EVD reached the human population through close contact with the blood and other body fluids of ill and dead animals. In humans, EVD is transmitted via direct contact through damaged skin and mucous membranes from infected individuals and via fomites. Burial ceremonies involving direct contact with the deceased are also thought to be an important source of infection. Numerous cases of transmission to health workers have been reported.

Successful treatment depends on rehydration and intensive supportive care. In 2019 a vaccine became available and in late 2020, two monoclonal antibodies (Inmazeb™ and Ebanga™) were approved by the US Food and Drug

---

Box 13.2   Community intervention package to prevent and control Ebola virus disease

Case management
Infection prevention and control wherever healthcare takes place
Surveillance with contact tracing
Safe and dignified burial
Vaccination programmes
Support for women wishing to breastfeed

Administration. Pregnant women who recover from Ebola can still carry the virus in breast milk and must be tested if they wish to breastfeed.

Prevention and control of EVD require strong community engagement programmes (Box 13.2).

Lassa Haemorrhagic Fever

Lassa haemorrhagic fever is caused by an arenavirus identified in the 1960s. Eighty percent of those infected do not develop symptoms but severe disease occurs if the virus affects the liver, spleen or kidneys. LHF spreads to the human host through contact with the urine and faeces of rodents belonging to the genus *Mastomys* (multimammate rat). It can be spread between humans by contact with blood and other body fluids. Person-to-person transmission has been reported via contaminated needles and other fomites in community and healthcare settings. Sexual transmission has also been reported.

The variable course of the infection complicates diagnosis and the implementation of public health measures. When a case of LHF is confirmed, prompt isolation, good infection prevention and control and rigorous contact tracing can prevent outbreaks. Treatment with ribavirin is effective if given early in the course of illness.

Public health measures depend on good 'community hygiene' to discourage rodents from entering homes, storing grain and other food in rodent-proof containers, disposing of garbage promptly, maintaining clean households and keeping felines.

Marburg Disease

Marburg disease is caused by a filovirus. It is extremely virulent, with mortality exceeding 80%. The first cases were reported in 1967 when seven animal handlers in the German town of Marburg died after contact with infected laboratory monkeys imported from Uganda. In recent years, a number of cases and outbreaks have been reported, often linked to exposure to bats or entering caves where they roost. No treatment is currently available but recovery is possible following vigorous supportive treatment.

Reducing Risk of Exposure to Blood-borne Viruses

Recommendations to reduce the risks of exposure to BBVs include:

- use of personal protective equipment (PPE), including non-sterile disposable gloves (NSDGs)
- safe sharps handling and disposal
- dealing with spillage of blood and other body fluids safely.

Use of Personal Protective Equipment

There is confusion regarding the use of PPE and concerns that NSDGs are often used at the expense of hand hygiene (Jain et al. 2017). Nevertheless, there is general consensus that exposure to BBVs should be reduced by wearing NSDGs when contact with blood or other body fluids is anticipated following risk assessment. The decision to use NSDGs should be based on the procedure about to be undertaken, not on the patient, as it is impossible to determine whether an individual is carrying a BBV. Fluid-resistant aprons or gowns and face/eye protection should be worn to prevent contamination when splashing is likely.

Sharps Handling

All staff employed in settings where healthcare is delivered are at risk of sharps injury even if they are not engaged in clinical practice. Ancillary staff can sustain injury when the correct procedure for sharps disposal has not been followed. Strategies to reduce sharps injuries are shown in Box 13.3.

Dealing with Sharps Injury, Splashing, and Spillage of Blood and Other Body Fluids

The UK Health and Safety Executive provides comprehensive information (Health and Safety Executive n.d.). If a sharps injury is sustained, the immediate priority is to implement first aid measures to reduce the risk of infection. The incident should then be documented and reported to the occupational health department. Health workers who have sustained a sharps injury are likely to be distressed and must be referred to assess the need for tests to detect seroconversion and postexposure prophylaxis (Riddell et al. 2015).

Outside hospitals, other health and social care settings must have policies and arrangements in place to ensure that staff can access immediate advice, intervention and follow-up. First aid following sharps injury is shown in Box 13.4.

Box 13.3 Strategies to reduce sharps injuries

- Ensure that all sharps containers comply with British Standards regulations. They should be rigid and impermeable to leakage and puncture. Other types of container should not be used.
- Minimise sharps handling events and always avoid passing sharps from hand to hand.
- Never resheath, bend or cut needles: these are the events most likely to cause injury (Wormser et al. 1984).
- Never disconnect syringes and needles after use.
- Provide sharps containers in all clinical areas. In critical care units, they should be placed at every bedspace; in wards and units, they should be placed on the drugs trolley and in treatment rooms.
- Dispose of the device into a designated sharps container as soon as possible. Disposal is the responsibility of the individual who has used the device.
- Never retrieve items from a sharps container.
- Never empty sharps containers.
- Replace sharps containers when they are two-thirds full. Discarded containers must be sealed and arrangements made for collection and incineration.
- Provide sharps containers of the appropriate size. Accidents are more likely when attempting to force large items into small containers.
- Patients who handle sharps at home (e.g. to administer insulin) should be supplied with a sharps container. Small, portable containers suitable for home use are available.
- Use needle-free devices where available.
- Keep sharps and sharps containers out of the reach of children and vulnerable adults (e.g. patients who may be confused).

Source: Wormser et al. (1984).

Box 13.4 First aid following sharps injury

- Encourage the wound to bleed. Hold it under running water if possible. Do not suck or squeeze it.
- Wash the injured area thoroughly with warm running water and soap.
- Apply a waterproof dressing.
- Complete an accident form, recording the patient's identity if known, and report the incident according to local policy.
- First aid following contamination of the conjunctivae and mucous membranes should involve:
  - irrigation of the area with water
  - documenting and reporting the incident.

Follow-up After Sharps Injury

Good practice includes the following.

- Testing for HCV infection at six weeks, three months and six months. Tests for HBV should be undertaken at the same time unless there is evidence of adequate vaccination. HIV tests should be performed after one month and repeated to exclude later seroconversion.
- Reassurance that seroconversion is very rare. Counselling should be available; sustaining a sharps injury is recognised as very distressing.
- Documenting events leading up to the injury to determine the need to review procedures, equipment or staff training to reduce the risk of further occurrences.
- Postexposure prophylaxis: antiretroviral medication and active or passive immunisation for hepatitis B.

Blood and Body Fluid Spillage

Spillages should be dealt with immediately using sodium dichloroisocyanurate (NaDDC) powder, granules or hypochlorite solution to cover the spillage (Box 13.5).

Box 13.5 Dealing with blood and body fluid spillages

- A plastic apron and NSDGs should be worn.
- If using NaDDC:
  - Pour the powder/granules over the spill and leave in contact for two minutes.
  - Scoop up the debris with disposable wipes.
  - Discard everything in a yellow bag to be incinerated.
  - Clean the area with water and detergent.
  - Ensure that ventilation is optimal during this procedure as NaDDC can release chlorine gas, which is toxic.
- If using hypochlorite solution:
  - Cover the spillage with paper towels to absorb excess fluid.
  - Pour the hypochlorite solution over the towels. Use a 1% solution containing 10 000 ppm of available chlorine.
  - Leave for at least two minutes.
  - Scoop all the debris into a yellow plastic bag for incineration.
  - Clean the area with water and detergent.
- In domiciliary settings:
  - Employ the same procedure using a solution consisting of one part household bleach to 10 parts water.

Suggested Activities

Exercise 13.1 Self-assessment

1 Blood-borne infection can arise through which of the following?
 A Touching
 B Splashes
 C Puncture injuries
 D All the above

2 Which of the following should be avoided?
 A Resheathing needles
 B Using sharps boxes more than two-thirds full
 C Carrying sharps around the ward/clinic
 D All the above

3 Hepatitis D is a blood-borne infection.
 True/False

4 What does the acronym SOE stand for?

5 Complete the sentence: 'The number of needlestick injuries reported annually is probably an underestimate because . . .'

6 Risk of developing a blood-borne infection after a sharps injury is high.
 True/False

7 Which of the following offer confidential HIV testing?
 A Pop-up stations in supermarkets
 B Genitourinary medicine (GUM) clinics
 C High street pharmacies
 D Private clinics

8 Which of the following body fluids can transmit hepatitis B?
 A Blood
 B Semen
 C Cerebrospinal fluid
 D Respiratory secretions

9 Which patient group is most at risk of contracting hepatitis C?

10 Ebola virus disease is not an occupational health risk for nurses and doctors in high-income countries.
True/False

Exercise 13.2

What arrangements are in place for dealing with and auditing exposure to blood and body fluids in the organisation where you work? Are these arrangements satisfactory? How difficult was it to find this information? Is it clear and up to date? Can you suggest any changes? If so, how should they be implemented?

Exercise 13.3

Obtain the paper by Nguyen et al. (2016) from the reference list. Read the paper and address the following questions.

- What type of study was conducted?
- What data were collected?
- Do you believe the study findings?
- Do you agree with the recommendations suggested by the authors for preventing future outbreaks of blood-borne infections?

References

Beltrami, E.M., Williams, I.T., Shapiro, C.N., and Chamberland, M.E. (2000). Risk and management of blood-borne infections in health care workers. *Clin. Microbiol. Rev.* 13: 385–407. https://doi.org/10.1128/CMR.13.3.385.

British Association for Sexual Health and HIV (2017). BASHH Guidelines. www.bashh.org/guidelines

Castella, A., Vallino, A., Argentero, P.A., and Zotti, C.M. (2003). Preventability of percutaneous injuries in healthcare workers: a year-long survey in Italy. *J. Hosp. Infect.* 55: 290–294. https://doi.org/10.1016/j.jhin.2003.08.013.

Coltart, C.E.M., Lindsey, B., Ghinai, I. et al. (2017). The Ebola outbreak, 2013–2016: old lessons for new epidemics. *Phil. Trans. R. Soc. B* 372: 20160297. https://doi.org/10.1098/rstb.2016.0297.

Elder, A. and Paterson, C. (2006). Sharps injuries in UK health care: a review of injury rates, viral transmission and potential efficacy of safety devices. *Occup. Med.* 56: 566–574. https://doi.org/10.1093/occmed/kql122.

Elseviers, M.M., Arias-Guillén, M., Gorke, A., and Arens, H.-J. (2014). Sharps injuries amongst healthcare workers: review of incidence, transmissions and costs. *J. Ren. Care* 40: 150–156. https://doi.org/10.1111/jorc.12050.

Health and Safety Executive (n.d.) Sharps injuries. www.hse.gov.uk/healthservices/ needlesticks

Jagger, J., Hunt, E.H., and Pearson, R.D. (1990). Sharp object injuries in the hospital: causes and strategies for prevention. *Am. J. Infect. Control* 18: 227–231. https://doi. org/10.1016/0196-6553(90)90163-m.

Jain, S., Clezy, K., and McLaws, M.-L. (2017). Glove: use for safety or overuse? *Am. J. Infect. Control* 45: 1407–1410. https://doi.org/10.1016/j.ajic.2017.08.029.

Lewis, J.D., Enfield, K.B., and Sifri, C.D. (2015). Hepatitis B in healthcare workers: transmission events and guidance for management. *World J. Hepatol.* 7: 488–497. https://doi.org/10.4254/wjh.v7.i3.488.

Liaw, Y.-F. and Chu, C.-M. (2009). Hepatitis B virus infection. *Lancet* 373: 582–592. https://doi.org/10.1016/S0140-6736(09)60207-5.

Lifson, A.R. (1988). Do alternate modes for transmission of human immunodeficiency virus exist? A review. *JAMA.* 259: 1353. https://doi.org/10.1001/jama.1988.03720090 043032.

Main, J. (1991). Therapy of chronic viral hepatitis. *J. Hosp. Infect.* 18 (Suppl A): 335–340. https://doi.org/10.1016/0195-6701.

Mast, E.E. (2004). Mother-to-infant hepatitis C virus transmission and breastfeeding. In: *Protecting Infants through Human Milk: Advances in Experimental Medicine and Biology* (ed. L.K. Pickering, A.L. Morrow, G.M. Ruiz-Palacios and R.J. Schanler), 211–216. Boston, MA: Springer https://doi.org/10.1007/978-1-4757-4242-8_18.

Nguyen, D.B., Gutowski, J., Ghiselli, M. et al. (2016). A large outbreak of hepatitis C virus infections in a hemodialysis clinic. *Infect. Control Hosp. Epidemiol.* 37: 125–133. https://doi.org/10.1017/ice.2015.247.

Pozzetto, B. (2014). Health care-associated hepatitis C virus infection. *World J. Gastroenterol.* 20: 17265. https://doi.org/10.3748/wjg.v20.i46.17265.

Riddell, A., Kennedy, I., and Tong, C.Y.W. (2015). Management of sharps injuries in the healthcare setting. *BMJ.* 351: h3733. https://doi.org/10.1136/bmj.h3733.

Rogers, G. and Campbell, L. (2003). Hepatitis C virus: its prevalence, implications and management. *Nurs. Times* 99: 30–31.

Venkatakrishnan, B. and Zlotnick, A. (2016). The structural biology of hepatitis B virus: form and function. *Annu. Rev. Virol.* 3: 429–451. https://doi.org/10.1146/ annurev-virology-110615-042238.

Ward, P. and Hartle, A. (2015). UK healthcare workers infected with blood-borne viruses: guidance on risk, transmission, surveillance, and management. *Contin. Educ. Anaesth. Crit. Care Pain* 15: 103–108. https://doi.org/10.1093/bjaceaccp/mku023.

World Health Organization (2014). *Supplement to the 2013 Consolidated Guidelines on the Use of Antiretroviral Drugs for Treating and Preventing HIV Infection: Recommendations for a Public Health Approach.* Geneva, Switzerland: World Health Organization.

Wormser, G., Joline, C., and Duncanson, F. (1984). Needle-stick injuries during the care of patients with AIDS. *N. Engl. J. Med.* 310: 1461–1462. https://doi.org/10.1056/ NEJM198405313102213.

14

Sexually Transmitted Infections

Sexually Transmitted Infections and Public Health

Sexually transmitted infections (STIs) are an enduring public health challenge. They are among the most common acute infections, but are neglected in terms of research and practice development (Unemo et al. 2017). The World Health Organization estimates that every day, almost a million people globally develop one of the four most commonly diagnosed STIs (Table 14.1).

Although treatable, STIs are responsible for a considerable burden of disease and are associated with stigma. Many people delay seeking treatment through embarrassment, fear or because they do not know where to seek help. The problem is compounded because symptoms are often vague, disappear spontaneously or patients remain asymptomatic and unaware that they are infected. Untreated STIs can result in pelvic inflammatory disease (PID), fertility problems and vertical transmission to the foetus if a pregnant woman is infected.

Antimicrobial resistance has become a serious problem in the treatment of gonorrhoea and vaccination is not yet possible for most STIs. Contact tracing and partner notification are central to management because many STIs are highly infectious and asymptomatic infection promotes rapid transmission. Sexual health services are provided free of charge in the UK to encourage people to come forward and seek help, prevent transmission and avoid reinfection.

Diagnosis and treatment are available in genitourinary medicine (GUM) clinics. General practitioners and some family planning clinics and pharmacies also provide services. A number of professional organisations contribute to service development and standards for sexual health across the UK. These include the Faculty of Sexual and Reproductive Healthcare (FSRH), the Terence Higgins Trust, NICE

Infection Prevention and Control in Healthcare Settings,
First Edition. Edward Purssell and Dinah Gould.
© 2023 John Wiley & Sons Ltd. Published 2023 by John Wiley & Sons Ltd.

Table 14.1   Sexually transmitted infections.

Infection	Causative organism
Chlamydia[a]	*Chlamydia trachomatis*
Gonorrhoea[a]	*Neisseria gonorrhoeae*
Syphilis[a]	*Treponema pallidum*
Trichomoniasis[a]	*Trichomonas vaginalis*
HIV disease	Human immunodeficiency virus[a]
Genital warts[a]	Human papillomavirus virus
Genital herpes	Herpes simplex
Candidiasis	*Candida* spp.
Mycoplasma genitalium	

[a] Most commonly reported STIs globally.

and the British Association of Sexual Health and Human Immunodeficiency Virus (BASHH).

The prevalence of STIs is increasing globally, with a marked increase for specific infections. The UK Health Security Agency collects data about service uptake and diagnosis in GUM clinics and other clinical and community-based settings to plan infection prevention and control campaigns and health promotion aimed at particular groups (Box 14.1). Young people (15–24 years) are at greatest risk but all age groups can be affected. Older people no longer concerned about contraception may overlook the barrier protection offered by condoms. When evaluating epidemiological data, it is important to remember that under-reporting occurs through missed cases, asymptomatic infection and failure to access the health services.

Box 14.1   Addressing the Increase in Syphilis. The Public Health England Action Plan

Official figures reported to the UK Health Security Agency indicate a recent, marked increase in the incidence of syphilis. Most cases are reported among men who have sex with men (MSM) but there has also been an increase in the heterosexual population. In 2019, Public Health England launched a campaign to increase awareness targeted at groups at high risk and clinicians. The campaign emphasises the importance of testing and using condoms to avoid transmission.

Patients and clinicians also need to be aware that for some STIs, other routes of transmission are possible and is particularly common for some groups. For example, *Candida* spp. frequently affects men and women with diabetes and those receiving antimicrobial treatment. Human immunodeficiency virus (HIV), hepatitis B and hepatitis C are sexually transmitted but can also be transmitted via contaminated blood and other body fluids.

Sexual Health and the Role of Genitourinary Medicine Clinics

The public health focus on STIs dates from the early twentieth century. The Venereal Disease Regulations (1916) required all local authorities to provide clinics where diagnosis and free treatment were available in confidence. Contact tracing became an essential feature of the service and has contributed to its success. A further advance was made in 1924 with the establishment of the Venereal Disease Reference Laboratory which made it possible to standardise methods of diagnosis and treatment and collate statistics.

Today, a broad view of sexual health is taken, integrating physical, emotional, intellectual and social components. Sexual health is regarded as an integral part of overall health and involves a great deal more than helping people avoid infection. Clinicians working in GUM clinics provide information and advice as well as diagnosing infection and providing treatment. Their work plays a central role in meeting government health targets through efforts to reduce the incidence of STIs and HIV. GUM clinics provide the following.

- A confidential self-referral service without a waiting list for anybody wanting to discuss sexual health matters.
- Examination and testing for genital infections.
- Health education and counselling.
- Partner notification.
- Free prescriptions.

GUM clinics offer a number of advantages over other venues where sexual health services are available. Many are equipped with satellite laboratories able to process specimens immediately, allowing swift, accurate diagnosis and treatment commenced at the same visit. The organisms causing many STIs are 'fastidious'. They have complicated growth requirements and do not survive for long in transport media so diagnosis is more accurate if the specimen is examined at once. The reception that attendees receive in the GUM clinic and the attitude of staff play an important role in securing adherence to treatment, advice and willingness to reattend (Box 14.2).

Box 14.2   The Patient Experience in GUM Clinics

Attending a GUM clinic can require considerable courage. It is essential for attendees to feel comfortable and understand that strict confidentiality is always maintained. Challenges in busy clinics are establishing rapport with attendees, emphasising the importance of completing the course of antimicrobials even if symptoms have disappeared and of returning for follow-up tests to ensure that the infection has resolved. Attendees need to be informed about the importance of co-operating with contact tracing. STIs often co-exist in the same individual (e.g. gonorrhoea and chlamydia) and they need to be aware that they will be screened for a range of STIs.

Sexually Transmitted Infections

Chlamydia

Chlamydia trachomatis is an intracellular pathogen responsible for the most commonly diagnosed STI globally. Incidence in the UK is increasing, especially in young people aged 15–24 years. Although infection can be serious and highly destructive, the natural history of chlamydial infection is poorly understood.

Infection is primarily through penetrative sexual intercourse, but the organism can be detected in the conjunctiva and nasopharynx without concomitant genital infection, and any chlamydial infection can resolve spontaneously. In heterosexual men, *C. trachomatis* infects the urethra, giving rise to urethritis. Complications include prostatitis and epididymitis. In MSM, rectal infection is possible. *C. trachomatis* is carried asymptomatically in 80% of women who have become infected and not received treatment, usually on the cervix. It can also cause discharge and may ascend the genital tract, leading to salpingitis, PID and impaired fertility. Some women develop chronic pelvic pain. Infection during pregnancy often results in preterm delivery. Repeated infection is common and in women is more likely to result in serious complications although the reason is unknown. The UK and many other high-income countries recommend annual screening for young, sexually active people with partner notification.

Diagnosis is by PCR testing. The patient needs only to supply a urine sample; uncomfortable clinical examination is unnecessary. Treatment is with doxycycline 100 mg twice daily for seven days (contraindicated in pregnancy) or azithromycin 1 g orally as a single dose, followed by 500 mg once daily for two days.

Gonorrhoea

Gonorrhoea is an enduring public health problem (Unemo et al. 2019). *Neisseria gonorrhoeae*, the causative organism, is a Gram-negative diplococcus. It attaches to the delicate urethral and cervical mucosae by minute surface filaments (pili) and is able to survive inside neutrophils once phagocytosed. The adult vaginal wall is inhospitable to gonococci because of its tough squamous epithelium. *N. gonorrhoeae* is rapidly inactivated by cold and drying and is unable to survive long outside the host, explaining why transmission is primarily via the sexual route. The eyes of infants can become infected during passage down the birth canal if cervical secretions contain gonococci, causing ophthalmia neonatorum (pus discharging from the infant's eyes). Infection usually becomes apparent within 21 days of birth.

In men and women, acute gonococcal infection presents as urethritis accompanied by discharge and dysuria following an incubation period of 2–10 days. It is thought that 50% of women and 10% of men remain asymptomatic. The consequences of infection are serious. Gonococci can migrate from the cervix to the uterus and fallopian tubes. In 10–20% of women, severe scarring follows, resulting in PID leading to occlusion, impaired fertility and occasionally peritonitis if the bacteria escape from the open fimbriated ends of the fallopian tubes. Women may also experience vague, debilitating chronic ill health and are highly infectious. Gonococcal vulvovaginitis in young girls can be a sign of sexual abuse. In men, untreated infection causes scarring, urethral stricture, epididymitis and prostatitis. Involvement of the joints results in gonococcal arthritis. This is a late occasional complication of infection in men and women.

Diagnosis is by PCR test or culture and microscopy. If treated promptly, gonorrhoea usually resolves without causing long-term problems. For uncomplicated infections, the treatment of choice in the UK is a single intramuscular dose of ceftriaxone. Penicillin-resistant strains were first reported in the 1970s and antimicrobial resistance is now a major challenge (Unemo and Shafer 2011). Alternatives to the cephalosporins are quinolones or azithromycin. Patients are advised to avoid sexual activity until the success of treatment is confirmed at a follow-up visit one week later, and partner notification is important. Infection does not result in immunity; it is possible to develop gonorrhoea more than once.

Syphilis

Syphilis is caused by the spirochaete *Treponema pallidum*. Transmission occurs sexually and vertically across the placenta, resulting in congenital infection. *T. pallidum* does not survive outside the tissues and cannot be grown in culture media but is highly infectious, evades host defences very effectively and is responsible for chronic infection that can be severe (LaFond and Lukehart 2006).

Syphilis can be viewed as a bygone example of a 'new' disease and there has been considerable speculation about its origins. It appeared suddenly in Europe in the late fifteenth century and two theories were suggested.

- *The Colombian theory*: syphilis endemic in the West Indies was brought to Europe by sailors returning with Columbus.
- *The Unitarian theory*: syphilis is a variant of the tropical treponemal infection yaws which is caused by a spirochaete indistinguishable from *T. pallidum*. Yaws is a skin condition transmitted via skin contact. It was widespread in the West Indies throughout the fifteenth century and reached Europe during slave trading. It was suggested that in colder climates where skin contact seldom occurs, the bacteria became dependent on sexual transmission.

Syphilis most commonly affects MSM aged 25–34 and of these, about 40% are co-infected with HIV. The site of entry in heterosexual patients is often via the genitalia but in a third of MSM, transmission is extragenital (mouth, anus, rectum). About a third of sexual contacts develop infection. Syphilis can result in a wide range of symptoms. Incidence is rising in the UK and other countries, especially among MSM (see Box 14.1).

Stages of Syphilitic Infection
The incubation period is usually about 20 days but can be much longer.

- *Primary syphilis*: a chancre (ulcer) appears at the site of infection on the genitals, rectum, mouth or, rarely, a finger. The early signs of infection are easily overlooked as chancres are painless and often develop at sites where they are likely to be undetected. Without treatment, chancres heal within 3–8 weeks but the spirochaetes spread rapidly to other parts of the body, probably within a few hours.
- *Secondary syphilis*: about 4–10 weeks after the primary infection, the individual may experience a vague, influenza-like illness with malaise, fever, aching joints and lymph node enlargement. Symptoms are often dismissed because they are mild and non-specific, although some people develop a rash. The surfaces of the lesions team with treponemes and the individual is highly infectious. Other manifestations of secondary syphilis include elongated ulcerated lesions ('snail-track' ulcers) and flattened warty growths (condylomata lata) usually affecting mucous membranes or other sites that are moist. These are easily overlooked or their significance is not appreciated. Secondary syphilis usually resolves spontaneously within 3–12 weeks.
- *Tertiary syphilis* arises 20–40 years after the initial infection. Manifestations include gummata formation, cardiovascular effects and neurosyphilis.
  Chronic ulcers (gummata) are lesions developing anywhere on the skin, in the tissues or internal organs. They are particularly damaging if they involve bone, cardiovascular or nervous tissue.
  - Inflammation of the lining of the aorta leads to the formation of an aneurysm, damage to the aortic valve or angina.

- Neurosyphilis leads to tabes dorsalis (lack of co-ordination with disturbed sensation in the legs) and dementia (general paralysis of the insane).
- The mechanism by which *T. pallidum* causes damage is unknown. It does not produce toxins and evokes only a weak immune response.

Congenital Syphilis

Congenital (prenatal) syphilis is transmitted vertically from mother to foetus via the placenta, causing miscarriage, stillbirth or delivery of an infant with the signs and symptoms of syphilis (Table 14.2). The earlier that maternal infection occurs during pregnancy, the more serious the outcome for the infant. All women in the UK are offered a prenatal blood test to screen for syphilis and as a result, congenital syphilis is now extremely rare (Townsend et al. 2017).

Table 14.2 The hallmarks of congenital syphilis.

Early (within two weeks of delivery)

- Skin lesions: a weeping, crusted rash principally affecting the peripheries followed by a maculopapular rash and condylomata lata reminiscent of adult secondary syphilis. Scarring may occur in areas where friction occurs (e.g. the mouth)
- Mucous membranes: discharging lesions develop in the nose, mouth, throat, larynx and pharynx, interfering with feeding. Fissures appear around the mouth, nose and anus
- Enlarged lymph nodes
- Rhinitis and nasal discharge
- Enlarged liver and spleen, altered plasma protein levels
- Meningitis
- Inflammation of the choroid layer of the eye
- Bone lesions: osteochondritis and inflammation of the periosteum

Late effects

Late effects and stigmata result from maldevelopment of the tissues resulting from the damage caused by the treponemes at birth or soon afterwards. They include:

- A perforated nasal septum
- Saddle nose
- Maldeveloped, notched, peg-shaped teeth (Hutchinson's incisors)
- Scarring (rhagades) from rashes around the nose, mouth and anus
- Keratitis leading to corneal scarring
- Effusion of the joints (Clutton's joints)
- Bony deformities, especially of the palate, maxilla and long bones (e.g. tibia). Bossing of the parietal and frontal cranial bones
- Eighth cranial nerve (auditory or vestibulocochlear nerve) deafness
- Any of the conditions arising during the adult form of tertiary syphilis

Treponema pallidum is diagnosed by PCR test or a laboratory technique called dark ground microscopy. Serological tests are used to monitor response to treatment. Treatment depends on the stage of the disease and the specific body systems affected if the patient presents late. For primary and secondary syphilis and the early stages of tertiary infection, a single dose of intramuscular benzathine penicillin is given. For later stage disease with cardiovascular involvement, three doses of intramuscular benzathine penicillin are given over three weeks. Neurosyphilis is treated with procaine penicillin or benzylpenicillin. Patients allergic to penicillin are usually given doxycycline, a tetracycline or erythromycin.

Once treatment has been completed, the infection is eradicated but exposure does not result in immunity. Asymptomatic contacts also require treatment.

Human Immunodeficiency Virus

The HIV is an RNA retrovirus that uses an enzyme called reverse transcriptase to convert its RNA into DNA to infect host cells. Two species have been identified: HIV-1 and HIV-2. HIV-1 was the species first identified, is the most widespread globally and the most virulent. HIV-2 is mostly confined to West Africa. Unless treated, both species eventually cause acquired immunodeficiency syndrome (AIDS), a condition in which the immune system is progressively weakened, resulting in opportunistic infection and cancers. Without treatment, most people die within 9–11 years.

The virus infects cells of the immune system, especially CD4 helper cells. Once the number of CD4 helper cells falls below a critical level, cell-mediated immunity is lost and the individual becomes progressively more susceptible to opportunistic infections and cancer.

The first case of HIV disease was reported in Africa in the 1950s. Initially, it appears to have been a zoonotic infection, probably transmitted to the human host by exposure to blood when hunting chimpanzees and other primates and butchering the meat. High rates of infection have been reported from people engaged in bush practices. Global spread was possible because of changes in sexual practices, international travel and migration from rural areas to the cities. HIV infection first attracted attention in the late 1970s when increasing numbers of cases were reported in the homosexual community, first in the US, then the UK.

The Human immunodeficiency virus is a STI but can also be transmitted via blood and other body fluids (e.g. breast milk, semen, vaginal secretions) and vertically from mother to foetus during pregnancy or delivery. Health workers are at occupational risk of blood-borne infections but risk of seroconversion after exposure to HIV is very low and depends on viral load (the amount of HIV particles in the blood). Other risk factors are shown in Table 14.3.

Risk is especially high for MSM but women are also at risk through unprotected sexual intercourse and needle sharing.

Table 14.3 Risk factors for HIV.

- Unprotected anal or vaginal sex
- Having another sexually transmitted infection (e.g. syphilis, herpes, chlamydia, gonorrhoea)
- Sharing contaminated needles, syringes and other injecting equipment and drug solutions
- Exposure to contaminated blood and blood products during transfusion, tissue transplant or medical procedures that involve unsterile cutting or piercing
- Occupational exposure through needlestick injury for health workers

Tests for HIV measure the viral load in a blood sample and play an important role during management of the condition. With effective antiretroviral infection treatment (ART), 'undetectable viral load' in the blood is achieved and the individual ceases to be infectious. Without treatment, the trajectory of the disease involves four stages.

- *Primary HIV infection* usually occurs within 28 days and lasts 3–4 months. Some individuals experience a short illness when they seroconvert (begin to generate HIV antibodies) but symptoms are often mild and non-specific and are dismissed or overlooked. Occasionally, an influenza-like illness with pyrexia and malaise occurs. The individual is most infectious during seroconversion.
- The *asymptomatic stage* begins once seroconversion is over and lasts for several years. Most people are asymptomatic but the virus replicates and infects new immune cells, and the ability of the immune system to resist infection declines.
- *Symptomatic HIV* results when the individual develops opportunistic infections (e.g. *Candida* spp., *Pneumocystis jirovecii*) or cancer. Some cancers (AIDS-defining cancers) are closely associated with HIV infection (e.g. Kaposi's sarcoma, invasive cervical cancer, non-Hodgkin lymphoma). A number of other cancers are also common in people with HIV (e.g. anal cancer linked to infection with human papilloma virus, liver cancer associated with co-infection with hepatitis B or C). The longer the individual goes without receiving treatment, the greater the risk of developing symptomatic HIV.
- *Late-stage HIV.* The immune system is severely damaged and the individual develops serious infections (e.g. pneumonia, tuberculosis) and cancers. These are called AIDS-defining illnesses. Most people never develop late-stage HIV but if this stage is reached, progress is influenced by lifestyle and how soon ART is commenced. Smoking, high levels of alcohol consumption, obesity and having another STI exacerbate late-stage HIV.

There is no cure or vaccine for HIV infection but since the availability of ART, it has become a manageable chronic health condition. The aim of ART is to reduce the number of virus particles in the blood to levels that are undetected by blood test. ART suppresses viral replication and allows the immune system to regain its ability to fight opportunistic infections and some cancers. The individual is no longer infectious although very small numbers of virus particles are still present.

Early diagnosis and treatment are important for individuals and to prevent transmission. The HIV virus can become embedded in the tissues, causing latent reservoirs. These viruses can become reactivated if treatment is stopped. Different antiviral therapies have been developed, classified according to the stage in the viral life cycle they inhibit. Several drugs are usually prescribed in combination therapy. Information about healthy lifestyle and the importance of adhering to medication is essential.

Human immunodeficiency virus disease is a global health challenge (World Health Organization 2021). It is estimated that, worldwide, about 38 million people live with HIV, mostly in low-income countries. Prevalence is highest in Africa where access to diagnosis and treatment is poor and mortality is still very high. Public health strategies to prevent HIV are discussed in Chapter 13.

Trichomoniasis

Trichomoniasis is caused by the highly motile, flagellated protozoan *Trichomonas vaginalis*. Symptoms usually develop within a month of infection. Women have an offensive, frothy, yellow-green vaginal discharge. Speculum examination reveals an inflamed cervix and vaginal walls. In severe cases, the vulva, perineum and insides of the thighs become sore. Men develop dysuria, penile discharge and soreness. Asymptomatic carriage is possible in men and women but they are still infectious. Complications seldom occur but there is growing evidence that infection increases the risk of HIV transmission and the infection will not resolve without treatment.

Diagnosis is by PCR test or inspecting a wet preparation of vaginal secretion under the low power of the microscope. In men, the organisms may be present in prostatic fluid or cause mild urethral discharge but diagnosis is much harder.

Sexual transmission is considered the most usual mechanism of transmission because partners often show evidence of infection if examined thoroughly and it is sometimes possible to identify chains of infection between multiple partners (Lewis 2014). *T. vaginalis* forms cysts under adverse environmental conditions and non-sexual transfer has been suggested but never demonstrated.

Treatment is administered orally with metronidazole (either as a large single dose or a seven-day course) or tinidazole (large single dose). Both partners should be treated but this may be difficult because routine partner notification is not undertaken.

Genital Warts

Genital warts are caused by the human papilloma virus (HPV). The incubation period is 2–3 months. Contract tracing and partner notification are not practical as the virus can remain latent for years. HPV is spread by skin-to-skin contact and is usually found on the fingers, hands, mouth and genitals. Entry is thought to occur via minor abrasions in the mucous membranes arising through trauma during sexual intercourse.

Genital warts are a source of distress because they are unsightly and catch on clothing. Many patients feel angry and depressed and perceive genital warts to be socially unacceptable and a source of shame (Clarke et al. 1996). Different types of HPV exist and some (types 16 and 18) have oncogenic potential. They are important causative agents of cervical cancer and of some head and neck cancers.

Annual cervical smears are recommended for patients with genital warts. In the UK, girls and boys aged 12–13 are offered vaccination for HPV. Substantial reduction in cervical cancer and precancerous lesions has been reported in young women since the introduction of the immunisation programme in England (Falcaro et al. 2021). Cervical screening is still important because vaccination has only been available since 2008 and many women have not received it.

Although approximately 30% of genital warts disappear spontaneously, most patients prefer treatment. Options include:

- application of topical creams (e.g. podophyllotoxin 0.15%, imiquimod 5%, trichloroacetic acid)
- cryotherapy
- laser
- surgical removal.

Podophyllotoxin and imiquimod are the most successful topical treatments for soft, non-keratinised lesions. Both are readily obtainable online. Application is not always easy, depending on where the lesions are located, and there is a temptation to apply too much product or apply it too often, resulting in damage to the local tissues. For keratinised lesions, trichloroacetic acid or physical removal tend to be more successful but treatment failures and relapses are common. Trichloroacetic acid is extremely corrosive and should only be used with great caution, protecting the surrounding area with petroleum jelly.

Herpes Simplex

Herpes simplex (HSV) is a DNA virus affecting the oral mucosae and also causing genital ulceration. By the age of five years, over 60% of the population are infected. There are two types.

- HSV-1 primarily isolated from oral lesions
- HSV-2 primarily isolated from genital lesions

There is an increasing tendency for HSV-1 to be isolated from genital lesions. People already infected with HSV-1 can become infected with HSV-2 and vice versa.

Primary oral herpes infection usually occurs early in life from contact with an asymptomatic salivary carrier or someone who has an actively discharging lesion. Characteristic vesicles appear around the mouth or eyes, sometimes associated with febrile illness. Encephalitis is a rare complication that can be fatal. Many infections are mild and often overlooked. Recurrent oral herpes infection occurs throughout adulthood. After primary infection, virus particles migrate along the sensory nerves to their associated ganglia where they remain dormant, occasionally becoming active through some challenge to the immune system (e.g. a cold, influenza, exposure to sunshine, menstruation). Virus particles travel back down the nerves and as these supply a localised area on the face, crops of vesicles develop at the same site, usually around the nostrils or lips.

Primary genital herpes infection is acquired sexually, probably through small breaks in the mucosae. Incubation is 2–14 days. The main reservoirs of the virus are the cervix and male genital tract. Painful ulceration develops on the glans and shaft of the penis or vulva, interfering with micturition.

Genital herpes infection recurs although episodes tend to decline over time. Treatment of the primary infection and recurrence is with the antiviral drugs aciclovir, valaciclovir or famciclovir. Delivery during primary infection acquired late in pregnancy may result in the baby developing fatal encephalitis unless elective caesarean section is performed.

Neonatal herpes results from contact with infected secretions during delivery. It is rare but extremely serious with a high mortality rate. Manifestations are:

- localised skin infection
- infection involving the central nervous system
- disseminated infection with organ involvement.

Health professionals are well placed to offer general advice and support to people with genital herpes (Box 14.3). Individuals feel most unwell during the prodrome (time between infection and the onset of symptoms) before the lesions have fully developed.

Candidiasis

Candidiasis is caused by the spore-forming yeast *Candida*. A number of species cause infection, the most common being *Candida albicans*. It causes a white, highly irritant vaginal discharge, often most troublesome just before

---

Box 14.3   Advice and Support for People with Genital Herpes

A diagnosis of genital herpes can have emotional and social implications in addition to the physical effects of infection. Individuals report feeling 'dirty' and, as herpes is recurrent, may feel that their sex life is at an end.
Advice and support include the following.

- Providing information about treatment, recurrence, risk to sexual partners, pregnancy and support from self-help groups.
- Health education to enable individuals to recognise the 'early warning' signs of a recurrent episode of herpes.
- Advice about simple symptomatic remedies (e.g. paracetamol for the systemic illness that occurs with primary infection), the importance of resting and taking fluids.
- Giving information about keeping the lesions clean and dry.
- Advice about when to stop having sexual intercourse; during the primary infection, for example, this would be until the lesions have healed and all other symptoms of genital herpes have resolved.
- Emphasising the importance of women informing health professionals about pregnancy or plans to conceive in the future.
- Encouraging patients to attend follow-up consultations and making sure that tests for other STIs are completed.
- Encouraging sexual partners to visit the clinic.

---

menstruation. *Candida* occasionally causes balanitis in men. It can be carried asymptomatically in both sexes. Transmission is not always by the sexual route but symptoms are most common in sexually active women, especially during the childbearing years and pregnancy. Some women experience repeated attacks which may be the result of reinfection. Incidence is high among diabetics and is often a sign of undetected diabetes. Episodes are frequently triggered by taking antibiotics. The personal, social and economic consequences of vulval and vaginal *Candida* infection tend to be overlooked: recurrent inconvenience, embarrassment and discomfort. Irritation is often most intense at night, interfering with sleep and the following day's activities, and micturition can be painful (Odds 1988).

Treatment is usually possible with tablets, vaginal creams or pessaries (e.g. clotrimazole, econazole, miconazole) with a vulval cream to control itching. Many over-the-counter products are conveniently single dose. Women should be warned that many preparations can damage latex contraceptive diaphragms or condoms. If self-treatment is unsuccessful, they can be given fluconazole or itraconazole orally. Contraception is vital during treatment with fluconazole, as it is teratogenic and high-dose long-term use has been associated with multiple foetal abnormalities. Recurrent vaginal candidiasis may require longer-term treatment. Sexual partners who are symptomatic should be treated.

Candida can cause invasive disease in the immunocompromised host and has been responsible for healthcare-associated outbreaks, mainly among the critically ill (Kullberg and Arendrup 2015). Infection often develops in the mouth or large bowel in response to antibiotic therapy. Transmission can occur via health workers' hands.

Mycoplasma genitalium

Mycoplasma genitalium is carried asymptomatically in the genital tract of men and women for months or years. Prevalence in the general population is estimated at 1–2%. Most people never develop symptoms but some men experience urethritis. Women can develop PID, dysuria, postcoital bleeding or heavy intramenstrual bleeding (Pinto-Sander and Soni 2019). Diagnosis is by PCR test. Screening is not undertaken routinely.

Treatment options are limited because mycoplasmas lack cell walls and antimicrobials that operate by inhibiting cell wall synthesis are ineffective. The first line of treatment is doxycycline 100 mg twice daily for seven days or azithromycin 1 g administered immediately, then 350 mg daily for two days. Patients with PID are prescribed moxifloxacin.

Bacterial Vaginosis

Bacterial vaginosis is often diagnosed in conjunction with other STIs but may occur in women who are not sexually active. It is thought to occur in up to 30% of women aged 15–44 years (Livengood 2009). The adult vagina has a pH of 4.5 and is colonised by lactobacilli. Bacterial vaginosis develops when an imbalance in pH occurs and there is overgrowth of anaerobes including *Gardnerella vaginalis*, *Bacteroides* spp. and genital mycoplasmas (Gardner and Dukes 1955).

Bacterial vaginosis can be a distressing condition and is most commonly diagnosed among women during the reproductive years, especially if they have had several partners or a recent change of partner (Temple 1994). Affected women are more likely to experience late miscarriage or preterm delivery (Hay et al. 1994). The most commonly reported symptom is an unpleasant, fishy odour from the genital area, not linked to poor hygiene and often most marked after sexual activity or during menstruation when the pH of the vagina tends to increase. Some women also complain of a frothy, non-irritant grey discharge but approximately 50% are asymptomatic. Treatment is with metronidazole or tinidazole.

Suggested Activities

Exercise 14.1 Self-assessment

1 Which of the following cause infections exclusively by the sexual route?
   A *Treponema pallidum*
   B Herpes simplex
   C *Neisseria gonorrhoeae*
   D None of the above

2 The organisms responsible for many sexually transmitted infections are described as 'fastidious'. Explain.

3 Which of the following are often carried asymptomatically?
   A *T. pallidum*
   B *Candida* spp.
   C *N. gonorrhoeae*
   D All the above

4 Which of the following can be transmitted from mother to foetus?
   A *T. pallidum*
   B *Candida* spp.
   C *N. gonorrhoeae*
   D *Trichomonas vaginalis*

5 Complete the sentence: 'Primary syphilis is often overlooked because . . .'

6 HIV can be described as:
   A A DNA retrovirus which uses an enzyme called reverse transcriptase
   B A chronic condition
   C A sexually transmitted infection
   D Spread by vertical transmission

7 What type of organism is *Trichomonas vaginalis*?
   A Gram-positive bacterium
   B Fungus
   C Protozoan
   D Gram-negative bacterium

8 Complete the sentence: 'Contract tracing and partner notification for genital warts are not practical because . . .'

9   Herpes simplex is carried asymptomatically in the nerve ganglia.
    True/False

10 *Candida* never causes infections in men.
    True/False

Exercise 14.2

What sexual health services are available in your local area? Where are they located? How easily are they accessed? How did you find out what was on offer? What are the implications for people who wish to access these services?

Exercise 14.3

Obtain the paper by Falcaro et al. (2021) in the reference list at the end of this chapter. Read the paper and address the following questions.

- What type of study was conducted?
- What data were collected?
- Do you believe the study findings?
- Do the study findings have implications for policy and practice at international level?

References

Clarke, P., Ebel, C., Catotti, D.N., and Stewart, S. (1996). The psychosocial impact of human papillomavirus infection: implications for health care providers. *Int. J. STD AIDS* 7: 197–200. https://doi.org/10.1258/0956462961917618.

Falcaro, M., Castañon, A., Ndlela, B. et al. (2021). The effects of the national HPV vaccination programme in England, UK, on cervical cancer and grade 3 cervical intraepithelial neoplasia incidence: a register-based observational study. *Lancet* 398: 2084–2092. https://doi.org/10.1016/S0140-6736(21)02178-4.

Gardner, H.L. and Dukes, C.D. (1955). Haemophilus vaginalis vaginitis: a newly defined specific infection previously classified non-specific vaginitis. *Am. J. Obstet. Gynecol.* 69: 962–976.

Hay, P.E., Lamont, R.F., Taylor-Robinson, D. et al. (1994). Abnormal bacterial colonisation of the genital tract and subsequent preterm delivery and late miscarriage. *BMJ.* 308: 295–298. https://doi.org/10.1136/bmj.308.6924.295.

Kullberg, B.J. and Arendrup, M.C. (2015). Invasive candidiasis. *N. Engl. J. Med.* 373: 1445–1456. https://doi.org/10.1056/NEJMra1315399.

LaFond, R.E. and Lukehart, S.A. (2006). Biological basis for syphilis. *Clin. Microbiol. Rev.* 19: 29–49. https://doi.org/10.1128/CMR.19.1.29-49.2006.

Lewis, D. (2014). Trichomoniasis. *Medicine* 42: 369–371. https://doi.org/10.1016/j.mpmed.2014.04.004.

Livengood, C.H. (2009). Bacterial vaginosis: an overview for 2009. *Rev. Obstet. Gynecol.* 2: 28–37.

Odds, F.C. (1988). *Candida and Candidosis*, 2e. London: Baillière Tindall.

Pinto-Sander, N. and Soni, S. (2019). *Mycoplasma genitalium* infection. *BMJ* 367: l5820. https://doi.org/10.1136/bmj.l5820.

Temple, C.A. (1994). Patient education. Diagnosis and treatment of bacterial vaginosis. *Nurs. Times* 90: 43–44.

Townsend, C., Francis, K., Peckham, C., and Tookey, P. (2017). Syphilis screening in pregnancy in the United Kingdom, 2010–2011: a national surveillance study. *Br. J. Obstet. Gynaecol.* 124: 79–86. https://doi.org/10.1111/1471-0528.14053.

Unemo, M. and Shafer, W.M. (2011). Antibiotic resistance in *Neisseria gonorrhoeae*: origin, evolution, and lessons learned for the future. *Ann. N.Y. Acad. Sci.* 1230: E19–E28. https://doi.org/10.1111/j.1749-6632.2011.06215.x.

Unemo, M., Bradshaw, C.S., Hocking, J.S. et al. (2017). Sexually transmitted infections: challenges ahead. *Lancet Infect. Dis.* 17: e235–e279. https://doi.org/10.1016/S1473-3099(17)30310-9.

Unemo, M., Seifert, H.S., Hook, E.W. et al. (2019). Gonorrhoea. *Nat. Rev. Dis. Primers* 5: 79. https://doi.org/10.1038/s41572-019-0128-6.

World Health Organization. 2021. HIV/AIDS. www.who.int/news-room/fact-sheets/detail/hiv-aids

15

Epidemiology and the Role of Public Health in the Prevention and Control of Infectious Disease

Introduction to Epidemiology

Epidemiology is the study of diseases and their distribution within populations. Traditionally, epidemiologists studied infectious disease but their remit has expanded to include all diseases irrespective of whether they are transmissible or not. Today, epidemiology is multidisciplinary; large teams comprising epidemiologists and experts in public health, infection prevention and other disciplines work closely together. During the 2020 COVID-19 pandemic, the input of experts with backgrounds in engineering and physics was particularly important when elucidating mechanisms of spread and the importance of good ventilation to reduce risks of infection (Greenhalgh et al. 2021). Throughout the outbreak of Ebola virus disease in West Africa in 2014–2016, lay people gave invaluable information about traditional local customs to help develop preventive measures (Garritty et al. 2017). Data scientists, computer and machine learning experts contribute to epidemiological investigations by using internet search data ('big data') to identify outbreaks, looking at the number and geographical distribution of symptoms.

The Epidemiology of Infectious Disease

Throughout the nineteenth and early twentieth centuries, infectious diseases were the leading cause of mortality. Once antimicrobials became available in the 1940s, it was anticipated that the burden of infectious disease would decline but it is now clear that it will remain a major source of morbidity and mortality for the foreseeable future (Selwyn 1991).

Infection Prevention and Control in Healthcare Settings,
First Edition. Edward Pursell and Dinah Gould.

The ageing population and increasing survival of people with chronic conditions have increased the number of those with weakened immune systems who are highly susceptible to infection. Poor standards of living and poor hygiene are also closely associated with susceptibility to infection and in low-income countries, millions of people continue to die from malaria, tuberculosis and other infectious diseases every year. The speed of air travel means that many apparently healthy individuals incubating infections develop symptoms after arriving at their destination, importing infectious disease to the western world. Pathogens depend on a supply of new victims and consequently, transmission occurs more rapidly when large numbers of susceptible people are gathered together in enclosed spaces, especially if ventilation is poor. In temperate climates, coughs, colds and other respiratory infections are more common throughout the winter months because people collect together indoors.

The impact of COVID-19 in nursing homes in 2020 highlighted the threat of infection to frail older people sharing communal living spaces. Many recent pandemics are thought to have been caused by viruses previously only found in animals which, after mutating, have become able to infect the human host (e.g. HIV, 'swine flu,' severe acute respiratory syndrome, COVID-19).

Emerging Infectious Diseases

An emerging infectious disease is recognised when:

- an infection appears in a population for the first time
- a previously existing infection begins to spread rapidly, either infecting large numbers of people for the first time or moving into one or more geographical areas where it had not previously been reported.

Emerging infectious diseases usually arise through changes in the behaviour of existing organisms, changes in antimicrobial resistance or breakdown in public health measures (McArthur 2019). They pose serious public health threats globally because the human host has little or no natural immunity against them. The impact on health, society and the economy is often marked and can be difficult to predict. Most emerging infectious diseases are caused by zoonotic pathogens and many are vector borne. The numerous biological, social and environmental drivers of these diseases interact to generate outbreak situations (Table 15.1). The work of epidemiologists is to investigate new infections and unexpected increases in the number of cases.

Clusters of Infection

A cluster is defined as two or more cases of the same infection linked in time where there is evidence of a common source or if the existence of a common

Table 15.1   Drivers of emerging infectious disease.

Microbial adaptation (e.g. genetic drift of influenza viruses, coronaviruses)
Changing host susceptibility (e.g. ageing population)
Increased density of the human population
Poverty and inequality (e.g. tuberculosis)
Environmental stress arising through expansion of farmland
Globalisation of food production and transport
Environmental contamination
Climate change
Population growth
Movement of populations, especially air travel
Breakdown in public health measures (e.g. following natural disasters)
Intentional biological attacks

---

source of infection is suspected. Suspicion might arise because a spate of infections caused by the same organism is identified or because a number of the same type of infections appear to be linked to the same locality or event (e.g. several people developing enteric infection after eating at the same restaurant).

Epidemics

An epidemic is an increase in the number of cases of an infection that exceeds the number usually expected in a given population or locality, especially if the increase occurs suddenly. The terms 'epidemic' and 'outbreak' are used interchangeably but an outbreak is often taken to indicate an increase in cases within a limited geographical area.

Pandemics

Pandemics are global epidemics involving large numbers of people across many countries. COVID-19 was responsible for a global pandemic declared in 2020. Historical examples are the Black Death (bubonic plague), which swept across Europe in the fourteenth century, and the influenza pandemic in 1918 which killed 20 million people globally.

Endemic Diseases

An endemic infection is an infection that is always present in a population. The number of cases varies depending on factors that allow the organism to multiply and the susceptibility of potential hosts. Malaria is endemic throughout Africa but this may change following the creation of a new vaccine in 2021. The virus responsible for the influenza pandemic in 1918 is believed to have persisted in the population in small numbers, giving rise to sporadic cases of infection.

Epidemiological Patterns of Infectious Disease

Epidemiological studies provide information about the ways in which infectious agents are spread and the types of people most likely to be affected, identify risk factors and inform public health strategies to reduce risk. The progress of an outbreak is followed by plotting the number of cases on a graph against time.

Classic Epidemiological Curve

The classic epidemiological curve is depicted in Figure 15.1. On the left-hand side of the graph, the number of people (shown as a proportion of the population) infected rises gradually until it reaches a peak at the midpoint. On the right-hand side, recovery proceeds more rapidly than the emergence of new cases until eventually the epidemic wanes. In a closed population infections eventually die out when there are no further susceptible people to become infected.

Much of our early knowledge of the behaviour of contagious disease has come from studying patterns of infection in geographically remote areas. Spitzbergen, a small island on the edge of the Arctic Circle, has been used to explore the way in which respiratory infections behave. Until the 1930s, Spitzbergen received no visitors throughout the winter months. In spring, colds began to appear in the population following the arrival of the first trade ship, brought by the crew. The epidemic curve gradually rose to a peak as the infection was transmitted throughout the local population. Numbers began to decline as the season progressed and everybody had been infected.

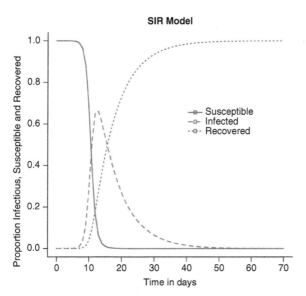

Figure 15.1 The classic epidemiological curve.

Single-Point Epidemiological Curves

The curve shown in Figure 15.1 is a single-point epidemiological curve. Its shape depends on the speed with which new cases appear and resolve. Figure 15.2 illustrates the typical curve following a cluster of cases of food-borne illness when the food was consumed at the same event and the outbreak developed and resolved over a short period of time. Note that there may be a delay in some cases being reported.

Secondary Spread with Longer Incubation Period

When the incubation period is longer (weeks or months) with the possibility of secondary spread within a population, the curve is flatter and a second peak appears (Figure 15.3). This is typical for an outbreak of *Salmonella* throughout an organisation. The first steep peak reflects the large number of people developing infection and recovering after eating the same food. The smaller curve appearing later illustrates person-to-person spread from the individuals who originally consumed the food to other people (probably via fomites and the environment) not infected during the initial peak.

Cyclical Epidemiological Curves

Some infectious conditions appear cyclically within a population, making their appearance every few years (Figure 15.4). Before the introduction of childhood vaccination for measles, mumps and rubella (MMR), these infections recurred cyclically. Outbreaks were possible when a cohort of children lacking immunity had built up and waned when they had all been infected. Cases occurred sporadically between outbreaks.

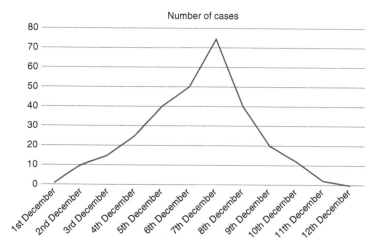

Figure 15.2   The single-point epidemiological curve typical when clusters of food-borne illness occur.

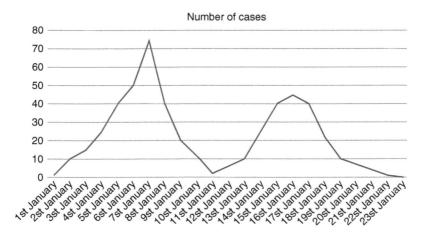

Figure 15.3   Secondary spread of infection with a longer incubation period.

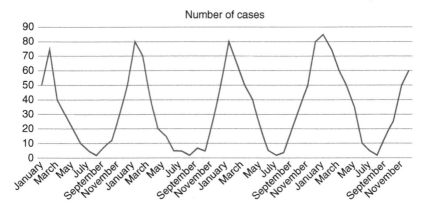

Figure 15.4   Cyclical epidemiological curves.

Screening

Screening is used in asymptomatic populations to identify people who are at high risk of having a particular condition. Particularly high risk is often age related or associated with specific co-morbidities (e.g. the increased risk of experiencing severe respiratory illness in older age groups and those with pre-existing cardiac or renal conditions).

Diagnosis

Diagnosis detects the presence (or absence) of disease in individuals who present with symptoms.

Surveillance

Surveillance is the systematic, ongoing collection, collation and analysis of health-care data and feedback to staff to prompt appropriate action (World Health Organization 2005). The main purposes of surveillance are shown in Table 15.2. The aim is to understand the extent, nature and trends of a condition within a population, not to diagnose illness in individuals. Surveillance is usually undertaken with large groups to identify trends in the data, often over time, or to compare different groups.

Surveillance Data

Data used in surveillance are obtained from individual case reports, individuals (passive surveillance), by actively seeking cases (active surveillance) or reported from a small number of localities or clinics extrapolated to the wider population (sentinel surveillance). Laboratory reports are frequently used as a source of surveillance data (Farrington 2003). Serological surveys are sometimes conducted to quantify the proportion of the population positive for a particular antibody or the titre (concentration) of antibodies in a population (Metcalf et al. 2016). Some surveillance systems are described as 'enhanced' which means that the data are derived from more than one source and combined. In the UK, enhanced surveillance is undertaken for tuberculosis. Clinical teams provide information on the number of cases and the data are matched against laboratory isolates (Public Health England 2020).

Comparisons between populations and between studies collected on the same populations over time are only valid if they are collected in the same way, using

Table 15.2 Purposes of surveillance.

Establish infection rates
Understand patterns and trends of infection within a population
Detect outbreaks or the emergence of a new pathogen
Estimate the magnitude of an infection
Identify the resources needed during and after a public health emergency
Evaluate public health programmes and infection prevention measures
Determine the nature and history of a disease
Monitor changes in infectious agents
Set research priorities
Support public health planning
Monitor changes in public health practice

Source: Adapted from Thacker and Berkelman (1988).

the same case definition (specific criteria used to determine whether an individual has a condition or not).

Surveillance is undertaken using one of two study designs.

- Prevalence studies
- Incidence studies

Prevalence Studies

Prevalence is the number of people with an infection at a specific point in time (point prevalence) or over a specified period of time (period prevalence). Prevalence studies include both new and existing cases and are influenced by the speed of recovery.

Incidence Studies

Incidence is the number of new cases of a condition arising over a specified period of time in a population. Incidence studies provide more comprehensive information about the risk of developing infection than prevalence studies and are used to identify increases in transmission. The findings help determine which interventions should be undertaken to reduce spread. Incidence studies are more expensive and challenging to conduct than prevalence studies and therefore less often conducted.

The incidence proportion ('attack rate') is the number of new cases of a condition as a function of the number of individuals in a given population. The population can refer to all the people living in a particular country or locality or can be much more specific, for example the number of men or women of a particular age within a locality. The secondary attack rate is the number of new cases among the contacts of the infected individual expressed as a percentage of the total number of contacts.

Modelling Infectious Diseases

Mathematical models are used to:

- study how infectious diseases spread
- predict the course of outbreaks
- evaluate strategies for control.

Different types of models exist (Mishra et al. 2011). The main categories are shown in Box 15.1.

One of the most widely used models is the Susceptible-Exposed-Infective-Recovered (SEIR) model. This is a compartmental model used to analyse data during the different stages of an outbreak. Decisions are based on knowledge of

---

Box 15.1   Epidemiological Models

- *Compartmental* models assign individuals into groups according to the stage of infection, e.g. those susceptible, infected but not infectious, infectious and recovered. Individuals move between groups as the infection process proceeds.
- *Deterministic* models are mathematical equations showing how individuals go through the infection process, illustrating the typical or average pathway of infection.
- *Stochastic* models allow randomly occurring events to be incorporated into the model.

---

the infection and equations reflecting how quickly and how likely people are to move through the different states.

Models are always simplified representations and, although regarded as important, are also recognised as an inevitably imperfect means of understanding and making predictions about infections. Much depends on the assumptions put into the model and it is generally accepted that the more complex the model is, the more imperfect it is likely to be because of the large number of assumptions made.

Modelling was extensively undertaken during the COVID-19 pandemic with widely varying conclusions between different research teams at different stages.

Three key parameters are considered to be instrumental in determining how well public health measures are likely to control infection (Fraser et al. 2004).

- *The basic reproductive number – R_0*. This is the average number of people who become infected as a result of one infectious person entering a completely susceptible population when there is no intervention. It can be used to model the impact of vaccination on progress of an outbreak and when herd immunity is likely to be achieved. An R of >1 means that more cases of the infection will occur. An R of 1 means that the numbers infected will remain approximately the same, while an R of 0 means that the number of cases will decrease.
- *The disease generation time – Tg*. This is the average time between one person becoming infected and the subsequent infection of other people in turn from that individual.
- The *proportion of transmissions* occurring asymptomatically or before the infection is detected.

The estimated R_0 for three childhood infections is shown in Table 15.3.

A relatively infectious disease with a high R_0 may be controllable with appropriate infection control and public health measures if it can be detected before transmission occurs. The control of COVID-19 was particularly challenging

Table 15.3 Estimated R_0 for three childhood infections.

Disease	Estimated R_0	Latent period (days)	Incubation period (days)	Infectious period (days)
Chickenpox	7–12	8–12	13–17	10–11
Measles	11–15	6–9	8–13	6–7
Mumps	11–14	12–18	12–26	4–8

Source: Anderson and May (2010); Keeling and Grenfell (2000).

because transmission frequently occurred from people who were asymptomatic, unaware of their infectious status and unaware that they needed to alter the behaviour.

Example of an Endemic Infection – Malaria

Malaria is endemic throughout many tropical countries. It has been eradicated from many temperate countries, including the UK and Europe, but remains a leading cause of mortality and morbidity in tropical countries. Nearly half the global population is at risk, particularly infants, young children and pregnant women. The nation most seriously affected is Africa.

Malaria is a major global problem and is responsible for enormous suffering and economic loss. According to the 2021 World Malaria Report, there were estimated to be 627 000 deaths due to malaria, from 241 million malaria cases around the world in 2020. This represents an increase of around 14 million more cases in 2020 compared to 2019, and 69 000 more deaths. Most of these additional deaths (47 000) were thought to be associated with disruptions in the provision of malaria prevention, diagnosis and treatment during the COVID-19 pandemic (World Health Organization 2021a).

Infection is caused by protozoal parasites belonging to the genus *Plasmodium* (Table 15.4). Traditionally, it was thought that there were four types of malarial parasite in humans, but with the addition of *Plasmodium knowlesi*, five are now recognised (Daneshvar et al. 2009). The insect vector responsible for transmission is the female *Anopheles* mosquito which breeds in stagnant water and is most active at night. Malaria is spread via the mouthparts of the mosquito.

Person-to-person infection does not occur and isolation is unnecessary unless a patient arriving from overseas with pyrexia and a presumptive diagnosis of malaria is also considered to be at risk of harbouring an additional tropical fever. Most cases of malaria reported in the UK are contracted abroad, although

Table 15.4   Malarial parasites.

Genus	Distribution	Severity	Fever
Plasmodium falciparum (malignant malaria)	Tropics	+++	Every 2 days
Plasmodium knowlesi	South East Asia	+ to +++	
Plasmodium vivax	Temperate zones	++	Every 2 days
Plasmodium malariae	Subtropics	++	Every 3 days
Plasmodium ovale	Variable and patchy	++	Every 2 days

travellers incubating the infection may not exhibit symptoms until after arrival (Chiodini 2006). Occasionally, malaria is reported in people with no recent history of overseas travel. These cases are the result of 'airport malaria' contracted when mosquitoes imported in aircraft escape on arrival (Isaäcson 1989). People in temperate countries are at risk of malaria if they do not take appropriate preventive measures when travelling to areas where it is endemic (Hill 2006). There are rare cases of infection spread through blood transfusions, organ transplant, sharing contaminated needles and vertically from mother to foetus.

After the mosquito has bitten, the plasmodia enter the bloodstream and are carried to the liver but soon re-enter the blood and invade the erythrocytes where they grow and multiply. At regular intervals (usually every 48–72 hours), the erythrocytes burst, releasing the plasmodia, and the victim experiences chills and fever. The symptoms of malaria usually develop 7–18 days after becoming infected, depending on the specific parasite, but in some cases may not become apparent for over a year or may be dismissed if the illness is very mild. Symptoms include:

- pyrexia
- fever
- headaches
- vomiting
- myalgia
- diarrhoea.

Malaria may not be easy to diagnose if the symptoms are mild and non-specific. However, once suspected, laboratory diagnosis is rapid as the plasmodia are easily detected by examining a blood film under the microscope.

The consequences of malarial infection can be very serious. Destruction of the erythrocytes results in loss of haemoglobin and haemolytic anaemia, respiratory distress arising through reduced oxygen-carrying capacity of the blood, liver failure and jaundice, shock and, rarely, cerebral malaria leading to seizures, coma and permanent cerebral damage. The most serious form of the disease is caused by *P. falciparum*, especially in young children who can develop severe respiratory problems and organ failure very quickly. Malaria in pregnancy can result in maternal mortality, stillbirth, premature birth or low birthweight.

Malaria is preventable through:

- protection against mosquito bites
- mosquito control
- chemoprophylaxis.

Transmission of malaria occurs mostly at night because of the nocturnal feeding habits of *Anopheles* mosquitoes. Protection from bites involves using mosquito nets over beds, air conditioning, wearing loose clothing to cover the skin and using insect repellents. Mosquitoes are controlled by draining standing water where they multiply and insecticide sprays to destroy the adult insects or larvae.

Choice of antimalarial medication for chemoprophylaxis when travelling to malaria-endemic countries depends on the area visited, duration of potential exposure to the parasite, its pattern of resistance to antimalarial drugs and age. Pregnant women are usually advised to avoid travelling to malarial endemic areas. The drugs used for prevention and treatment include chloroquine, amodiaquine, primaquine, mefloquine, atovaquone-proguanil, quinine and doxycycline.

Developing effective vaccines has been challenging because the plasmodia are protected inside the erythrocytes but in 2021, Oxford University announced that a new, effective vaccine had been created (Datoo et al. 2021).

The Changing Patterns of Infectious Disease

Meningitis

Meningitis is inflammation of the membranes surrounding the brain and spinal cord. Infective meningitis is caused by a range of micro-organisms (Table 15.5).

Viral meningitis is generally milder than bacterial infections and most people recover spontaneously. Bacterial meningitis has a mortality rate of 3–6%, is much more severe and can have an extremely rapid rate of onset (Kornelisse et al. 1995). Patients, especially infants and children, can deteriorate and die within hours of first feeling unwell. The symptoms and signs of bacterial meningitis are listed in Table 15.6.

Table 15.5   Some micro-organisms causing meningitis.

Bacterial meningitis	Viral meningitis	Fungal meningitis	Protozoal meningitis
Streptococcus pneumoniae	Echovirus	*Candida*	*Toxoplasma*
Haemophilus influenzae type b	Coxsackie virus	*Cryptococcus*	
Neisseria meningitidis	Mumps virus	*neoformans*	
Escherichia coli	Epstein–Barr	*Histoplasma*	
Group B streptococci	virus	*Coccidioides*	
Listeria monocytogenes	HIV		
Mycobacterium tuberculosis	Influenza		
(usually insidious onset)	Herpes simplex		
	Varicella zoster		

Table 15.6   Signs and symptoms of meningitis.

Children and adults

Non-specific, influenza-type symptoms at early onset
Fever but cold extremities
Heightened respiratory rate
Headache
Nausea and vomiting
Confusion
Increasing drowsiness
Altered consciousness
Neck stiffness
Abdominal pain
Painful joints and muscles
Photophobia (intolerance of bright light) and phonophobia (intolerance to noise)
Seizures

Infants and babies

Irritability, not wanting to be handled
Poor feeding, rejecting feeds
Abnormal cry: whimpering or high-pitched
Poor muscle tone and 'floppiness'
Bulging fontanelle ('soft spot') as pressure increases in the skull
Reduced responses
Pallor or skin mottling
Retraction of the neck with an arched back

Prompt treatment with antimicrobials is usually effective but complications can result in permanent disability (e.g. brain damage, epilepsy, hearing loss).

Meningococcal Meningitis

Neisseria meningitidis is a Gram-negative, aerobic coccus. It is an exclusive human pathogen – there is no animal reservoir. The bacteria colonise the nasopharynx and are transmitted person to person in nasopharyngeal secretions and respiratory droplets spread most readily between members of the same household through close contact (e.g. kissing, sharing crockery and cutlery). Most infections result through close contact with an individual who is carrying the bacteria asymptomatically. Rates of carriage vary; approximately 2% of children under two years are carriers but rates of 25% have been reported in teenagers. If the bacteria gain access to the bloodstream before immunity develops, meningococcal septicaemia results. The bacteria gain access to the meninges via the bloodstream, resulting in meningitis. The incubation period is usually 3–4 days and in children often follows a sore throat or other mild respiratory illness.

Meningococcal disease is most common in infants and young children and among young adults living in close proximity (e.g. college halls of residence, barracks). In addition to the symptoms shown in Table 15.6, approximately 50% of patients develop a rash.

Most cases occur sporadically in the community in high-income countries but outbreaks are occasionally reported. Numerous serotypes of *N. meningitidis* have been identified based on the polysaccharide molecules on the outer capsule of the bacteria. The most common serotypes are A, B, C, D, X, Y, 29E and W135. Serotypes A, B, C and Y are responsible for most meningococcal disease. In the UK, a vaccine offering protection against serogroup C was introduced in 1999 and the incidence of meningococcal disease it causes has declined. Most infections are now caused by serotype B with some increase in other serotypes, notably W. The childhood vaccination schedule has been amended to offer protection against these serotypes and the MenACWY vaccine is offered to teenagers.

Meningococcal disease is still common in low-income countries, especially sub-Saharan Africa. Suspected infection should always be taken very seriously because potentially it is fatal. Antimicrobial therapy should commence before laboratory confirmation because the patient is critically ill and the bacteria may be hard to grow in culture. A range of antibiotics may be used for treatment, including penicillin, ampicillin, chloramphenicol and ceftriaxone. Risk of person-to-person transmission from somebody who is infected is low but in hospital patients are usually nursed in isolation for the initial 24 hours after commencing antibiotics. Chemoprophylaxis is recommended for close contacts (e.g. members of the same household).

Haemophilus influenzae

Haemophilus influenzae is a Gram-negative bacterium often carried in the healthy throat. It causes respiratory infections, epiglottitis and otitis media. Infection is most damaging in young children and before the introduction of vaccination in 1992, it was the principal cause of bacterial meningitis in those under five years of age. Infection was also associated with neurological deficits including deafness, learning disabilities and poor motor co-ordination. Onset is insidious. Infection often follows a cold and the symptoms are non-specific, so parents may not be aware that their child is becoming seriously ill. Currently, Hib vaccine is administered as part of the combined vaccine given at two, three and four months with a booster combined with meningococcal group C around 12 months of age.

The Hib vaccine, which protects against *Haemophilus influenzae* type b, was developed in the early 1970s. Since the introduction of vaccination in 1992, the incidence of this infection has declined sharply in the UK.

'New' Infections

Creutzfeldt–Jakob Disease

Creutzfeldt–Jakob disease (CJD) is an example of a 'new' disease which is much less common than originally feared. It belongs to a group of diseases called the transmissible spongiform encephalopathies which progress slowly as the brain develops minute perforations, eventually assuming a spongy appearance. CJD is inevitably fatal. It destroys neural tissue through the accumulation of abnormal prion proteins in the cells of the nervous system, disrupting function. Diagnosis is made on clinical grounds. CJD is differentiated from other forms of presenile dementia by its rapid onset and progression, death usually occurring within a year of diagnosis. The typical spongiform changes in the cerebral cortex are seen at post mortem. No treatment is currently available.

The main risk of transmission is through surgical procedures involving neurological tissues and the posterior eye. A number of other tissues are associated with medium levels of infectivity (e.g. anterior eye, cornea and lymphoid tissues such as the thymus, tonsils and spleen). Other tissues including blood and blood products are considered to have low levels of infectivity.

All prions are very hard to destroy, presenting challenges when decontaminating potentially infectious items.

Middle Eastern Respiratory Syndrome

Middle East respiratory syndrome (MERS) is a respiratory infection caused by a coronavirus called COVID-12 first identified in Saudi Arabia in 2012. Some people develop very mild symptoms or remain asymptomatic but others are severely affected and a third die as a result of MERS, especially those with pre-existing illness. The incubation period is 2–14 days. Symptoms include:

- fever
- cough
- shortness of breath
- diarrhoea.

The virus is believed to have originated in bats and at some point to have crossed the species boundary and infected camels. Dromedary camels appear to be the main reservoirs and handling them is a risk factor. Infection is also thought to occur after consuming camel-based food products and by person-to-person spread among people in close direct contact with one another. Outbreaks have been reported in Saudi Arabia and Korea and health workers have contracted infection. All known cases have been traced back to Saudi Arabia.

The infection is diagnosed by a PCR blood test. No specific treatment is available but vaccines are being developed. The WHO advises washing hands thoroughly, avoiding the consumption of camel-based food products and contact with sick camels. MERS is extremely uncommon in the UK. Over the last ten years, only five cases have been reported. At present, MERS is attracting considerable research attention because of the similarity between the virus and SARS-CoV-2 (Zhang et al. 2021).

Severe Acute Respiratory Syndrome

Severe acute respiratory syndrome (SARS) originated in China in 2002, probably as a mutation from a virus previously infecting small mammals. It causes a highly contagious form of pneumonia which can be life-threatening. Two outbreaks of SARS occurred in 2002 and 2004 respectively. They spread from China to other Asian countries. There were four cases in the UK and a small outbreak in Toronto, Canada. The epidemiological pattern was strongly influenced by air travel and super-spreading events (Shen et al. 2004). SARS was controlled in 2003 by isolating individuals suspected of infection and screening all air passengers travelling from affected countries. During the pandemic, there were 8098 reported cases and 774 deaths. Mortality rate was 15–20% and most of those who died were over 65 years.

Since 2004, no new cases have been reported but the World Health Organization continues to undertake international surveillance to detect the appearance of further cases. SARS is spread by the air-borne route and probably by direct and indirect contact with fomites and contact with an individual who is infected.

The signs and symptoms of infection begin 2–10 days after exposure to infection and include:

- malaise
- pyrexia
- extreme fatigue
- chills
- myalgia
- diarrhoea
- dry cough
- breathing difficulties.

There is no vaccine for SARS. During the pandemic, patients received supportive treatment and steroids to suppress pulmonary inflammation. Antiviral treatment appears to be effective if given in the early stages of infection.

Zika Virus Disease

Zika virus disease is caused by a flavivirus first identified in Uganda in 1947 in monkeys. The vector is the *Aedes* mosquito which bites during the day. The virus was first reported in the human host in 1952 in Uganda. Most people are asymptomatic or experience mild symptoms including fever, rash and conjunctivitis lasting for only a few days but infection during pregnancy can result in miscarriage, premature birth or an infant with congenital malformations, including microcephaly. Infection has been associated with the later development of Guillain–Barré syndrome. Outbreaks of Zika virus disease have been reported in French Polynesia, the Pacific islands and Brazil (Baud et al. 2017). Pregnant women are advised not to travel to affected regions. Other protective measures include use of loose clothing and insect repellents.

COVID-19

Coronavirus disease (COVID-19) is an infectious disease caused by the SARS-CoV-2 virus. It is an RNA virus with the ability to mutate quickly and numerous variants have been identified. The pandemic it caused in 2020–2021 commenced with an outbreak of unknown origin in Wuhan, Hubei Province, in China in December 2019. Cases were linked to a seafood market in Huanan and were caused by a novel respiratory virus named the severe acute respiratory syndrome coronavirus virus (SARS-CoV-2). Rapid spread led to thousands of deaths and the WHO declared a pandemic situation on 12th March 2020. The subsequent global impact has been immense in terms of lives lost and economically.

The origin of SARS-CoV-2 has been much debated. According to one theory, the virus was the product of laboratory manipulation but it has also been suggested that COVID-19 is a naturally occurring zoonosis with bats as the reservoir host. SARS-CoV-2 has been isolated from a variety of body fluids and survives for prolonged periods on many different types of surface but is thought to spread predominantly by the air-borne route. Throughout the pandemic, there was intense debate on the main route of spread, reawakening interest in the airborne mode of transmission, particularly the relative importance of droplet versus aerosol spread and precise requirements for personal protective equipment (PPE) for health workers, especially when undertaking aerosol-generating procedures. National and international guidance has been constantly updated (World Health Organization 2021b).

Most people infected with SARS-CoV-2 experienced mild to moderate respiratory illness and recovered spontaneously but serious illness was also widespread. It occurred most frequently in those with underlying health conditions (e.g. cardiovascular disease, diabetes, chronic respiratory disease, cancer), those who were overweight and some ethnic groups. Throughout the pandemic, the sickest patients required positive pressure ventilation and were isolated with full use of PPE. Infections were linked to super-spreading events likely to generate aerosols (e.g. shouted conversation, singing) and prolonged contact between members of the same household. Asymptomatic carriage was estimated to occur in 46% of cases. Children and young people were very likely to remain asymptomatic or to develop mild illness. Large numbers of nosocomial outbreaks were reported with staff and patients operating as super-spreaders, especially if they were asymptomatic (Jung et al. 2021). The incubation period was estimated as typically 5–6 days and up to 14 days following exposure.

The most frequently experienced symptoms were:

- fever
- cough
- fatigue
- loss of smell and taste.

Less commonly experienced symptoms included:

- sore throat
- myalagia
- headache
- diarrhoea
- red, irritated eyes
- skin rash or discolouration of the fingers and toes.

Seriously affected patients deteriorated rapidly. They develop respiratory difficulties, loss of speech and mobility and chest pain. Risk of death was high and caused by multiple organ failure. Suspected cases were confirmed by PCR test.

Public health measures varied between countries. Typical measures adopted are shown in Table 15.7. The speed of implementation and the effectiveness of response varied between countries and between states in federal countries. Those which had suffered the brunt of the SARS epidemic in 2002–2004 were most agile in their initial reaction.

Table 15.7 Public health measures adopted during the COVID-19 pandemic.

Quarantine ('self-isolation') of those exposed to infection
Curfews, lockdowns
Travel restrictions within countries and internationally
Mask wearing
Hand hygiene
Closure of premises where mass gatherings occur (e.g. entertainment and sports venues, places of worship)
School closures
Working at home, avoiding face-to-face meetings
Closure of non-essential retail outlets, offices
Advice to avoid seeking non-emergency healthcare
Advice to ventilate homes and work premises
Temperature screening at airports, when entering communal buildings
Vaccination

A number of effective vaccines were developed in 2020 followed by rapid 'roll-out', usually commencing with older people and those with underlying health problems. Throughout the pandemic, there was a massive influx of critically ill patients to acute hospitals, seriously delaying elective treatment. Societal upheaval resulting from the pandemic was enormous and obliged those responsible for policy to make swift and hard choices to balance the containment of infection against the wider negative effects on society (e.g. psychological stress leading to mental illness, failure to identify other conditions requiring health intervention, interrupted education, loss of employment) (Douglas et al. 2020).

Infections and Vaccine Hesitancy

Reluctance to be vaccinated and to have children vaccinated is not a new phenomenon although it attracted particular attention during the COVID-19 pandemic. There have been resurgences in other infections which could in theory be controlled by vaccination and cases of vaccination failure.

Measles

Measles is a highly contagious infection caused by an RNA virus belonging to the paramyxovirus family. It is transmitted in respiratory secretions through the air and by direct and indirect contact with contaminated fomites. The virus infects the respiratory tract and then spreads throughout the body. Symptoms appear 7–10 days after exposure: pyrexia (as high as 40 °C), malaise, a cold-like illness accompanied with sore, red eyes which may be sensitive to light and a characteristic reddish-brown maculopapular rash. White spots (Koplik spots) sometimes appear on the oral mucosae. The infection usually resolves after about 10 days. Measles can cause serious complications in children under five years of age, particularly if they are undernourished or suffering from an immunosuppressive condition (e.g. HIV). The most serious complications are blindness, encephalitis, severe diarrhoea and the resulting dehydration, middle ear infections and pneumonia which can result in mortality.

There is no specific treatment but an effective vaccine became available in 1963 and is given as part of the routine childhood vaccination schedule in combination with mumps and rubella. Before the vaccine became available, major epidemics of measles occurred every 2–3 years, resulting in an estimated 2.6 million deaths per annum. Although theoretically preventable, outbreaks of measles have since been reported in the UK, mainly because of parental reluctance to have children vaccinated through concerns about serious side-effects which are now considered to be unfounded. An outbreak in the Swansea area in 2012–2013 resulted in 664 cases, 88 hospitalisations and one death from associated pneumonia in a man of 25 years. Since 2016, there has been a further increase in measles infections in the UK.

Mumps

Mumps is caused by an RNA virus belonging to the paramyxovirus family spread by the air-borne route and contact with fomites contaminated with the salivary secretions of an infected person. Spread from individuals who are asymptomatic is common. The virus is inhaled and then moves from the respiratory tract to the parotid (salivary) glands which swell as it replicates in large numbers. Other parts of the body can become infected including the pancreas, testicles and ovaries. The incubation period is 15–24 days. Symptoms include headaches, joint pain and pyrexia usually developing a few days before painful swelling of the parotid glands appears. Serious complications following infection are rare. Orchitis and oophoritis may result in adults who become infected and there have been reports of pancreatitis and meningitis if the virus gains access to the central nervous system.

The MMR vaccination is estimated to give 80% protection against mumps. Most infections occur in young people who have not been vaccinated, particularly those living in shared residential accommodation such as college halls of residence. Occasional outbreaks have been reported, mainly from the American Mid-West and the Netherlands (Hviid et al. 2008).

Rubella

Rubella (German measles) is caused by an RNA virus belonging to the Maltonoviridae family transmitted by the air-borne route and contaminated secretions. Since the introduction of vaccination, it is rare in the UK and other high-income countries. Most cases are imported from parts of the world where vaccination has not been introduced but occasional outbreaks are reported. In 1996, there were over 3000 cases of rubella in England and Wales. Symptoms are usually mild and many people do not realise that they have been infected. Symptoms include a pinkish rash lasting 2–3 days, swollen lymphatic glands, pyrexia and a cold-like illness. Adults who become infected often reported aching joints. The most infectious period occurs 1–5 days after exposure to infection.

Rubella contracted during the first trimester of pregnancy can result in miscarriage, stillbirth or congenital rubella syndrome which is associated with congenital defects: impaired hearing, eye and heart defects, diabetes and thyroid dysfunction. Before the introduction of rubella vaccine in 1970, children in the UK usually acquired infection between 4 and 9 years of age but it was estimated that approximately 18% of women of childbearing age were susceptible to infection, and congenital rubella was a significant problem: about 200–300 births occurred in non-epidemic years, and many more during epidemics.

Rubella vaccination was introduced in the UK in 1970. Initially, it was offered to schoolgirls and susceptible women as the aim was to reduce the tragic consequences of infection during pregnancy rather than eradication. By 1990, only 2–4% of pregnant women were susceptible to rubella compared with 10–15% before 1970. Congenital infections were still reported and as unvaccinated children operated as a reservoir, the vaccine was offered as part of the routine childhood immunisation programme.

Prevention and Control of Infectious Disease at International Level

A number of organisations are involved in the prevention and control of infectious disease internationally.

World Health Organization

The World Health Organization (WHO) is a United Nations agency founded in 1948 to promote global health and safety and co-ordinate the world response to emergencies. It has responsibility for administering international programmes to control disease, including infectious disease. The WHO has exclusive authority to declare global health emergencies and directs efforts to overcome them at international level. Successful initiatives have included the eradication of smallpox in 1979, management of the Ebola virus disease outbreak in sub-Saharan Africa in 2014–2016 and management of the epidemic of SARS in 2003. More recently, the WHO has been criticised for its advice during the COVID-19 pandemic in 2020 (Greenhalgh et al. 2020).

On a day-to-day basis, the WHO provides advice about controlling infection by:

- supporting individual nations to collect and analyse data to share with other countries
- operating as a resource for health workers by collecting, consolidating and publishing epidemiological data from different countries

- providing technical assistance and training to encourage countries to standardise the methods they use to collect and present epidemiological data to allow meaningful national comparison.

The WHO requires countries to report any 'event that may constitute a public health emergency of international concern'. The criteria used when assessing need include:

- the seriousness of the event in terms of impact on public health
- the unusual or unexpected nature of the event
- the risk of international spread
- the risk that travel or trade restrictions will be imposed by other countries (World Health Organization 2005).

The WHO is closely involved in the prevention and control of healthcare-associated infection. Its 'SAVE LIVES: Clean Your Hands' global campaign launched in 2009 seeks to maintain the global promotion, visibility and sustainability of hand hygiene in healthcare. Its hand hygiene guidelines and associated toolkit published in 2009 have been implemented in over 100 countries.

Control of Communicable Disease in the UK
The UK Health Security Agency (UK HSA) was established in 2021. It assumed responsibility for health protection formerly held by Public Health England, including responsibility for the prevention and control of infectious disease. The UK HSA works closely with Public Health Wales and Health Protection Scotland which perform similar functions. Among its many responsibilities, the UK HSA provides advice about infection prevention and control to health provider organisations, oversees public health functions (e.g. testing water, food, milk) and contributes to the control of communicable disease through surveillance, investigating outbreaks and formulating policies for control. Sudden increases in the number of infections caused by a specific organism are reported to the UK HSA which monitors and helps control it. The early recognition of a problem and prompt action by the public health bodies enable emerging outbreaks to be contained.

Notifiable Infections
Infectious diseases are of concern at the individual, local, national and international level. The exact arrangements for how clinicians work in conjunction with wider public health bodies varies but in many countries specific infections (notifiable diseases) considered to offer particular threat must be notified to government authorities by law. Notifiable infectious conditions in the UK are shown in (Table 15.8). They must be reported to the proper officers of the local authority

Table 15.8 Notifiable infections in the United Kingdom.

Acute encephalitis
Acute infectious hepatitis
Acute meningitis
Acute poliomyelitis
Anthrax
Botulism
Brucellosis
Cholera
COVID-19
Diphtheria
Enteric fever (typhoid or paratyphoid fever)
Food poisoning
Haemolytic uraemic syndrome
Infectious bloody diarrhoea
Invasive group A streptococcal disease
Legionnaires' disease
Leprosy
Malaria
Measles
Meningococcal septicaemia
Mumps
Plague
Rabies
Rubella
Severe acute respiratory syndrome
Scarlet fever
Smallpox
Tetanus
Tuberculosis
Typhus
Viral haemorrhagic fever
Whooping cough
Yellow fever
Other diseases that may present significant risk to human health

Source: Adapted from Public Health England (2021).

under the Health Protection (Notification) Regulations 2010. Notification enables the public health authorities to trace the contacts of those who might have been exposed to infection so they can be monitored and receive treatment. For food- or water-borne infections, it is important to determine and eliminate the source. The data generated at local and national level are used to monitor fluctuations in the incidence of infection, identify potential outbreaks, take preventative action and determine when health promotion campaigns are necessary. Responsibility for notification falls to local authorities which have a statutory responsibility to control infectious conditions within their boundaries.

Control of Communicable Disease in Other Countries

Other high-income countries have also developed public health systems to manage communicable and other disease. In the US, the Centers for Disease Control (CDC) is responsible for controlling the introduction and spread of infectious diseases and provides consultation and support to other nations and international agencies to help improve prevention and control, environmental health and health promotion initiatives.

European Centre for Disease Prevention and Control

The European Centre for Disease Prevention and Control (ECDC) is a European Union agency established in 2005 to strengthen defences against infectious diseases throughout Europe. The ECDC works closely in association with the WHO and collects data on an international basis. Both organisations work together to develop a single European reporting and response system, and to implement the 2005 International Health Regulations. The ECDC undertakes surveillance, identifies threats and outbreaks and provides public health training. In 2019, following its departure from the European Union, the UK ceased to contribute data to the ECDC.

Suggested Activities

Exercise 15.1 Self-assessment

1   Which of the following might be included in a large team of epidemiologists investigating a 'new' disease?
    A Public health expert
    B Lay person
    C Laboratory technicians
    D All the above

2   Explain what is meant by the term 'emerging infectious disease'.

3   An epidemic involves a large number of people across many different countries. True/False

4 Cyclical epidemiological curves are typical of which of the following?
   A Rubella prior to introduction of the MMR
   B Norovirus
   C Gonorrhoea
   D Seasonal influenza

5 Complete the following sentence: 'Surveillance is. . . .'

6 Modelling of infectious diseases is used for which of the following?
   A Study how infectious diseases are spread
   B Predict the course of outbreaks
   C Determine the prevalence of infection
   D All the above

7 Malaria is never reported in temperate climates.
   True/False

8 Which of the following can cause meningitis?
   A *Haemophilus influenzae* type b
   B Prions
   C Coxsackie virus
   D None of the above

9 Severe acute respiratory syndrome (SARS) was last reported in 2007.
   True/False

10 SARS-CoV-2 frequently causes mild illness.
    True/False

Exercise 15.2

Which types of infections are currently/have recently been reported in the media as causing specific threats to health? Look up details of one of these infections online. What parts of the world are affected and which sectors of the population? Who is at risk and why? What arrangements are in place for surveillance? Do you believe these figures? What public health measures are in place and how effective are they proving?

Exercise 15.3

The vaccination coverage necessary to achieve herd immunity is calculated thus: $1-1/R_0$ (multiplied by 100 to give a percentage). Calculate the vaccination targets for each of the diseases in Table 15.3. Looking at these values, and the other parameters given in this table, what are the benefits of vaccination over other strategies such as isolation of infectious or particularly vulnerable people, or simply letting children catch the infection?

References

Anderson, R.M. and May, R.M. (2010). *Infectious Diseases of Humans: Dynamics and Control*. Oxford: Oxford University Press.

Baud, D., Gubler, D.J., Schaub, B. et al. (2017). An update on zika virus infection. *Lancet* 390: 2099–2109. https://doi.org/10.1016/S0140-6736(17)31450-2.

Chiodini, J. (2006). Malaria in UK travellers: assessment, prevention and treatment. *Nursing Standard* 20: 49–58. https://doi.org/10.7748/ns.20.34.49.s52.

Daneshvar, C., Davis, T.M.E., Cox-Singh, J. et al. (2009). Clinical and laboratory features of human plasmodium knowlesi infection. *Clin Infect Dis* 49: 852–860. https://doi.org/10.1086/605439.

Datoo, M.S., Natama, M.H., Somé, A. et al. (2021). Efficacy of a low-dose candidate malaria vaccine, R21 in adjuvant matrix-M, with seasonal administration to children in Burkina Faso: a randomised controlled trial. *Lancet* 397: 1809–1818. https://doi.org/10.1016/S0140-6736(21)00943-0.

Douglas, M., Katikireddi, S.V., Taulbut, M. et al. (2020). Mitigating the wider health effects of covid-19 pandemic response. *BMJ* 369: m1557. https://doi.org/10.1136/bmj.m1557.

Farrington, P. (2003). *Infectious Disease*. Milton Keynes: Open University.

Fraser, C., Riley, S., Anderson, R.M., and Ferguson, N.M. (2004). Factors that make an infectious disease outbreak controllable. *Proceedings of the National Academy of Sciences* 101: 6146–6151. https://doi.org/10.1073/pnas.0307506101.

Garritty, C.M., Norris, S.L., and Moher, D. (2017). Developing WHO rapid advice guidelines in the setting of a public health emergency. *Journal of Clinical Epidemiology* 82: 47–60. https://doi.org/10.1016/j.jclinepi.2016.08.010.

Greenhalgh, T., Schmid, M.B., Czypionka, T. et al. (2020). Face masks for the public during the covid-19 crisis. *BMJ* 369: m1435. https://doi.org/10.1136/bmj.m1435.

Greenhalgh, T., Jimenez, J.L., Prather, K.A. et al. (2021). Ten scientific reasons in support of airborne transmission of SARS-CoV-2. *Lancet* 397: 1603–1605. https://doi.org/10.1016/S0140-6736(21)00869-2.

Hill, D.R. (2006). The burden of illness in international travelers. *N. Engl. J. Med.* 354: 115–117. https://doi.org/10.1056/NEJMp058292.

Hviid, A., Rubin, S., and Mühlemann, K. (2008). Mumps. *Lancet* 371: 932–944. https://doi.org/10.1016/S0140-6736(08)60419-5.

Isaäcson, M. (1989). Airport malaria: a review. *Bull World Health Organ* 67: 737–743.

Jung, J., Lim, S.Y., Lee, J. et al. (2021). Clustering and multiple-spreading events of nosocomial severe acute respiratory syndrome coronavirus 2 infection. *Journal of Hospital Infection* 117: 28–36. https://doi.org/10.1016/j.jhin.2021.06.012.

Keeling, M.J. and Grenfell, B.T. (2000). Individual-based perspectives on R0. *J. Theor. Biol.* 203: 51–61. https://doi.org/10.1006/jtbi.1999.1064.

Kornelisse, R.F., de Groot, R., and Neijens, H.J. (1995). Bacterial meningitis: mechanisms of disease and therapy. *Eur. J. Pediat.r* 154: 85–96. https://doi.org/10.1007/BF01991906.

McArthur, D.B. (2019). Emerging infectious diseases. *Nurs. Clin. North Am.* 54: 297–311. https://doi.org/10.1016/j.cnur.2019.02.006.

Metcalf, C.J.E., Farrar, J., Cutts, F.T. et al. (2016). Use of serological surveys to generate key insights into the changing global landscape of infectious disease. *Lancet* 388: 728–730. https://doi.org/10.1016/S0140-6736(16)30164-7.

Mishra, S., Fisman, D.N., and Boily, M.-C. (2011). The ABC of terms used in mathematical models of infectious diseases. *J. Epidemiol. Commun. Health.* 65: 87–94. https://doi.org/10.1136/jech.2009.097113.

Public Health England (2020). Reports of cases of TB to UK enhanced tuberculosis surveillance systems. www.gov.uk/government/statistics/reports-of-cases-of-tb-to-uk-enhanced-tuberculosis-surveillance-systems

Public Health England (2021). Notifiable diseases and causative organisms: how to report. www.gov.uk/guidance/notifiable-diseases-and-causative-organisms-how-to-report

Selwyn, S. (1991). Hospital infection: the first 2500 years. *J. Hosp. Infect.* 18: 5–64. https://doi.org/10.1016/0195-6701(91)90004-R.

Shen, Z., Ning, F., Zhou, W. et al. (2004). Superspreading SARS Events, Beijing, 2003. *Emerg. Infect. Dis.* 10: 256–260. https://doi.org/10.3201/eid1002.030732.

Thacker, S.B. and Berkelman, R.L. (1988). Public health surveillance in the United States. *Epidemiol. Rev.* 10: 164–190. https://doi.org/10.1093/oxfordjournals.epirev.a036021.

World Health Organization (2005). International Health Regulations (2005) 3. www.who.int/publications-detail-redirect/9789241580496

World Health Organization (2021a). *World Malaria Report 2021*. Geneva: World Health Organization.

World Health Organization (2021b). Country and technical guidance - Coronavirus disease (COVID-19). www.who.int/emergencies/diseases/novel-coronavirus-2019/technical-guidance-publications

Zhang, A.-R., Shi, W.-Q., Liu, K. et al. (2021). Epidemiology and evolution of Middle East respiratory syndrome coronavirus, 2012–2020. *Infect. Dis. Poverty.* 10: 66. https://doi.org/10.1186/s40249-021-00853-0.

Suggested Activities: Responses

Chapter 1

1 A microbial pathogen is defined as a micro-organism able to cause disease.
2 c
3 Direct contact
Indirect spread via fomites
Air-borne spread
Contaminated food and water
Inoculation via skin or mucous membranes
Vertical transmission from mother to foetus
Zoonotic spread from animals
4 b
5 False
6 Endogenous (self) infection results in the transfer of micro-organisms from one anatomical site to another on the same person. Exogenous (cross) infection occurs when micro-organisms are transferred between different people, for example on the hands of health workers or via fomites.
7 False
8 b and c
9 c
10 False

Infection Prevention and Control in Healthcare Settings,
First Edition. Edward Purssell and Dinah Gould.
© 2023 John Wiley & Sons Ltd. Published 2023 by John Wiley & Sons Ltd.

Chapter 2

1 Intervention studies are positioned higher up the hierarchy because if rigorously undertaken, they are associated with a very low risk of bias and validity is high.
2 True
3 b
4 True
5 Two-armed cluster randomised controlled trial: the intervention group and the group exposed to usual practice (control). In this study, the clusters were the wards where data were collected.
6 Seasonal trends are cyclical and recurrent. Secular trends do not recur and are not cyclical.
7 True
8 False
9 d
10 Grading of Recommendations, Assessment, Development and Evaluation (GRADE)
2b. The concentration of alcohol used in the handrub evaluated was not great enough to kill to exert a bactericidal effect.

Chapter 3

1 Any substance able to stimulate an immune response.
2 a, c
3 d
4 False
5 Erythema, swelling, heat, pain, loss of function.
6 It is the same for everybody.
7 a, b
8 a) anatural active immunity – immunity gained by exposure to the organism
   b) acquired active immunity – vaccination
   c) natural passive immunity: maternal immunoglobulin/antibodies transferred from mother to child
   d) acquired passive immunity: immunoglobuin/antibody transfusion
9 False
10 Two

Chapter 4

1 e
2 True
3 This will vary according to your clinical area, but might include multiply resistant or newly resistant organisms such as *Enterococcus faecium*, *Staphylococcus aureus*, *Klebsiella pneumoniae*, *Acinetobacter baumannii*, *Pseudomonas aeruginosa* and *Enterobacter* spp.; viruses or bacteria that spread very quickly, such as *Cryptosporidium*; or are new or re-emerging, such as COVID-19 and monkeypox.
4 True
5 Point-of-care testing improves the patient experience because it can be undertaken at the location where healthcare is delivered, patients can test themselves in privacy, the results are available very rapidly enabling treatment to begin at once, and the results are highly reliable.
6 Blood, lower airways, urine, cerebrospinal fluid
7 No. Routine sampling is pointless because the clinical environment is contaminated with large numbers of organisms that are mostly harmless.
8 The patient is very likely to have a urinary infection. Neither *E. coli* or Enterococci are likely to be contaminants in this case, and there are quite large numbers of white blood cells seen. Both organisms are covered by nitrofurantoin, which is a first-line antibiotic for urinary tract infections.
9 Good practice involves: obtaining the specimen only if there is good reason to suspect infection (inflammation, pyrexia, purulent exudate); aspirating pus from the wound if possible; if it is impossible to aspirate pus, obtaining 2–3 swabs and sending them to the laboratory in special transport media. All specimens should be sent to the laboratory as soon as possible and refrigerated if not possible.
10 Stool specimens and vaginal swabs should not be refrigerated because the types of pathogens likely to be causing infection/infestation become sluggish at low temperatures and are more difficult to identify. Specimens of blood and cerebrospinal fluid should not be stored in ward refrigerators because these patients are likely to be very ill. These specimens should be sent to the laboratory at once.

Chapter 5

1 a) Any drug used to treat an infection
   b) A natural product that is used to treat an infection. This means that it is a substance produced by a living organism
   c) Antibiotics are natural products; antimicrobials include natural and synthetic products

2   a) True
    b) False
    c) True
    d) False
    e) True
    f) False
    g) True

Chapter 6

1   True
2   Reduce risk of transferring infectious agents from recognised and unrecognised sources of infection
3   d
4   Cleaning, disinfection, sterilisation
5   a, b, d
6   False
7   Control of Substances Hazardous to Health
8   False
9   Before patient contact; before clean or aseptic procedures; after exposure to blood/body fluids; after patient contact; after touching the close patient environment; between activities involving the same patient that could lead to contamination.
10 Source isolation is necessary when a patient is known to be infected or colonised with a specific pathogen requiring transmission precautions and when infection or colonisation is suspected.

Chapter 7

1   Healthcare-associated infection can be acquired as a result of healthcare in all the following settings: nursing homes; acute hospitals; community clinics; private hospitals; the domiciliary setting.
2   True
3   Prevalence is the number of people with an infection at a specific point in time (point prevalence) or over a specified period of time (period prevalence). Prevalence studies include both new and existing cases and are influenced by speed of recovery; prevalence appears greater if data collection occurs over a long period of time. Incidence is the number of new cases of a

condition arising over a specified period of time in a population. Incidence studies provide more comprehensive information about the risk of developing the condition than prevalence studies.

4   a, b, d
5   False
6   a, c
7   a, d
8   a, b, c, d
9   a, c, d
10   a, b, c, d

Chapter 8

1   Being female, age over 65 years, pregnancy, recent sexual activity, being obese, immunocompromised, diabetic and having a renal abnormality or a chronic wound.
2   a, c, d
3   b, d
4   Bacteria can gain access to the bladder of a patient with an indwelling urinary catheter when the catheter is inserted, by migrating from the drainage bag. Migration occurs upwards along the inside of drainage tubing (interluminal route) or via the periurethral space between the outer wall of the catheter and the bladder (intraluminal route). Access can also be gained when the 'closed' system of drainage is opened (e.g. to empty the bag or change it).
5   False
6   a, b, c
7   Trial without catheter
8   a, c, d
9   True
10   Fluid intake generates larger volumes of urine and dilutes the nutrients within it necessary to support bacterial growth.

Chapter 9

1   Healing by primary intention occurs when tissue loss is minimal (e.g. surgical wounds). Healing by secondary intention takes place when tissue loss has occurred and tissue heals through granulation (e.g. pressure ulcers, leg ulcers).

2 A surgical site infection is defined as an infection arising within 30 days of undergoing surgery or within one year if the patient has received an implantable device (e. g. prosthetic joint replacement).

3 a, b, c

4 a, c, d

5 d

6 True

7 Studies have evaluated different patient populations with different degrees of risk; there are differences in the interventions included in different bundles and the type of procedure evaluated varies. The ability of bundled interventions to reduce surgical site infections is further complicated because adherence by staff is often poor.

8 The aim of national surveillance schemes for surgical site infections is to improve the quality of patient care by encouraging health providers to compare their own infection rates over time against a national benchmark and use the data to review and support practice.

9 d

10 a, b

Chapter 10

1 True

2 Ventilator-associated pneumonia (VAP) and non-ventilator-associated pneumonia (nVAP)

3 d

4 False

5 Person-to-person transmission of *Legionella pneumophila* has never been documented.

6 b

7 b, c, d

8 Aerosol-generating procedure

9 b, c

10 False because although it is caused by *Bordetella pertussis*, this is a Gram negative, not Gram positive bacterium.

Chapter 11

1 Bacteraemia is the presence of pathogens in the bloodstream. Septicaemia is the multiplication of bacteria in the blood.

2   Secondary bloodstream infections are seeded from another site of infection elsewhere in the body.
3   b, c
4   True
5   False
6   a, b, d
7   c
8   True
9   There is no evidence for their use in this situation, so it is not possible to state for sure, although it is likely to be false.
10   a, b, c

Chapter 12

1   c, d
2   The signs and symptoms of *Staphylococcus aureus* food-borne illness appear rapidly because it is caused by toxins released by the bacteria and no incubation period is necessary.
3   a, b
4   In hospital: inform the infection prevention team. In nursing homes: inform the manager. In both cases, implement infection prevention precautions.
5   False
6   b, c
7   b
8   b
9   Widal reaction
10   a

Chapter 13

1   b, c
2   d
3   True
4   Significant occupational exposure
5   Audit is not mandatory and it is likely that many incidents are omitted from the official figures.
6   False
7   b, d
8   a, b
9   Intravenous drug users who share needles
10   False

Chapter 14

1 d
2 They have complicated growth requirements and do not survive for long in transport media.
3 d
4 a, c
5 Chancres (first lesion to appear) are painless and often develop at a site difficult to see.
6 b, c, d
7 c
8 The virus can remain latent for years.
9 True
10 False

Chapter 15

1 d
2 An emerging infectious disease is one that has appeared in a population for the first time or a previously existing infection that begins to spread rapidly, either infecting large numbers of people for the first time or moving into one or more geographical areas where it has not previously been reported.
3 False
4 a, d
5 Surveillance is the systematic, ongoing collection, collation and analysis of healthcare data and feedback to staff to prompt appropriate action.
6 a, b
7 False
8 a, c
9 False
10 True

Index

Infection Prevention and Control in Healthcare Settings,
First Edition. Edward Purssell and Dinah Gould.
© 2023 John Wiley & Sons Ltd. Published 2023 by John Wiley & Sons Ltd.